GIVING BIRTH IN CANADA, 1900–1950

In G ... ...orical study of childbirth in Canada,
Wen ... ...a fascinating account of childbirth rituals in the first half of ...ntieth century. Thorough and comprehensive, the work is based on a rich variety of sources, including medical
textbooks, the medical periodical press, popular medical advice books,
literature published in women's magazines, patient records, and interviews with women who gave birth and physicians who practised during the period.

Mitchinson follows the birthing experience from the initial diagnosis
of pregnancy, through prenatal care, and childbirth – who was present
and where it took place – to obstetrical intervention, postnatal care, and
the definition of what constituted a normal birth, much of which changed
significantly through those years. She explores physicians' responses to
the needs of pregnant women, developments in medical practices, and
the increasing medicalization of childbirth.

While the book focuses on conventional medical practices, the author's
survey of midwifery and Aboriginal birthing practices provides a counterpoint to the approach taken by Western medicine and permits valuable discussion about the dynamics of gender and race as they relate to
childbirth and, more broadly, to early-twentieth-century Canada.

(Studies in Gender and History)

WENDY MITCHINSON is a professor of history at the University of
Waterloo.

STUDIES IN GENDER AND HISTORY

General editors: Franca Iacovetta and Karen Dubinsky

GIVING BIRTH
IN CANADA
1900–1950

Wendy Mitchinson

UNIVERSITY OF TORONTO PRESS
Toronto Buffalo London

© University of Toronto Press Incorporated 2002
Toronto Buffalo London

Printed in Canada

ISBN 0-8020-3631-7 (cloth)
ISBN 0-8020-8471-0 (paper)

Printed on acid-free paper

National Library of Canada Cataloguing in Publication Data

Mitchinson, Wendy
Giving birth in Canada, 1900–1950

(Studies in gender and history)
Includes bibliographical references and index.
ISBN 0-8020-3631-7 (bound)   ISBN 0-8020-8471-0 (pbk.)

1. Childbirth – Canada – History – 20th century.   2. Obstetrics –
Canada – History – 20th century.   I. Title.   II. Series

RG518.C3M58 2002   618.2'00971'0904   C2001-903023-1

University of Toronto Press acknowledges the financial assistance
to its publishing program of the Canada Council for the Arts
and the Ontario Arts Council.

This book has been published with the help of a grant from the
Humanities and Social Sciences Federation of Canada, using funds provided
by the Social Sciences and Humanities Research Council of Canada.

University of Toronto Press acknowledges the financial support for
its publishing activities of the Government of Canada through the
Book Publishing Industry Development Program (BPIDP).

For Frances Mitchinson
and in memory of
Cameron Mitchinson

Contents

CONTENTS

Illustrations follow page 180.

Preface

I always seem to be writing books I don't intend to write. Certainly this is the case for *Giving Birth in Canada, 1900–1950*. My aim was to write an overview of the medical treatment of women in early-twentieth-century Canada, a sequel to *The Nature of Their Bodies: Women and Their Doctors in Victorian Canada*. However, during a sabbatical year it quickly became clear that if I wanted to get even a very rudimentary first draft written, I would need to narrow my focus. I was in the enviable position of having too much research data. So I decided to concentrate on childbirth, and what follows is the result. The only part of the book previously published was a somewhat shorter version of chapter 2, which appeared as 'The Sometimes Uncertain World of Canadian Obstetrics, 1900–1950,' *Canadian Bulletin of Medical History* 17, 1–2 (2000): 193–208.

Although I am the author of the book, I could not have written it without the help of many others. Funding agencies are crucial for research, and while many of us criticize what we see as the lack of funding and a sometimes eccentric decision-making process, I have certainly benefited from research support provided by the Social Sciences and Humanities Research Council of Canada (SSHRC), Associated Medical Services through the Hannah Institute for the History of Medicine, and the University of Waterloo. I was privileged during the period of researching and writing to be awarded a Thérèse Casgrain Fellowship (1993–4), to be a scholar in residence at the Rockefeller Study Center in Bellagio,

Italy, for one month in 1994, thanks to the generosity of the Rockefeller Foundation, and to spend a month as scholar in residence in southern Spain through the Danish Fundación Valparaiso in 1997.

None of the above would have been possible without the sources to research, and it is in making them available to researchers that librarians, archivists, and holders of collections are central to the process. I would like to thank Dr Badley and Lynn Molloy from the Victoria General Hospital, Halifax, the former for giving me permission to look at the hospital's records and the latter for helping me do so. Philip Hiscock, who was then at the Memorial University of Newfoundland Folklore and Language Archive, was particularly generous in sending me material on midwives from the folklore collection. I also appreciate the work of his successor, Patricia Fulton, who checked note references. The Igloolik Oral History Project was a wonderful source, and I especially wish to thank the Inuit elders involved in it, as well as their translators. For making the material available, I appreciate the generosity of the Science Institute of the Northwest Territories and the Government of the Northwest Territories, in particular John MacDonald of the Science Institute. McGill University Archives, the Public Archives of Nova Scotia, the Provincial Archives of British Columbia, Queen's University Archives, Women's College Hospital, Toronto, and the Kitchener-Waterloo Hospital were most accommodating to me, and I particularly appreciated the officials of the latter two institutions, who gave me access to their records and were generous in setting up research space for either myself or a research assistant. Kathryn Rumbold, too, made space available for photographing items from the University Health Network Artifact Collection. Susan Bellingham of the Doris Lewis Rare Book Room, Dana Porter Library, University of Waterloo, was always helpful and interested in what I was doing.

The generosity of other scholars in sharing their research has been gratifying. David Gagan and Suzann Buckley were particularly giving. David provided me with statistical runs of the patient records from his own work on the Owen Sound General and Marine Hospital, and Suzann did the same for the Ottawa Maternity Hospital. I cannot thank them enough. Dr Charles Hayter shared his research, as did Lesley Biggs, Jill Oakes, and Janet McNaughton. Judi Albright and her family lent me their Aunt Mary How's Cottage Hospital records from Abbey, Saskatchewan, and Sheila Joel the tapes of 'Traces,' a women's project devoted to collecting the remembrances of older women. Marlene O'Brien allowed me to relate the experiences of her mother in childbirth. Drs Stuart Houston and Robert Macbeth took an interest in what I was doing and regaled me with stories of their training and practice.

Over the many years that I was working on this project (in its larger manifestation), I was fortunate to have good research help. I would like to thank Linda Ambrose, Marlene Epp, Mona Gleason, Susan Johnston, Barbara Holzmark, Megan Davies, Julia Roberts, and Mary MacDonald. These individuals helped find patient records and coded them for analysis, surveyed medical textbooks and input data. A special thanks is due to Helen Harrison, who interviewed many women about their health experiences. The women themselves are particularly deserving of gratitude. They gave of their time and they shared experiences that were not always happy. Although not named (for purposes of confidentiality), each one contributed to the making of this book, as did the several physicians I interviewed.

During the research and writing of this manuscript I was fortunate to work with a group of scholars as part of a SSHRC Strategic Research Network Grant. As participants in the Feminist Health Care Ethics Research Network, these women both stimulated and challenged me. I thank Françoise Baylis, Marilynne Bell, Maria DeKonick, Jocelyn Downie, Abby Lippman, Margaret Lock, Kathryn Morgan, Janet Mosher, Barbara Parish, Susan Sherwin, Peggy Spencer, and Ariella Pahlke. Colleagues and friends are often unaware of how they help simply by being there and showing some interest. I would like to thank Bonnie Shettler, Chris and Linda Dumbell, Alison and Jim Prentice, Franca Iacovetta, Ian Radforth, John English, Ken McLaughlin, and Patrick Harrigan. Family members, too, are central for maintaining sanity and keeping life in perspective. Over the years the joy given me by Leo, Misha, Georgia, Calder, and Bustopher will not be forgotten. I can't express enough appreciation to three individuals who with good grace took on my request to read a draft of the manuscript. Drs Murray Enkin and Charles Roland explained with endless patience the medical perspective and fortunately caught some of my more egregious faux pas. Janice Dickin, in her cheerful way, kept me focused on what it was I was trying to say. I appreciated (well, not always) the comments of the anonymous readers and those of Jill McConkey of the University of Toronto Press and the encouragement given by Karen Dubinsky of the Press's Studies in Gender and History series. Until he left University of Toronto Press, Gerry Hallowell continued to express interest in the project and kept reminding me to finish it. The editorial help provided by Carlotta Lemieux and Frances Mundy made the final work on the manuscript less stressful than it might have been. Production assistance by Len Husband also smoothed the process. Connected to producing the actual manuscript, my thanks to Nancy Birss, Irene Majer, Jill Willwerth, and Vic Neglia, all of whom remained calm when computer technology made me frazzled. Arthur Sheps suggested a working title for the book, and while it did not become the final title it lifted my spirits while I was writing.

I now feel like one of those recipients of an award who has thanked everyone. Of course that is never possible, and in writing the acknowledgments I am fearful that I may have left someone out. If that is the case I am sorry, but I trust that my oversight will be forgiven. One person I have not thanked, however, has not been forgotten. The best has merely been left for last. Rex, thank you for being in my life.

GIVING BIRTH IN CANADA, 1900–1950

Introduction

Maternalism, a belief that mothering is central to the lives of women, was an ideology that most Canadians shared with others in Western society in the first half of the twentieth century.[1] The ability to bear children was a physical act that separated women from men. It was crucial to the survival of the species and, more particularly, to the survival and strength of various national and racial groupings. But before a woman could become a mother, she had to give birth. This was and is the most fundamental of creative acts. This book is a history of that process in Canada from 1900 to 1950. These were the years in which the medicalization of childbirth, begun in the late nineteenth century, intensified. As a consequence, this book focuses on the regular medical profession and the views of its members about the nature of birthing, and, even more significant for the women concerned, on the way in which medical practitioners treated their patients. As such, the book is part of a wider historiography on the medical treatment of women, the history of childbirth, and gender and science.

The literature examining the medical treatment of women has not been particularly complimentary. Feminist activists, motivated by what they observed in the contemporary world – the problematic side effects of the pill, the dangers of breast implants, increased medical intervention in birthing, and the emergence of new reproductive technologies – concluded that medicine seemed to be targeting women's bodies.[2] In the last decade or so, the burgeoning field of feminist medical ethics has continued the activism, suggesting that something is missing in the way in which medicine was and is practised.[3] Historians followed suit, emphasizing the alienation from their bodies that women felt as a result of medical control.[4] One of the few exceptions to this was Edward Shorter's *History of Women's Bodies*, which was a homage to the medical profession as a saviour of women from the problems of their bodies. Although Shorter's work garnered much public attention, it was not reflective of the trend away from seeing the medical profession and its practitioners as the rescuers of women.[5] It is within that context that the early historical monographs on childbirth emerged.[6] Reproduction was central to sexual differences, and the feminist concern with the changes occurring in reproductive biology and technology made it important to understand the history of the process.[7]

No book has focused on the history of childbirth in Canada, though there are numerous studies incorporating aspects of it.[8] The international literature continues to be voluminous,[9] and its criticism of the medical profession has become much more nuanced than it had been. It now reflects anthropological and sociological as well as historical concerns about the process of birthing, the role of women in it, and the way in which birthing practices have changed as a result of pressure from both women and physicians. The literature in the field of gender and science also has been influential on childbirth studies, challenging our understanding of the nature of science in all its manifestations (including medicine) and its objectivity.[10] Nevertheless, the feminist activism of the earlier period still resonates in most of the work written.[11]

Feminist scholarship has made much about the difference between gender and sex, originally arguing that gender is socially constructed while sex is biologically grounded. This distinction was a major step forward in feminist analysis, since the focus on gender allowed a historical examination of the body and its treatment.[12] While the concept of the gendered nature of the body has been useful, it has not been without controversy. Some feminist theorists have reacted against the concept of gender as being too generalizing, not recognizing the diversity of women.[13] In addition, the stability of the sex/gender binary is somewhat illusory, as Ruth Hubbard has pointed out: 'The distinction between sex and gender ... [is] based on the implicit, but false, assumption that the effects of biology and society are discrete and separable, at least in theory if not in practice ... These effects are in fact inseparable. Every organism constantly transforms its environment while being transformed by it, and, in the case of people, the society in which we live is a major component of our environment.'[14] Nonetheless, the conceptual conceit of the gender/sex divide led to a wealth of research on the medical treatment of women. Within this literature two major issues emerged.

The first was that medicine was part of culture and, as such, was constrained by the norms of culture. Historically, the norms of our culture have defined and limited women, and medicine could not help but do the same. The second was modern Western medicine's mechanistic view of the body, which stemmed from its mechanistic view of the universe.[15] The mechanical model emphasized the body as a machine – regular, predictable – and favoured a technological response to it. But bodies are not predictable. Nevertheless, for physicians, the male body approached the mechanistic ideal better than the female did, and as a result it became the norm for what a healthy body should be. That most physicians were male also reinforced the view that the male body was the norm.

Because of the differences between a woman's body and a man's – the ability of women to menstruate, to give birth, to undergo menopause – physicians (and others) have long assumed that women are closer to and more readily identified by their bodies than men. Consequently, they saw women as closer to nature, or as not transcending nature. Men do not completely escape being body, particularly in the realm of sexuality (their sex drive is often viewed as uncontrollable or dominating). But physicians (as men) tended to view men as being outside their bodies rather than in them. Feminists have argued that in seeing women so closely aligned to and influenced by their bodies, medicine essentialized them – the woman's body became equated with a reproductive body.[16] The normative model of a woman was one who was young enough to be still menstruating and able to bear children. Physicians judged young women entering puberty by how well their bodies were approaching this ideal, and they judged older women by how much their bodies had deviated from it. Differences based on class, ethnicity, ability, and so on were secondary. Because physicians saw women's bodies as different from men's – as foreign – they tended to see what those bodies did as problematic, even though they acknowledged that for the vast majority of women they were not.

As physicians focused on differences between men's and women's bodies, so did historians and others. Feminist scholars have been interested in studying the repercussions that this view had on women. In the early monographs, the tendency was to see women as victims of the medical establishment.[17] However, delineating the areas in which women were victimized tells us very little about the women themselves. As the field developed, so too did interest in discerning how women patients were actors – how they exerted agency within the limits they faced. And the limits were considerable. Whether male or female, patients seldom negotiated with physicians from a position of strength. First, since the late nineteenth century, the power of science in our society has been so strong that any public challenge to it has been seen as irrational. Medicine shared in that power. By going to a doctor, the patient expressed his or her belief in the medical system. Patients have refused to follow medical direction, but medical literature, until very recently, viewed this as aberrant behaviour. Second, the difference in power between the patient and the physician compromised choice for the patient. Since the late nineteenth century, the status of medical practitioners in Canada has been high. Most were middle class (and, until recently) white males, and outside of Quebec, most were of British heritage. Third, physicians obfuscated medical information in a technical language, which made it next to impossible for patients to understand and lessened their ability to make informed judgments. Even when a decision was left to the patient, that person generally worked only with the information provided by the physician. Fourth, the patient was vulnerable compared with the physician; otherwise that person, would not be a patient.

Women were doubly disadvantaged in that as well as being patients, they were women and thus were constrained by their place in society – considered different from men, usually weaker, and often inferior. The male physician they faced was part of an influential profession, and his class position represented public power. Could such a man listen to his women patients as effectually as to his men patients, or would he see in women's bodies the concrete expression of female inferiority and subordination?[18] In the interaction between male (or even female) physicians and female patients, how much choice did the patients have? How much agency could they exert? While no general answer can be given – it certainly depended on the woman and the physician – patient agency did exist. Women often controlled whether and when they would see a physician, and they sometimes supported the increased medicalization of their lives. Just as physicians were a product of their society, so were the women they treated. Many regarded medicine as the rescuer of the ill; they believed in the objectivity of medical science and often subscribed to the social conventions that determined woman's role in society.[19]

Just as women exhibited agency, physicians experienced constraints in their practice, although feminist scholars have not been quite as willing to detail them. In Canada, most physicians were general practitioners who were overwhelmed by the demands of busy and varying practices. Many travelled long distances to see their patients and were not always paid well for doing so. They worked within the context of a professional culture that demanded that they act in a certain way. If affiliated with a hospital, they needed to respond to its regulations. Legal obligations also constrained their actions, as did their personal and moral views.

Many of the themes in the wider literature are present in this study of childbirth. I argue that reproduction itself was (and is) in part socially constructed and that it tells us much about the culture in which it occurred.[20] Even the most 'natural' childbirth had rituals surrounding it that changed greatly over the first half of the century: who was present at the birth, what constituted a normal birth, how long a woman stayed in bed after giving birth, and so on.[21] Doctors had a very specific view of pregnant women, which stemmed from the wider view of women in society. Their medical training emphasized the problematic nature of women's bodies, a reflection of the more general societal belief in the inferiority of women. Both views influenced the medical treatment of women experiencing childbirth.

As well as being partly socially constructed, childbirth is a physiological process, and an understanding of it is necessary in order to appreciate physicians' response to it. Pregnancy lasts approximately nine months, although variations from that average can be considerable. Spontaneous labour begins with one or more of the following signs: a 'show,' or passage of small quantities of blood-stained mucus from the vagina; rupture of the amniotic sac (or bag of waters); and 'true' labour contractions. Physicians tend to see this as the beginning of the first stage of labour. During this stage, the uterine muscles contract and the cervix becomes thinner and more open. The length of this process of dilation varies considerably from patient to patient. What doctors refer to as the transition to the second stage of labour is characterized in general by the woman's urge to bear down and may also be accompanied by symptoms of nausea and temperature fluctuations. The second stage is when the most intense contractions occur, the cervix is fully dilated, and the woman bears down with each contraction to help expel her child. Once the baby has been expelled, the placenta becomes detached from the uterine wall and is also expelled.[22]

In addition to emphasizing the social interpretations of birth over its physiological nature, two other themes are central to this book. First, there is the contingent meaning of words such as *science*, *natural*, *normal*, and even *body*. But to signify this by the frequent use of quotation marks would introduce a visual messiness to the page, so I have not done so. What I have done is to point out the apocalyptic language that physicians sometimes used when trying to convince pregnant women that they should follow medical advice. Physicians' use of binaries to emphasize the value of what they had to offer – civilized as opposed to primitive birth; educated as opposed to midwife care – was an additional language stratagem. Second, as with much of the literature on childbirth, I have had to recognize how and in what ways childbirth became more medicalized in the years under study. Pregnancy itself came under close scrutiny, and this affected the relationship between a pregnant woman and her physicians and indeed created that relationship through the various prenatal visits.

As I was researching and writing, my fascination with the medical profession increased, not just with what it was doing and how it viewed childbirth but why it did so. In many respects my work is part of a continuum of studies on the medical profession in Canada. Early studies viewed the subject very much from within the profession, emphasizing the heroic aspects of early medicine, the rise of professionalization, the great medical discoveries, the histories of medical institutions, and the biographies of medical practitioners.[23] With the emergence of social history in Canada in the 1970s and 1980s, historians became more critical of the profession, and in studies on women and their contact with medicine they emphasized the way in which medicine saw and treated women. In other words, they examined medicine from without. In recent years, historians have been at pains to find women's agency.[24] In some respects my work is a reflection of the older studies that focused on the medical profession and its treatment of women. However, I do not see the profession as a monolithic group. Indeed, I am intrigued by the internal debates that took place within it. While I recognize the constraints on medical practitioners, I do so not as an apologist for them but in order to further an understanding of why they believed what they did and why they acted the way they did. As part of the research process I became aware of the diversity of doctors, the contradictory nature of some of their beliefs, and their efforts to come to some consensus. They seemed at the same time very uncertain about what they were doing and convinced that they knew best. As Gerald Grob has argued,

As human beings we generally inhabit two different worlds simultaneously. The first is characterized by contingency, indeterminacy, and an inability to comprehend or control the numerous variables that shape our environment; our judgements, analyses, and actions often represent a pragmatic response to a seemingly intractable and partially incomprehensible universe. The second is an imaginary and idealized world – one characterized by certainty and clarity, and where pure and precise knowledge leads to a kind of understanding that enables human beings to cope with or solve perennial problems. The static nature of this idealized world fosters the illusion that the creation of a veritable utopia is within reach.[25]

Doctors sought certainty in a field in which little existed, and they did so in several ways, including the above-mentioned use of language.

In looking at childbirth, I am analysing the structure of medicine rather than the motivation of individual physicians. The treatment that physicians gave varied, depending partly on when and where they trained and where they practised.[26] Nevertheless, the physician represented the point of contact between the individual and the medical system, although he (and most physicians throughout the first half of the century were male) may not represent the contact between the individual and health care. The purpose of this book is not to blame anyone but to point out the consequences of certain types of perspectives. There were particular ways in which medical practitioners examined issues, saw problems, and described what they did. My aim, in part, is to illuminate some of these and to make the reader more aware of how doctors as a group worked. I am not suggesting that physicians in the past should have renegotiated a new type of medicine; there is no value in taking such a position; it would be redolent with historical presentism and arrogance. Rather, my purpose is to see how physicians worked in their world. Our distance from that world allows us to be aware of what they may have been unaware of. All of us have a view of life that allows us to cope with complexity, but sooner or later this view comes against the reality of the complexity, and that is when change is possible and – in the case of medicine – when criticism of it occurs.

And it is very easy to criticize. Yet it seems to me that often historians have created a new binary with their criticism. We have juxtaposed Western medicine against a romanticized view of how we think medicine should be. With respect to childbirth, we have romanticized midwives in particular. Certainly, many of the women who assisted other women in birth were deserving of admiration. They worked long hours for little pay. They provided care, comfort, and tangible support, and they intervened in childbirth less than physicians did. But some midwives intervened considerably and dangerously. Too often we have compared the best midwives to the worst physicians.[27] Too often we have overly dichotomized (bad) intervention and surveillance and (good) natural birth.

In the introduction to *The Nature of Their Bodies: Women and Their Doctors in Victorian Canada*, I tried to address the reason for doing a study of Canadian medicine when it could be argued that Canada was part – and perhaps not a particularly important part – of the Western medical world. There is no doubt that Canadian physicians were influenced by trends elsewhere. Their reading of the international literature was considerable. Nevertheless, to see what they were doing only within an international context is, I think, a rather provincial and limited view. It ignores the importance of place, and as the narratives of many Canadian practitioners reveal, their place of practice was a crucial factor in the medical care they could offer. Yet the call to compare the Canadian situation with that of the United States and Britain refuses to disappear. For that reason I have made some effort to tell readers what was happening elsewhere. Perhaps, as a result, some future anonymous reader of a British or American study will offer the novel critique that it should go beyond its national boundaries and take Canada into consideration!

I do not consider *Giving Birth in Canada* a definitive work by any means. To understand the nature of medical and patient choice, we need to know much more about what alternatives to medical care existed and what understanding women had of their own bodies. Rather than detailing all the variations and shifts in treatment, I have tried to illuminate some of the trends and processes underlying treatment. In examining the first half of the twentieth century, I have chosen to focus on years that most historians of childbirth have not examined. These were years of tremendous change. In medicine, the century began with a profession practising very much as it had in the latter years of the nineteenth century. However, more rigid standards in medical education were soon implemented, and expectations of the ability to deliver curative health care increased with the discovery of insulin in the 1920s and the introduction of antibiotics by the 1940s. Nevertheless, practitioners were hard-pressed to meet those expectations. The influenza epidemic at the end of the First World War revealed the weaknesses of the health system in Canada and led to the establishment of the federal Department of Health in 1919. No medical response could offset the broader attacks on health caused by the Great Depression of the 1930s or the challenges of the Second World War – which, at least for Canadian service people, was not as horrific as that of the Great War of 1914–18.

For women's lives, the changes that would come in this half-century were difficult to imagine when the twentieth century dawned. In 1900 Canadian women did not have the vote, very few married women worked in paid employment, birth control was illegal, and while birth rates were generally in decline they were still significantly higher than they later became. A woman's prestige was very much linked to her maintaining an image of moral rectitude. Her status was closely aligned to her maternal role – indeed, motherhood was deemed to be her primary purpose. Canadians believed that the urge to mother was instinctive; it was natural for women to want to be mothers. In 1911, Lucy Maud Montgomery's reaction on discovering that she was pregnant for the first time was perhaps overly romanticized, but it was one with which many Canadian women would have identified: 'I want to have a child – something to link me with the future of my race. I want to give a human soul a chance to live this wonderful life of ours. I want something of my very own – bone of my bone, flesh of my flesh, to love and cherish.'[28] Motherhood was women's defining social role. It was the source of their prestige; and to be worthy of it, their commitment to mothering had to be total. Other aspects of their lives and experience had to either take second place or be eliminated altogether.

In the early years of the century, higher education, women's rights activism, and women's labour were all suspect.[29] For example, critics argued that education raised women's sights to something other than their maternal responsibilities. Some physicians feared not only that educated women were more likely than their uneducated sisters to reject maternity, but that education altered the experience of maternity and made it more difficult.[30] The First World War caused some, but certainly not all, to change their views about these matters. The war brought most adult Canadian women the right to vote; it even forced Canadians to accept the significant involvement of women – including many married women – in the workforce. However, the return of peace, the desire to forget the war, and the urge to make up for the lives lost in the conflict and in the influenza epidemic that followed meant that women's childbearing role was re-emphasized.

Throughout the period under study, many people continued to see having children as the purpose of marriage. A 1935 medical text argued that women who made a conscious decision not to have children or could not have children should not have the right to marry.[31] Emily Murphy, one of Canada's leading advocates for women's rights, told her women readers in *Chatelaine* that without children a marriage was no more than 'an agreement between a flirt and a philanderer.'[32] The United Church of Canada believed that no marriage 'built on the refusal to bear children [was] a complete marriage.'[33] Childless marriages were unhappy marriages. When in 1947 a woman wrote an article in *Chatelaine* claiming that she did not want to have a child, readers greeted her words with consternation and then with relief when she later recanted.[34] By emphasizing the natural or instinctual aspect of motherhood, commentators aligned it with the biological. In doing so, they removed it from women's agency. In motherhood, women became grouped, generalized, essentialized.

But such essentialism was not of concern to most Canadians. While they had learned to accept higher education for women and the desire of single women to work, they were still uneasy about the employment of married women. Statistics showed that infant mortality was higher for children whose mothers worked than for those whose mothers did not.[35] During the Depression of the 1930s, many Canadians raised the concern about women, especially married women, taking jobs away from men. And, of course, the issue of working mothers became especially cogent during the Second World War, when the government of the day recruited mothers into the war effort and expected future mothers to engage in work traditionally done by men. While Canadians acknowledged the necessity of both, they expressed concern that in order to win the war they might be squandering their future.[36] After the war, although the government as well as the opinion makers in society encouraged women to withdraw from the workforce, by the 1950s labour-force participation rates for married women were increasing.

The irony is that, at the same time, birth rates were rising, with the beginning of the baby boom. The boom was particularly obvious because birth rates had been in a continuous decline since 1900. This decline had been accentuated by the economic woes of the 1930s, to which Canadians had responded by not getting married, by delaying marriage, or by not having large families. The decline ended with the Second World War, which brought full employment and caused a psychological shift away from delaying personal gratification. The end of the war simply emphasized this trend, which was strengthened by the desire of Canadians to focus on home and family.

Despite the decline of the birth rate from 1900 to the early years of the Second World War and its subsequent rise and then explosion, the legality of controlling fertility had altered very little. True, by the interwar period a birth control movement had emerged, and it had achieved some success in the courts. But the law of the land was unchanged – birth control was illegal. Childbirth remained a central experience for the vast majority of Canadian women.

What follows is a description of how physicians treated women in childbirth. The first chapters set the context by providing the reader with an overview of medicine and obstetrics. Because so much of the historical literature has juxtaposed midwife-directed birth and physician-directed birth, I thought that a chapter on midwives would be appropriate; it provides a comparative basis for those that focus on regular medicine. The latter follow a woman's birthing experience from the diagnosis of pregnancy, through childbirth and its complications, to the postnatal period.

My focus is on the English-speaking regular medical profession in Canada, and the sources used for this study consisted of the following: textbooks assigned to medical students in the major Canadian medical faculties; the Canadian medical periodical press; popular medical advice books written specifically for nonmedical people and read in Canada; popular medical literature published in women's magazines; the patient records of a number of hospitals; interviews with women who gave birth during the period under study; and interviews with a number of physicians who were trained or who practised medicine during these years. As with any source material, each has its strengths and weaknesses.

One characteristic of the medical textbooks is that most were not Canadian. Canadian medical schools assigned predominantly American and British texts to their students. There were few textbooks written by Canadians, and those that did exist were not always under a Canadian imprint. The textbook authors tended to assume that their readers either were or would be urban practitioners, although occasionally they recognized the specificity of rural practice. Nonetheless, the textbooks are a central source, for they represent what Canadian medical teachers chose to have their students read. Textbooks represent the orthodoxy of the medical profession. As Nelly Oudshoorn has argued, they reflect not only the latest research but also the 'representation [of] a new reality.'[37] The evidence indicates that most physicians practised according to that reality.

The articles in the Canadian medical periodical press support this evidence. They are full of communications from Canadian physicians across the country, summaries of conferences attended, editorials on the major medical issues of the day, and reviews of the latest publications, as well as articles reprinted from other medical journals which the editors believed to be of interest to their readers. Unlike the textbooks, the articles allowed the average practitioner to have his say, and it is remarkable how many physicians from rural and small town practices found the time to describe their medical beliefs and work. Nevertheless, there is little doubt that the urban medical elite, predominantly from teaching hospitals, had pride of place. Yet regardless of who the authors were, the communications provide detailed descriptions of cases, which enable the reader to compare what some practitioners were doing with what they had been taught to do, as represented by the medical textbooks. The periodical medical press was impressively energetic during the first half of the twentieth century – there were more than seventy English-language publications. Many did not last long; some were continuations of others under a different name; still others were very specialized in their perspective.[38] The value of this literature is that it was the major forum for physicians in Canada to communicate with one another and to raise issues about what concerned them. It was written by and for physicians.

The difficulty with both the medical textbooks and the medical periodical press is that they were public forums, even if the public was only other physicians. Consequently, they tended to describe the unusual case rather than the usual, to put forward new ways of doing a procedure, or to debate the old ways. It is not always easy to get a sense of what practitioners were actually doing in their practises. The cases related in the periodical press do help overcome this problem, but even more valuable are the patient records of hospitals (both large and small) and private practices. These records represent a treasure trove for the historian of medicine, for they allow her to get closer to what physicians actually did in the past, rather than relying on what they said they did or what they recommended to others. I was very fortunate in being given access to records from several hospitals, but there is little doubt that, for some administrators, the issue of access was a difficult one. Final agreement was reached only because I made it clear that I was not interested in using the names of patients. Instead, I have invented names that reflect the patient's ethnicity, keeping the same initials. In doing so, I have maintained confidentiality without making the new mothers appear anonymous.

Another source that helped focus more attention on the patient was the popular medical literature: books written with patients in mind, and medical articles published in women's magazines. Both sources were excellent reminders of the relationship that always existed between the patient and her physician. They provided me with the opportunity to see what women were reading about pregnancy and childbirth, and how the advice was couched when they, rather than medical professionals, were the recipients of it. This literature is popular because, in the words of one historian, 'it does not have to persuade – it does not innovate– it addresses readers who are ready for it.'[39] This was particularly true for the women's periodical press. The circulation figures of the women's press was impressive. The *Canadian Home Journal*, for example, had a circulation of over 52,000 in the mid-1920s and over 250,000 in 1940. *Chatelaine*, the premier Canadian women's magazine, had a circulation of over 70,000 in its first year of publication (1928) and over 252,000 by 1940.[40]

What was particularly rewarding about doing the research for this project, compared with my previous work on the nineteenth century, was the opportunity to conduct interviews. There was no pretence of doing so in any systematic manner. Rather, what sociologists refer to as the snowball effect (using word of mouth, etc.) was the 'method' utilized. The physicians interviewed were always open about their own training and that of others. They appreciated the changes that had occurred over time and believed that most had been for the better. At times, they suggested areas where their own practice of medicine had deviated from what they had been taught, thereby emphasizing a central tension in the profession. Hearing the accounts of women about their birthing experience was a constant reminder of the patient's view, a needed counterpoint to the medical perspective that dominated most of the published literature on birthing. The women's memories were insightful, often ironic, and sometimes funny, but always heartfelt. They reminded me, as nothing else could, of the centrality of the childbirth experience for their lives.

While my focus is on regular medical practice, I have attempted to introduce the experience of other birthing models (whether First Nations or midwifery) to remind the reader that there is always another way of doing things – even of having a baby. Physicians were aware of these models but saw them as something more than different. They created a hierarchy of birth practices, which at times they racialized. They differentiated between 'civilized' and 'primitive' women in childbirth and attached significant meaning to those differences. In doing so they too acknowledged, at least in part, the constructed nature of childbirth.

CHAPTER ONE

The Uncertain World of Medicine
and Medical Practitioners

We look with condescension on mere empirical knowledge as differing in kind from scientific dicta. Actually 'science' tells us nothing, but is itself integrated from empirically established facts. It changes constantly, both in scope and content.

F.B. Exner, 1951[1]

Medicine in Canada in the first half of the twentieth century was a profession full of tension. Its practitioners aligned themselves with science in their use of a specialized language, in their increasing dependence on technology, and in their insistence on standardization. Each of these provided an element of certainty to what physicians did, and many historians of medicine have recognized them as reflections of the development of the profession, for good or ill. Less acknowledged is that some physicians questioned the emphasis on science, at least in comparison with the art and practice of medicine. Nonetheless, the tension between medicine as science and medicine as art was negligible compared with the stresses caused by the world in which physicians worked, a world that was less than scientific and full of uncertainty. It is these stresses and uncertainties that historians of medicine, especially historians of the medical care of women, have generally overlooked. Yet they are significant if we are to understand why physicians acted in the way they did, why they emphasized the certainty of what they had to offer their patients, and why they were so categorical about their advice. In part, such behaviour was a reflection of their belief in science and its validity. In part, it was a way of overcoming their own uncertainties and the challenges facing them as practitioners.

In addition to the perennial science-versus-art debate in medicine, several other issues confronted physicians. First, the growing dominance of hospitals in the medical care system challenged the individual physician and his ability to control his practice and his status within the profession. At least in the medical literature, hospitals were becoming a focus of attention: they were where exciting medicine took place. Second, while medical history has emphasized the way in which the allopathic approach gained a monopoly over who could call himself doctor, alternative forms of health care and caregivers still existed. Their continuance was a constant reminder of competition, but it also evinced the unwillingness of Canadians to embrace Western medicine as the only acceptable health modality. Third, many doctors believed they had received insufficient training as medical students: when they entered practice they became aware of how much they did not know. Fourth, within medicine itself various practitioners were sensitive to how their own colleagues competed with them. Of particular note was the rise of specialists and the overwhelming emphasis which the published medical literature directed at them. In reading the literature, rural practitioners could easily become aware of the gap between a well-serviced urban practice and their own.

Finally, the very nature of medical practice had its own difficulties, and many practitioners believed themselves to be overworked and underpaid. The relations between physicians and patients were always challenging, and although critics of medicine have emphasized the discrepancy in power between physician and patient, patients were not without agency; in expressing it, they could appear to be rejecting what physicians had to offer them. The patient-doctor relationship was a site of contestation and negotiation. When the patient was a woman, the power of the physicians loomed even larger. Even so, some physicians were sensitive to the power their women patients held over their practices and were aware that the women could pose a threat to their image of respectability. This chapter introduces the world of medicine and the physician in Canada – on the surface a secure world, but one that was changing, often presenting medicine's practitioners with doubts and uncertainties.

Physicians worked within two worlds. The first was the construct of science. Positivist in nature, it reduced reality in order to study it through experimentation, and it formalized knowledge into cause and effect relationships. The second consisted of the physician's medical practice, where on a day-to-day basis he faced the vagaries and contradictions of human lives.[2] D.W. Cathell preferred the former world and criticized patients, especially women, who apparently rejected it. In his turn-of-the-century book *The Physician Himself and Things That Concern His Reputation and Success*, he contended: 'The real secret why so many truly scientific physicians ... very often decidedly lack popularity, and fail to get much practice, is that cold, unemotional, impassive logic ... [is] often associated with a deficiency of the qualities of head and heart which appeal to the weak side of woman – *her emotions*.'[3] For Cathell, lack of emotion was the strength of scientific medicine. Yet there were problems. Dr D. Mackintosh from Pugwash, Nova Scotia, feared that the 'impassive logic' so esteemed by Cathell caused patients to have overly high expectations of medicine. Science endowed medicine with an aura of certainty which neither it nor its practitioners could meet. In trying to meet it, Adam H. Wright, professor of obstetrics at the University of Toronto, worried that too often the art of medicine suffered; the danger, he said, was that the science of medicine worked to the detriment of patient care.[4]

Despite such concerns, the science of medicine seemed to be winning out over the art of medicine. Medical faculties in the interwar period increased the scientific component necessary to enter medical school, and advertisers appealed to the science of medicine to sell their products.[5] Private citizens, too, recognized that they were living in a scientific age. In 1925, Lucy Maud Montgomery wrote in her diary about what she saw as the decline of the church and asked herself, 'But suppose it does die.

What matter? It has served its day as God's instrument. He is using another now – Science. Through Science the next great revelation will come.'[6]

Not everyone was happy with the way science was dominating medicine. In 1926 Dr Harold Atlee, professor of obstetrics and gynaecology at Dalhousie University, questioned the emphasis given to the theory of medicine over its practice. The practice of medicine was what doctors did, he said, yet in medical school the students seemed to shirk the practical clinics so that they could concentrate on book learning to pass their exams.[7] Atlee did not advocate teaching less theory but wanted more time devoted to the clinical side of medicine. Any suggestion to lessen theory would have appeared to be an attack on the science of medicine, which had become the watchword for progress and modernity in medical practice. F.B Exner, in his *The Nature of Medical Practice* (1951), caught the contradiction within medical science best: 'We live in a "scientific age" and we bow in abject worship at every invocation of the holy word "Science." We tend to forget that this sacred Frankenstein is a man-made and rather amorphous structure composed of all the things we think we know – and includes all the things we know that are not true.'[8] Long before the term was coined by social historians, Exner was arguing that science and thus medicine were socially constructed.

Twentieth-century medicine aligned itself with science in three ways: through language, technology, and insistence on standardization. Scholars have argued that specialized language exemplified scientific medicine in the twentieth century. It separated both the medical practitioner and his practice from the vast majority of patients who utilized health care. Medical language helped insulate physicians from the emotional world of patients, their friends, and relatives. It distanced them from the world outside medicine and helped make medicine a somewhat closed world in which contradictions were difficult to acknowledge. Patients and physicians spoke two different languages of the body. But as scholars have also suggested, even more than using a different language to explain the same thing, medical language constructed a different way of looking at and thinking about the body; it created 'a new world altogether.'[9] Ruth Hubbard has written revealingly on how science has deleted the person, the humanness of who did science. What was observed became more real than who did the observing.[10] What the scientist observed became a subject in its own right, and this removed it from attacks of bias. At the same time, the language of medicine was (and is) very rich metaphorically. Medical writers depicted medicine as coming to the 'rescue.' Physicians engaged in a 'war against disease.' Doctors used apocalyptic images and warnings to ensure that their patients followed recommended treatment.[11]

The use of technology also distanced the medical practitioner from his patient. Expensive technology, once purchased, demanded to be used, with the result that cheaper alternatives might disappear from practice.[12] The expansion of technology in medicine is easy to track. The coming of x-ray machines to small hospitals, such as the Owen Sound General and Marine Hospital in 1918, was a major event in their histories. The use of such machines generated money for hospitals, and they were ways in which individual institutions could distinguish themselves from one another and assure their patients that they had something special to offer. The availability of technology became the measurement of a good hospital.[13] As a result of technology such as x-rays, and through procedures that allowed surgeons to explore almost every cavity of the body, physicians became more intimate with some parts of their patients' bodies than their patients themselves were. Add to this the fact that patients did not have the specialized language to explain what it was they were experiencing, and the result was, in the words of one critic, that medical science 'owned' the study of the body.[14]

Western medicine viewed the body as a machine that should run properly. When it did not, that indicated illness or an unhealthy state. Even Dr Wilfred T. Grenfell, whose missionary work in Labrador and Newfoundland was renowned, could advise his readers in his 1924 book *Yourself and Your Body*: 'Remember that it is all machinery; and it is all the machinery that you have, and if you spoil it, you can never have another set.'[15] Such a perspective left little room for emotional or spiritual aspects –

which, given Grenfell's evangelistic persuasion, was ironic. But ironic or not, it underlined how physicians argued in books designed to be medical in orientation.

Linked to the mechanistic view of the body was the belief in the ability to measure its functioning. In Western medicine, the ability to measure what the body did through instrumentation is central, and it had become key to doing science by the mid-nineteenth century. What was important was what could be measured. This was true in the wider society as well.[16] Not just anyone could take measurements. For example, Dr Frederick Fenton, an associate professor in obstetrics at the University of Toronto in 1906, warned his colleagues not to depend on the pelvic measurements of women taken by nurses. Only someone familiar with the anatomy of the pelvis and abdomen – namely, a physician – could be trusted.[17] Measurements had to be accurate; decisions about treatment depended on them. Measurement established the standards of how healthy bodies worked – the average experience. But problems could arise when the average or normal experience became equated with the healthy experience.[18]

Measurements lent an element of certainty to what physicians did. Certainty, or at the very least a sense of confidence, was crucial for their ability to function, since they often worked in a very uncertain field. Much of a physician's skill came from experience and an intuitive sense of what might ail a patient or what might work for a patient. Each individual had his or her own responses to illness and to medication. Medication might work, but the reasons why it did were not always clear. What should work might not. Faced with such uncertainty, physicians tried to create a world of certainty or at least an aura of certainty. Measurements were hard facts, concrete indicators (once there was agreement on what they indicated). They took the art (uncertainty) out of medicine. The results of monitoring the body were dependable, whereas the patient's experience was not. Measurements allowed physicians to remove the responsibility from themselves as individual practitioners and to place it with the medical collective, which had agreed on what the measurements meant.

For some physicians, measurements became a substitute for the art of medicine and a means by which to 'read' a patient. An 1934 editorial in the *Nova Scotia Medical Bulletin* expressed concern that the medical student of the day was becoming too dependent on the 'accessory aids to diagnosis – the X-ray, blood tests, bacteriological examinations,' to the detriment of 'keen observation.'[19] Such aids constrained the medical imagination. They encouraged belief in certainty. Nowhere was this expressed more explicitly than by Montreal physician Dr A.H. Gordon:

> In the pursuit of pure science absolute accuracy is our goal, and a large part of science consists in *measurement*, and measurements of form, size, colour, density, length, breadth, strength, are the processes which occupy much of our time and energy in the premedical and primary medical years of our apprenticeship. Normals are established, and from these judgements are formed, and in the attempt to bridge the gap between pure science and its practical application in clinical medicine and surgery we presume to establish normals for man and for his various systems, and by the methods of clinical medicine we attempt to recognize the deviations from these normals. We recognize sensations of heat and cold, colour, sound and tension through our special senses, and assemble the results and adjudicate upon them. To these are then added other impressions through the special senses, conveyed by instruments of precision, and all of these together constitute our foundation in fact.[20]

The acceptance of and dependence on measurement, medical language, and machines resulted in conformity and standardization. This was not necessarily bad – standards protect patients. But once standards of health or illness were in place, they were difficult to shift. Also, associating health with what is normal or standard may not be advantageous, since what is normal in a society may not be healthy. Also what is normal for any one person is constantly shifting.[21] Nevertheless, standardization of treatment (or its encouragement) was part of medical culture. Trained one way as a medical student, it was not always easy for a physician to change.[22] If he did, it could call into question the treatment he had given patients in the past, resulting in heightened levels of uncertainty and insecurity.

The increasing importance of hospitals added to the push for standardization. The expansion of hospitals in the first half of the century was partly a response to the increased technological orientation of medicine – the hospitals housed the machines. Hospitals were also where the elite of the profession practised and set standards for private practice. In the nineteenth century, most hospitals had been started as charity institutions, designed to care for the poor. As a result, there were not many of them. In 1890, for all of Ontario, there were only twenty public general hospitals in fifteen communities. But by 1922 Ontario had 122 public hospitals, including 10 sanatoria for consumptives, and in 1944 it had 116 general and 25 Red Cross hospitals. In Saskatchewan before 1900 there were few hospitals except nursing homes. By 1920 the province could claim 35 hospitals, and 23 more were built by 1930. In Canada as a whole there were 481 public general hospitals in 1929; four years later the number was 589. By 1952 there were 730 (including paediatric), and the total number of hospitals of any kind was 924.[23] The hospitals also were becoming standardized. In 1921; a hospital accreditation program began. It originated with the American College of Surgeons, which defined the minimum standard to be met by all hospitals with which its members were affiliated.[24] This was a powerful incentive for Canadian hospitals to measure up. In addition, if specific hospitals wanted to maintain their ability to teach either interns or nurses, they had to conform to the interwar period's new demands for modernity and efficiency.[25]

Not only were there more hospitals, but they were increasing in size. The Royal Victoria Hospital, in Montreal, was fairly typical of a large urban hospital in its growth pattern. In 1901 it admitted 2,579 patients; in 1915, 5,421; and by 1934, 13,307. Although numbers were incredibly large in the 1930s, officers of the hospital were concerned about occupancy rates. In 1935 the hospital reported an occupancy rate of only 65 per cent, the lowest for several years. The Depression was having its effect as potential paying patients put off hospital care, which they felt they could no longer afford. Outpatient clientele, however, had increased. The low occupancy rates ended with the Second World War, when overcrowding became a problem for many hospitals.[26]

The expansion reflected the increasing use made of hospitals by the middle classes, for hospitals had widened their appeal. They were vocal in their insistence on aseptic conditions; they basked in the reflected glory of medicine's rise in status, a result of new discoveries such as insulin. The increase in surgery, and complex surgery at that, could best be done in an institutional setting that provided both technological and personnel support. The attractiveness of hospitals also reflected the decreasing size of homes large enough to care for the sick and the decline in the percentage of families with domestic servants who could help with the care. Some analysts have also speculated that the increasing emotional intensity of the twentieth-century family meant that illness within it became a dysfunctional factor that was lessened by removal to a hospital.[27]

Linked to middle-class use of hospitals was the rise in paying patients. In 1906 the Kingston General Hospital had 886 ward patients and 457 paying patients. In 1915 the numbers were 1,500 and 1,200, respectively. By 1917 paying patients constituted the majority – 1,663 compared with 1,473 ward patients. At times, the breakdown does not give the full impact of the shift. In looking at the number of paying patient days, the annual report for 1927 noted that they had increased 20 per cent from the previous year, whereas indigent patient days had increased only by 15 per cent. The Depression years saw a reversal of the trend. In 1934 there were 42,485 public ward patient days compared with 27,476 private and semi-private ward patient days. The annual report for that year warned: 'Since 1930 the public service has increased by over 30%. At the same time the private and semi-private service has decreased by about the same proportion.'[28] With the return of economic prosperity, the situation again reversed itself, so that by 1947 there were 39,061 public ward patient days and 85,601 private and semi-private ward patient days.[29]

Hospitals were not only growing in numbers and size; they were also becoming increasing complex, as reflected in the expansion of departments and the variety of ailments for which people were being admitted. As well, the orientation of the hospital had shifted. In the early years of the century, hospital care was generally divided between medical and surgical, the former being predominant. Soon the latter became the primary focus of hospital admissions, with medical perhaps being represented increasingly by outpatient departments and services. This followed a more general and wider sensibility within the profession, both in Canada and elsewhere, which adopted the surgeon's traditional focus on external diseases such as tumours as a model for internal diseases. As Ornella Moscucci has argued, 'Efforts were made in order to render internal diseases accessible to the senses, as was the practice in surgery, and increasing emphasis was placed on instrumental and surgical interference in diagnosis and treatment.'[30] At the turn of the century, the Victoria General Hospital, Halifax, divided its eight attending physicians and surgeons equally between the medical and the surgical divisions. In 1920–1, however, there were 424 admissions to the medical division but 1,650 to the surgical. This imbalance continued and by 1938–9 there were 982 admissions to the medical division, equally divided between the sexes, whereas there were 4,210 to the surgical with women numbering 2,278.[31] Surgery had become the predominant aspect of hospital practice. A 1917 text described it as follows:

> The performance of a surgical operation resembles the conduct of a military campaign. Special knowledge and prolonged training are required on the part of the principals – the surgeon and his assistants; the implements employed must be familiar to those who use them, and must be got ready with minute and scrupulous care; the environment must, if possible, be selected to the greatest possible advantage. The actual operation demands skill, courage, prudence, and resource; the campaign is not ended with the closure of the wound, but must be pursued without slackening until the decisive result, viz. the recovery of the patient, is assured.[32]

One consequence of the increase in surgery was a decrease in time spent in hospital, because diseases were not allowed to run their course. The push toward paying patients was also a factor, as was better nursing. Montreal General Hospital patients stayed an average of 21.2 days in 1901, 17.8 days in 1920, and 16 days by 1940.[33] Public patients stayed longer than paying patients. The difference between the two reveals that the nineteenth-century charitable legacy had not been forgotten. Non-paying patients may have arrived at the hospital sicker than paying patients and thus needed more time for care. And since they did not have the same access to supervised care at home, they stayed in hospital longer to ensure their recovery.

Hospitals added to the aura of medical practitioners because it was they who determined who could be accepted as a patient. Yet the rise of hospitals and their increasing dominance could increase an individual practitioner's anxiety. Was he good enough to receive hospital-admitting privileges? Hospitals helped create a medical elite: ambitious practitioners wanted to be on the staff of teaching institutions. In a hospital setting, the daring surgeon could find the support he needed as well as patients. Despite the fact that most medical care took place in private practice, the hospital practitioner, especially in teaching hospitals, became the focus of attention. He set the standard; he could train disciples. If that was not enough to make some in private practice feel somewhat insecure, there was also competition from other health providers who offered Canadians medical advice and assistance, challenging the hegemony over health care which doctors believed was their right.

Not everyone subscribed to the Western medical paradigm of medicine. In Canada, the First Nations had their own medical system. Franz Boas found that three types of healers existed among the southern Kwakwa Ka'wakw (Kwakiutl) people at the turn of the century: one healer could locate disease in the body but could do little about it; another could cure patients by building up their supernatural power; the third and most important could cure individuals and actually throw off or extract the disease from them.[34] Each First Nation or group had its own arsenal of medicine depending on where they lived and what was available. It is just as well that they did. Even though the health of First Nations people was a federal responsibility, Ottawa shirked its duty. In 1934 Ottawa's health costs spent on Native people amounted to $9.60 per capita; on non-natives, $31.00.[35]

Alternatives to regular medicine abounded in mainstream society. Folk medicine remained very popular even when regular medicine seemingly was increasing its sway. At the turn of the century, in Brigus and Brigus Gullies, Cape Breton, the local midwife, Mrs Hazel Way, recalled: 'If you wrapped a herring around your neck you could cure strep throat. The finbone of a haddock was supposed to charm away a toothache.'[36] A school-teacher in Quebec in 1939 noted a remedy for unwanted hair: 'Have someone give you a piece of fresh pork and rub it on the part where the hairs are to be removed and bury it in the ground (where it is left to rot) and say, "Cursed hair, remove yourself just as the devil removes himself from the sight of God and never come back again, never, never, never!"'[37] People learned to cope when doctors were not available. One woman recounted the situation on the Alberta frontier:

I can remember Homestead's little boy when he was born. He was only two pounds. Now what do you do with a premature baby back in those days? Well, this Mrs. Lind was a Swedish woman, and they lived about six miles from us. Mrs. Homestead was at her place when the baby arrived. They rolled him in oil, or maybe vaseline, and into a little white casing right up to his head. I can still see that little tiny head. They put him in a shoebox packed with blankets. Then they put him in the warming oven of the coal stove for an incubator, and kept the lid open for circulation of the air. Mom and Mrs. Lind took turns staying up at night and keeping the heat in the stove just right so that the baby's temperature wouldn't drop. They fed him with an eyedropper. They had him six weeks in that warming oven and Mrs. Lind didn't dare bake bread because the stove would get overheated. They built another stove outside with stones so they could save that one little baby. These two women working to save that little baby. And, by jingo, he a great big six-foot guy![38]

Women throughout the country treated their families with remedies proven by experience. Most homes had their medical manuals. Some were written by physicians; others not. But all emphasized that the mother was to be nurse and doctor, not only when there were no doctors nearby but even when there were. In 1932 an article in *Chatelaine* stated: 'It is of paramount importance that every woman, especially mothers, should know what remedies to use in the treatment of slight ailments – little matters for which a physician would not be consulted but which, if neglected, may lead to grave disorders.'[39] Only when the family could not care for sick members or did not know how to respond to illness was a physician called in.

Patent medicine was also readily available, advertised in newspapers, magazines, and Eaton's catalogue. A 1918 article signed 'A Medical Man' complained that for every dollar earned by a general practitioner an equal amount was spent on patent medicines or given to alternative practitioners.[40] While some physicians were concerned about the ingredients of patent medicine and their dangers (many contained cocaine, strychnine, opium, or alcohol), their popularity testified to people's belief in their efficacy. Throughout the 1920s Canadians could still purchase old standby tonics: Lydia Pinkham's Vegetable Compound, Dr Chase's Nerve Food, and Siegel's Syrup. Dr Pierce's Favourite Prescription made a special appeal to women who had 'ills peculiar to their sex.' It played on their fear of surgery by stating that women's ills could respond to 'remedies made of herbs [used] by the Indians, among whom operations are rare.' It assured them that the prescription was 'an old, reliable, reconstructive tonic.'[41] As hospital records show, doctors were well aware that their patients took such medicines. Gordon Stiles, thirty-eight years old and a married farmer, entered the Victoria General Hospital, Halifax, on 18 December 1920 complaining about poor digestion; from which he had suffered off and on for the last eight to ten years. His case record noted that he had taken 'numerous' patent medicines. Only when they seemed to fail him had he sought the help of physicians, one of whom sent him to hospital.[42] Since physicians usually saw people when the patent medicines did not work, it is not surprising that most opposed them.

Physicians were also concerned about the attraction that other healers had, especially among women. Spiritual healing, which became popular in the interwar period, directed attention away from regular practitioners.[43] In addition, more traditional alternative medical systems continued to thrive. Dr A.W. Paskins, director of the Associated Nature Cure & Physiotherapy Institute in British Columbia, wrote to the Royal Commission on State Health Insurance and Maternity Benefits (B.C.) in 1930 requesting that naturopathic medicine be covered. He reminded the commission that not everyone used allopathic medicine. To bolster his claim, he included a letter from a Mrs Byers, describing how she had gone to a physician in St Paul's in 1927 for breast lumps. The physician had provided her with ointment, but the lumps became worse, so he advised surgery. At this point Mrs Byers went to Paskins, who treated her successfully, apparently through diet. When she became pregnant with her fourth child, the physician who eventually delivered her complained that her Paskins diet was starving her child; but despite her doctor's misgivings she gave birth to a healthy 7½ lb. baby.[44] In trying to explain the allure of competing systems of medicine, regular physicians claimed that the public did not understand the rigour of science and associated medicine with 'hocus-pocus mixed with superstition' which, they said, appealed to the 'semi-educated, the credulous and superstitious.'[45]

Although supporters of regular medicine assumed that the physician should have authority, many Canadians wanted ways of improving their health without resorting to doctors. Women often relied on what they had gleaned over the years. Vera McNichol recalled being a child in Kitchener and having flu in February 1920. The doctor did not hold out much hope for her recovery, but her parents would not give up: 'I could not get my breath, so dad took the bedroom window out and mother stretched a white sheet across the opening. Mother, on her own initiative, brought the coal-stove into the hall and fried up onions, which she put into a poultice to wrap my feet in. She rubbed my chest with goose grease with a little turpentine added ... As Time went on I steadily improved until I was able to sit propped up on pillows.'[46] Women talked and wrote to one another, and news travelled quickly if one found something that worked. The Maple Leaf Auxilliary was a formalized neighbourhood network among the wives of Toronto's machinists, who aided each other in times of sickness.[47] Midwives, too, often offered more than birthing services. These alternative caregivers were competition for physicians, especially the local healers who seldom charged anything, or charged very little.

Even nurses were competitors, though they were not necessarily offering alternative medicine. Many physicians viewed nursing as an extension of the natural female role – mothering. Medical care was learned, rational, and skilled, but nursing care was domestic, intuitive, and considered menial. The fact that, once graduated, most nurses became private-duty nurses emphasized their role as domestic adjuncts. Despite this, some physicians saw nurses' training as a threat to their own status and therefore belittled it. When the University of British Columbia proposed opening a nursing department in 1919, the College of Physicians and Surgeons of British Columbia commented that 'overtraining of nurses is not desirable and results largely in the losing of their usefulness.'[48] In 1920, Eunice Dyke, director of public health nursing for Toronto's health department, told the story of Dr Bryce, chief medical officer for the federal Department of Immigration, who felt that public health nurses were taking too much credit for the decline in infant mortality in the city: 'He insisted recently upon extracting statements from us of other possible factors resulting in the reduction. Finally he remarked, "Don't you think that the weather may account for it?"'[49] Both Bryce's attitude and Dyke's response reflect the tension that at times could exist between physician and nurse. Not that all physicians were so dismissive. Many were more than willing to recognize the knowledge that nurses had. For example, a 1930s medical text pointed out that compared with interns, nurses were much more familiar with therapy and patients' responses to it.[50]

If the mother of the home was the gatekeeper to her family, nurses often were the gatekeepers to medical care. Those working in isolated areas might be the only medical personnel available. In some of the nursing hospitals on the prairies, the women in charge sometimes performed amputations, appendectomies, stitching, and tonsil and adenoid surgery.[51] Others could decide when a physician should be called. Some physicians' concern about keeping nurses deferential, and their fear of being usurped by them, was particularly strong with respect to public health nurses. These women were the most highly trained of all nurses and were accustomed to working on their own, unlike private-duty nurses and hospital nurses, who were far more under the supervision of physicians. Certainly, some physicians felt that public health nurses were unfair competitors – they were on salary and, unlike physicians, did not have to work as 'business-men.'[52] Even hospital nurses sometimes seemed to be encroaching on doctors' territory. One nurse working in Glace Bay in the late 1920s remembered that nurses used to deliver babies and give anaesthesia in the operating room.[53] To maintain the division of power between doctor and nurse (of any kind), physicians in the 1920s, through the College of Physicians and Surgeons, attempted to regulate nursing by defining nurses' duties and determining who could be registered as a nurse. They failed in their attempt, but not until the 1950s could nurses themselves fully regulate who could train and be certified as a nurse.[54]

Meanwhile, Canadians continued to use what they believed worked, though they incorporated scientific discoveries into their own medical treatment. Lucy Maud Montgomery, when carrying her first child, followed the exercise regime set down in a medical book for pregnant women. But at the same time she created her own positive-thinking program: 'I have ... a strong belief in the power which the subconscious mind can exert over physical functions. Every night, as I was dropping off to sleep, and frequently through the day I repeated over and over again the command to my subconscious mind "Make my child strong and healthy in mind and body and make his birth safe and painless for me."'[55]

The external challenges to the medical profession were not the only ones that physicians faced. Their own training and colleagues could add to their insecurity. Many felt that their medical education had been deficient in preparing them for practice. H.L. Burris considered his course and clinical training good but the practical aspects lacking. According to him, his teachers, who were trained under an apprenticeship system, had been better served.[56] In 1930 the Canadian Medical Association reported that 35 per cent of those responding to a questionnaire on medical education stated that they believed their training in preventive medicine had been inadequate. The deputy minister of health for the Province of Ontario blasted the medical schools for emphasizing 'sickness to such an extent that the student is not aware of the fact there is such a thing as health!'[57] Criticisms arose about the emphasis on testing and measuring, rather than observing, and on seeing patients not as people but as organs that did not work.

As physicians expanded their areas of influence, deficiencies in training became more noticeable. In the early decades, medical schools offered little training in psychiatry. Yet society expected doctors to judge whether a patient needed to be committed to an asylum.[58] Doctors gave guidance on infant feeding, but as child expert Dr Alan Brown pointed out in 1918, most students never came into contact with a normal, healthy baby and knew little about infant formulas.[59] Training varied from medical school to medical school and from teacher to teacher, and new courses were added as the need arose. In 1916 a course in medical ethics was begun at Dalhousie. It was also at Dalhousie that Harold Atlee, in the 1930s and 1940s, was willing to train his students in birth control, though it is unclear how formal the training was.[60] Considering that birth control was illegal, Atlee needed to be circumspect.

As medical schools responded to new needs in education, other requirements received less attention than previously. When this was criticized, the schools responded by rebalancing the curriculum. But by then an even newer need had emerged and the cycle began again. New graduates criticized older ones. Older ones felt that their education did not measure up to the modern medicine being taught, which they were expected to practice. The perceived deficiencies in training are important to keep in mind, since many of the physicians practising in the period under review trained in an earlier period. In 1931 almost one-quarter of the more than 10,000 physicians and surgeons in Canada were fifty-five years of age and over.[61] But quality of training did not translate directly into practice. In 1939 Carvell MacIntosh caught this well in the *Dalhousie Medical Journal*: 'It has always been rather amusing to me to think of the emphatic way in which we as students, in written examinations, graphically describe conditions which we have never seen; positively subscribe to the usefulness of treatments which we have never tried; and with just as much vehemence, damn others which we, from experience, know little or nothing about.'[62]

Too often, in the historical literature on the medical profession, scholars have made sweeping generalizations as if all physicians were alike. A normative model of medicine and its practice did exist, but individual physicians differed from one another, and specialists jealously guarded their respective territories. Adam Wright, professor of obstetrics at the University of Toronto, reported in the January 1910 *Saskatchewan Medical Journal* that on the issue of septic peritonitis, the obstetrician, gynaecologist, and general practitioner all held different opinions, and at times those differences of opinion were 'neither temperate nor dignified.'[63] One of the reasons for such tensions was the increase in medical specialties and the attempt of each to maintain exclusivity to particular arenas of practice. Yet the vast majority of physicians in Canada were general practitioners, who were somewhat overlooked by the medical literature. In addition to this tension between specialists and general practitioners there was that between state-paid health advisers and those in private practice. Local health officers, for example, often felt the need to tread warily to avoid impinging on the 'prerogatives of the private physician.'[64]

The general practitioner may not have had the status within the profession that a surgeon did, but when most Canadians heard the word 'doctor,' the local GP came to mind. The work of these physicians was onerous. William Victor Johnston recalled what a practice was like in the interwar period:

In my day, a rural and small-town doctor like myself was interviewing each week from Sunday to Sunday about two hundred people. This is at a rate of ten thousand a year. He met all the emotions from fright to lust. The average rural doctor had about twenty-five deaths a year and about twice as many births. He dealt with countless colds, much indigestion, many anemias, chronic bronchitis, and urinary infections. He was presented with an occasional suicide and abortion, a little madness, and much personal misery from worry and anxiety.[65]

Such physicians took well-deserved pride in what they did and were anxious that others in the profession appreciate it too. They tried to do the best they could in trying circumstances, and many made special efforts to keep up to date with the latest advances.[66]

Depending on the kind of practice a physician had, he could live quite well or be struggling. Some physicians carried a large roster of charitable patients, which limited their income. In the Depression, many found that even their paying patients could no longer afford their services. A Canadian life insurance advertisement in 1931 played on this by telling the physician-reader that a doctor needed to insure his life 'BECAUSE he is exposed to risks peculiar to his calling. BECAUSE he usually has no asset but his skill, and a life insurance policy capitalizes that ability for the family.'[67] Despite these problems, physicians as a group were able to make more than four times the average Canadian salary before the 1930s and, in the 1940s, about three times the national average.[68] This reality did not necessarily translate into a feeling of security, however. Some physicians considered that their financial situation was vulnerable to competition, that they were by necessity independent entrepreneurs having to sell themselves to the public and thus were at the mercy of the public. Harold Atlee, ever the caustic critic of his own profession, complained: 'In our eagerness to make money in private practice we have surgeons who snatch tonsils and uteri, gynaecologists who remove gall bladders, obstetricians who do general practice, and internists who do urology; all this is to the waste of their training and ability, and not always to the good of the people.'[69] One custom that upset some was lodge practice, whereby doctors worked under contract for lodge members at a discount rate. At the turn of the century, the Victoria Medical Society expelled any physician taking such a contract.[70]

Despite some feelings of vulnerability, physicians had more power and influence than most Canadians, because of their education and specialized knowledge and the fact that they dealt with life and death situations. Dr Charles J. Whitby, writing in the *Canada Lancet* in 1907, noted: 'The deference we are accustomed to expect, and upon the whole to receive, is not merely a personal deference, it is also the allegiance of uninstructed to expert opinion, to an impersonal authority whose mouthpiece we are or profess to be.'[71] Physicians had influence in society as experts on a wide variety of issues. The commission of inquiry into the Bell Telephone operators' strike in Toronto in 1907 called twenty-one women from Bell to testify about working conditions but invited thirty-three physicians to give their considered opinion on the relationship between the working conditions of these women and their health and future reproductive abilities.[72] The *Canadian Home Journal* in 1931 accorded Harold Atlee 'authority' to speak on the psychic disturbance of women because he was head of a department of obstetrics and gynaecology in a 'grade A. Canadian Medical School.'[73] Some physicians revelled in the authority they had. Alton Goldbloom of Montreal, one of Canada's best-known paediatricians, wrote a telling description of his specialty: 'The pediatrician to-day, particularly the older one is much in the relation to his patient that the priest is to the faithful. The consulting room is akin to the confessional. Many of my French patients address me as "mon père" with a little embarrassed laugh at their error not realizing how much they have unconsciously sensed the analogy.'[74] Another, however, was less enraptured by the personalities medicine attracted:

Physicians are above average intelligence ... They are individuals who want their own way even more than do other men. They are very sensitive and are inclined to be egoists, since many of them have a deep sense of inferiority and insecurity. They have a life of their own, mostly among their medical confreres ... [and] frequently do not have a very high regard for such extra-medical, non-scientific activities and interests – all of which often makes for a certain amount of narrowness and rigidity.[75]

As another critic pointed out, in 1950, the medical profession remained 'a closed corporation, or a trade union' where physicians governed themselves.[76]

Women physicians were not very visible within this corporation. When in 1902 the Toronto General Hospital decided to hire a woman on the regular visiting staff and to appoint two more as registrars, the *Canadian Practitioner and Review* found this significant enough to mention.[77] In 1911 there were 196 women physicians in Canada, representing only 2.6 per cent of the profession. By 1921 the numbers had declined to 152. After that, they increased, but at a very slow rate. In 1931 there were 203 women doctors, representing 2 per cent of all physicians; in 1941, 384 (3.2 per cent); and in 1951, 587 (4.1 per cent).[78] It wasn't easy to be a woman physician in Canada. Women medical graduates had difficulty finding residency appointments in Canada, and many took them in the United States. When Florence Murray (who later became a medical missionary in Korea) graduated in 1919, she was unable to obtain an internship at Halifax's Victoria General Hospital because the superintendent refused to give any internships to women. Murray took her internship in Boston. One of the earliest women to intern in Canada was Mabel Paterson, who in 1921, at the age of forty, graduated from Dalhousie Medical School and interned at the Saint John General Hospital despite the fears of some that she might not be able to do the work.[79]

Some male physicians, especially in the early years of the century, were suspicious of women who became doctors. How could such women do the training they did and remain respectable?[80] Even in later years, women physicians continued to face opposition. Some medical schools would not accept them, and others limited their numbers. Women medical students were often excluded from the formal activities provided to male students, and they found many of their professors hostile to them in the classroom. Their teachers advised them not to apply for certain residencies because patients would not go to women specialists in private practice; others encountered physicians who refused to work with a woman doctor; still others were confronted by patients who preferred the authority of a male physician. When the Second World War broke out, women physicians who enlisted discovered that they could not legally be commissioned in any of the three services. Meanwhile, women doctors in the civilian world were reaping the opportunities presented by the absence of many of their male colleagues.[81]

Medicine demanded a great deal from women. Marion Hilliard, in looking back on her medical training and her internship, asked: 'How a woman can undertake such an arduous, time-consuming course without a definite sense of mission and the beginning of a career, I do not know. And we take it for granted she must also have a strong body and stable nervous system.' But medicine demanded even more. Hilliard felt at times that medicine had taken her youth from her and had made having a normal life difficult. 'It also bans marriage ... If only I were a man, it would be so easy.'[82] For women such as Hilliard, Toronto's Women's College Hospital was a refuge – a supportive environment in which women physicians could practise and feel accepted.[83] But although the hospital received much support from men both within and outside the profession, it also faced opposition. J. Hunter, in a 1901 letter to the *Canadian Journal of Medicine and Surgery*, referred to the notion of having a women's hospital as 'a very dangerous experiment.'[84] The women who established the hospital, however, perceived that many women wanted access to a woman physician, who would not only treat them but would do so in a 'mothering' way.[85]

The latter point raises the central issue that physicians, male or female, had to address – the doctor-patient relationship. The differences in power between the two cannot help but colour the relationship. The doctor is an educated individual, and more often than not the patient does not have equivalent training.

Even if in everyday life the patient is a powerful man, he is seeing the physician because he is ill, fears he is ill, or is in need of something from the physician. Indeed, the word *patient* denotes someone in need. Physicians diagnose the patient and in so doing wield a powerful tool of control, a form of social labelling. Information about the individual is significant only in terms of how it enables a physician to do this. The life of the person, then, becomes objectified, summarized in a few brief paragraphs of the case record. The patient becomes a problem to be diagnosed.[86] Underlying the inequitable relationship between physician and patient is the prestige, power, and status that physicians have in our society.

But even in the past, all the power did not lie with the physician. One turn-of-the-century advice book for physicians cautioned new doctors establishing a practice about the importance of gaining the confidence of the women in the families they hoped to treat: 'No one can succeed fully without the favourable opinion of the gentle maids and acute matrons with whom he may be associated in the sick-room. They can be his best friends or his worst enemies. Women and children constitute four-fifths of all the population. Females have more sickness than males and the females of every family are the autocrats of the sick-room, and have a potent voice in selecting the family physician.'[87] Physicians have never been free agents. We often forget that the decision to go to a physician is not straightforward. Even after the decision has been made, the physician is not in total control. Both patient and physician have a cultural, personal, and professional history that limits what each can do. They negotiate with one another, and although the physician may be privileged in this negotiation, his power is not absolute. The negotiations go back and forth, forming a series of 'story tellings' until both patient and physician agree on a version.[88] Even then, the patient may not be compliant. She or he may not take the medicine prescribed or may seek other help at the same time.

We know very little about what the patient-doctor relationship was like in the past. Many Canadians fondly remembered acts of kindness. One woman on the Alberta frontier told of a physician, paid by the local miner's union, who purchased food for those in need and did not charge for almost half of the obstetrical work he did. Similarly, Eunice Jordon remembered that her physician was a family doctor, a friend, who didn't charge when her family could not afford to pay. Esther Thomas recalled that she seldom saw a physician because she could not afford one. Nevertheless, when she needed emergency surgery after the birth of her first child in the 1940s, she was impressed that her doctor came to see her at home in the middle of the night and then again in the morning to take her to the hospital. Mrs Annie L. Atkinson also fondly remembered her physician, Dr Harold Atlee. Writing to his biographer in 1980, she recalled: 'In May of 1940 I became his patient while seriously ill at Grace Maternity Hospital in Halifax. I found him a kind and considerate doctor who took the trouble to explain what was going on and how treatment would proceed.'[89] Not all were so fortunate. In 1908, Lucy Maud Montgomery was undergoing considerable nervous turmoil and wrote in her diary: 'I heartily wish I could see a competent doctor whom I could trust and discuss my condition with him.' Unfortunately, the local doctor went on 'sprees' and, while on them, told people about his patients' ailments. Quite apart from that, Montgomery did not think he was really able deal with nervous disorders.[90] But at least she had the choice of whether or not to go to a doctor. Many Canadians did not have access to one, either because none were nearby or because they could not afford a doctor's services.

For their part, some physicians worried about the emotional separation they saw developing between patients and doctors as medicine became more business oriented. In 1898 in Vancouver, 66 per cent of doctors lived where they worked, but by 1920 only 12 per cent did. There was less of a home atmosphere when a patient entered a physician's office. Going to a physician felt less personal, and they were more difficult to reach.[91] Alton Goldbloom blamed specialization; too often the specialist was a stranger rather than a 'familiar friend.'[92] Medicine's dependence on measurement and testing was also a factor in distancing physicians from their patients. Sydney Thomas, a fifty-six-year-old insurance agent, entered Halifax's Victoria General Hospital on 28 October 1930. The tests performed came back with a diagnosis of 'tape worm.' Thomas was 'very much wrought up over the statement that he had a tape worm. Insisted that he was "harboring no Intestinal Parasite" and said all and sundry who believed it were unexperienced and incompetent.' Thomas was right. Another page of his hospital record noted, 'By an unfortunate mistake the tapeworm found was in the faece of another patient ... [and] this report is to correct the previous and earlier report.'[93]

Physicians in teaching hospitals were concerned about how the emphasis on scientific medicine affected the care of individuals. Adam Wright in his 1908 textbook wrote that he had 'seen many acts of positive cruelty on the part of those who appear in aim [to be] treating the diseases and injuries, and not the patients.'[94] In 1934 the Montreal doctor A.H. Gordon wrote an article in the *Canadian Medical Association Journal* with the revealing title 'The Patient as a Person.' In it he told his readers: 'In the progress of our art the case of illness may by almost imperceptive stages pass from being a *person*, through the stage of being *a problem*, and end in being regarded as so much *material*.' However, Gordon believed that medicine was changing and that the 'case' was becoming a 'person' once again.[95] Some hoped that the trend to psychology and psychiatry would allow the individual to be seen as 'an indivisible whole each part affecting and being affected by the other parts.'[96] But James B. McClinton from Timmins, Ontario, was not so sanguine. He argued that the various tests that could be run (and not always by the patient's physician) on an individual could mean that the only patient a modern physician definitely had to see was a dead one, since a physician was not allowed to sign a death certificate without viewing the body.[97]

Of course, physicians were also aware of the problems that patients posed for them. Dr Walter Bapty in the interwar period observed: 'The best patients are those who set you up on a pedestal, always friendly, of course, but a certain reserve is maintained.'[98] The reserve was necessary to ensure distance when the physician treated the patient – scientific objectivity demanded this. Placing the physician on a pedestal also suggested patient compliancy. Non-compliance was frustrating for physicians, and the most antagonistic statements in case records were reserved for the non-compliant patient.

In 1913, when Letitia Danvers, age twenty-four and married only two months, wanted to leave Montreal's Royal Victoria Hospital despite suffering from double salpingo-oophoritis (inflammation of both uterine tubes and ovaries), her case record reveals the disdain of the recording person for this decision: 'Is of low mentality, hysterical and gives very foolish reasons for wanting to go.' Although some improvement in her condition had occurred, noted the record, the 'patient thinks that because she can walk about readily that she will be alright at home.' Physicians at the Royal Victoria may have been distressed by the prospect that a young woman, who was just married and was suffering from a severe and potentially sterilizing disease, would be leaving the hospital before she was well. But there was little attempt to understand why a bride of only two months would want to return home. Instead, she was a defaulter, someone who did not accept medical advice.[99] As Annette and Graham Scambler have pointed out, the sick are exempted from certain responsibilities, but in return they must want to get well and try to get well, and the latter meant following a doctor's advice.[100] The needs and concerns of patients and physicians could not always be reconciled.

Doctors often desired that patients would recognize their significance and acknowledge their status. In 1910 John Hunter, a Toronto physician, declared: 'The mission of medicine ... is the prevention, mitigation of the consequences, and cure of disease ... It stands for purity in morals; temperate and cleanly habits. It seeks the enactment of sanitary laws for the protection of private, social, industrial, civic and national life. It has to solve the many complex problems pertaining to heredity, education, climate, vocation, etc.'[101] Hunter believed that medicine was to protect 'private, social, industrial, civic and national life.' Other physicians agreed, and they advised Canadians on what they could and should do in almost every aspect of their lives. One bluntly summarized the physician's role as 'father confessor.'[102] An advertisement in a 1933 *Nova Scotia Medical Bulletin* showed a picture of a little girl with the heading 'This Little Girl Has Three Parents: Yes, this little girl has three parents. The third one is the family physician.'[103] All expressions reflected how some physicians wanted medicine to be and how they wanted Canadians to see them.

If at times the doctor-patient relationship was problematic, it was even more so when the patient was a woman.[104] Physicians and others in society viewed the adult male body as the norm against which they judged the female body and found it wanting. Physicians tended to see the female body as uncertain in terms of health. Women's bodies were more complex than men's, and consequently physicians deemed them more prone to disorders. Most physicians (at least as reflected in the medical literature) assumed that women could be healthy only if they remained within clearly defined social roles and that if women went outside these roles they would endanger their health – a variant on the 'biology is destiny' argument. Such an argument could apply to men as well, but in the period under study doctors did not fear this as much. Part of physicians' prestige centred in their being pillars of convention, acting conventionally and holding conventional attitudes. As a result, the gender of patients was of significance. Harold Atlee warned his male medical students that when they went out into practice they should not give a vaginal examination without a nurse being present.[105] Male physicians had to take care. Even as late as the interwar period, the prospect of a male physician seeing the female body in all its intimacies was disturbing to many Canadians, and the physician had to take all the precautions necessary to maintain an image of propriety and respect. While Atlee's suggestion was a sensible one, not all physicians had a nurse to call upon.

Despite the potentially problematic relationship between women and their physicians, women patients were not without choices. While we can talk about 'women' and 'doctors' and find the patterns of relationship between them, this does not mean that the individual outcome of the contact was predictable.[106]

After all, each woman had an embodied knowledge of herself that might not correspond to medical opinion. She had a memory of her body, and that memory was probably more real to her than what physicians told her was going on in her body. She could use physicians for her own purpose, adding what they told her to other sources of information – popular literature, other women, and other health advocates. As already seen, physicians were aware of this and were concerned about it.

The world in which physicians worked was full of tensions. The medical model with its attendant scientific trappings tried to comfort physicians with certainty, but the reality of their practices challenged this on a day-to-day basis. Many physicians could feel themselves vulnerable as a consequence of what they perceived as their lack of adequate training and the existence of alternative medical care and competition from other practitioners. The increasing importance of hospitals undermined their control over medicine and its direction. Even their patients challenged them in their unwillingness at times to follow the medical advice given to them. And in caring for their patients, many family practitioners expressed their sense of fatigue and the lack of recognition by their colleagues. Recognizing the problems and constraints they faced helps us understand some of the choices they made. The power of medicine was much more significant than the power of individual practitioners, and the power of the latter varied considerably. But while many physicians may have considered themselves at risk, the public stance they took seldom gave indications of this. They strode across the medical field confident in the public status they had achieved, believing that the science behind them made them deserving of it. In public they exhibited what Sir William Osler referred to as *aequanimitas*, 'coolness and presence of mind under all circumstances; calmness amid storm, clearness of judgement in moments of great peril.'[107] Only to one another would they suggest that all was not right with their profession or with their individual place in it. Nowhere could this tension be seen more than in obstetrics.

CHAPTER TWO

The Even More Uncertain World of Obstetrics

To a beginner in obstetric practice there is much that is embarrassing. The novel and intimate relations with his patient; her evident dread of the necessary examinations more or less revolting to every women; the doctor's keen consciousness of a lack of experience; mistrust of his capacity to recognize the stage of labor, the presentation and position of the fetus; the knowledge that his every movement is watched by critical friends or attendants of the patient, who possess, perhaps, just what he lacks, – practical experience, – all unite to produce a most unenviable frame of mind in the practitioner attending his first few cases of labor.

Barton Cooke Hirst, 1912[1]

All specialties in medicine in the early years of the twentieth century partook of the prestige of medical science, and their practitioners looked back to the past as a gauge of how far their specialty had progressed. Those who delivered children were not any different. The introduction to most obstetric textbooks and articles contained almost mandatory praise for the advances made. The emphasis was on the science of obstetrics, even though the writers acknowledged the art of obstetrics and at times gave it equal rhetorical standing. But as the above quotation from Barton Cooke Hirst's textbook hints, underlying the bravado there was unease that all was not well with the field. Several issues contributed to this sense of anxiety. The tension between the view of childbirth as natural and the view of it as pathological divided practitioners in where they placed their emphasis. The deficiencies in obstetrical education undermined the confidence of some, as did obstetrics' status vis-à-vis other medical specialties. Compared with gynaecology and other surgical specialties, obstetrics seemed to be the poor cousin. Yet not all practitioners who delivered babies were willing to acquiesce in their apparently secondary position, though maintaining confidence in the importance of what they did was not easy. The realities of practice, including the remuneration doctors received and their perception of competition from 'unqualified' individuals, could undermine the optimism of even the most committed. These concerns are important for the historians of childbirth to recognize. Too often in the vast literature of the field, scholars have portrayed physicians as powerful and exhibiting significant agency, if not autonomy.[2] When compared with the women who were their patients, this interpretation certainly has merit. But it is not the full story. Physicians treated their patients within the broader context of medicine, and their own sense of place within that context could not help but influence that treatment.

Seeing obstetrics as scientific was important for those in the field. They believed that their discourse, based as it was on scientific observation, was superior to any other knowledge base on the female body.[3] In the early decades of the century and in succeeding years, practitioners highlighted the science of obstetrics, in part by their insistence on keeping track of different aspects of the birth experience. Physicians and others believed in the value of information – eventually information would translate into knowledge. Information gathering was also part of the standardizing thrust of medicine. If physicians detailed the birth experience of different women, they would begin to glean what the average experience was and could transform it into the normal experience. Anything outside its limits became not just a minority experience but an abnormal one, signifying the need for medical concern and perhaps intervention. One aspect of a hospital's responsibility was to teach medical students, interns, and nursing students; to help in this, hospital records increasingly took on a data-collecting orientation. For example, in 1906 the

Burnside Lying-In Hospital, Toronto, directed its nurses and house physicians to record the following birth details: 'length of first stage, length of second stage, length of time before expulsive pressure is used over the fundus of the uterus [the part of the uterus above the opening of the uterine tubes], length of time of such pressure, total length of third stage, time of washing of vulva, time of application of abdominal binder, time of putting patient in bed, time of first weighing baby, time of first washing baby.'[4] The purpose was to take as much of the guesswork out of the management of childbirth as possible, thus lessening the uncertainty of medical practice. Some of the information became maxims, such as 'Older women had more difficulty delivering.'[5] Maxims became rules, and rules had the aura of scientific legitimacy behind them.

During the interwar period and the following years, the science of obstetrics took pride of place. Many physicians had come to believe that, with proper supervision, the dangers that had once shrouded pregnancy could be alleviated. John Puddicombe, the staff obstetrician at the Canadian Council on Child and Family Welfare, bragged in 1934: 'Great strides have been made in the knowledge and treatment of the more serious pathological conditions arising out of pregnancy and parturition,' although he had to admit that, for whatever reason, the death rate had not decreased correspondingly. At the end of the period, Toronto physician H.B. Van Wyck did not qualify his enthusiasm: 'No longer is obstetrics the despised practice of midwifery, but takes its place as a fully scientific branch of practice, a field in which modern concepts of medicine and surgery have a most beneficent application to the function of reproduction.'[6]

Physicians collected even more information on their patients than before. Obstetrical records in hospitals, where increasing numbers of women were giving birth, included the usual socioeconomic data, details of previous pregnancies, and the history of the present one. The latter involved the following: the last date of menstruation, the date of quickening, normal weight, urinary volume, position of fundus and its measurements, and type of pelvis; any experience of nausea or vomiting, headache, oedema (abnormal accumulation of fluid), heartburn, disturbance of vision, constipation, or evidence of leucorrhoea (a whitish or yellowish discharge), the results of a general physical exam (heart, lungs, breasts, abdomen), the results of a pelvic exam (perineum [pelvic floor], vagina, cervix, body structure, position and size of uterus), and much more. Also recorded was a detailed description of the actual labour, which included the size of the cervix, remarks on the first stage, when the membranes ruptured, the position of the child, and when it was born. Specific questions addressed the use of catheterization, the induction of labour, or the use of anaesthetic or medication. Remarks on the second stage included the condition of the cord, whether an episiotomy (incision of the perineum) was done, and whether a laceration occurred or the perineum remained intact. Recorded as well were descriptions of the expulsion of the placenta.[7] Simply filling out the forms forced physicians and hospital workers to see birth not as a continuous process but as a series of discrete segments which they had to detail. This segmentation reflected the efficiency and time-management process of the industrial world and challenged the view of medical care as an art. Specific questions emphasized that birth was anything but natural and could result in a physician second-guessing what he had done and what had occurred.

If hospitals wanted to gain certification, they had to keep complete records, have specific obstetrical technology available, ensure that surgical procedures occurred only after consultations, and follow an accepted standard definition of morbidity.[8] All such requirements emphasized professional standardized procedures of birthing, which distinguished good care from bad care. The benchmark for good care increasingly became hospital birth, where records and standards seemed easier to deliver and control. In private practice, the general practitioner often did not have the time or personnel necessary to maintain them. Even if he had, these accoutrements of scientific obstetrics did not provide all the answers. Doctors reminded one another that diagnosis was often difficult and what worked for one patient might not work for another.

Although there was a sense of progress in obstetrics, within the broader field of medicine it did not have the status that its practitioners wanted. In 1914 B.P. Watson, professor of obstetrics and gynaecology at the University of Toronto, argued that obstetrics deserved its low status: 'In no department of medicine is custom and routine so difficult to overcome as in obstetrics. We are afraid to step aside from the beaten path, lest if things go wrong, we be blamed.' Others apologized for even writing about childbirth, a 'commonplace subject,' lagging behind other specialities in medicine.[9] Defensiveness also existed with respect to what childbirth entailed. Most physicians delivering babies believed in the importance of what they did but were aware that others did not necessarily share their view. In 1917 S.P. Ford referred to a physician who had claimed 'that he would rather clean out a garbage can than attend a confinement, for he could use a shovel in the former case but would have to soil his hands in the latter.'[10] The traditional image of a physician was of someone who cured, but in childbirth women were not ill and the physician's responsibility was to wait and intervene only when something went wrong.[11] Compared with other medical specialties, the obstetric patient was more active (or could be), and this activity potentially lessened physician autonomy. The art of obstetrics loomed larger than the art of other medical specialties, and with the art came uncertainty. Similar concerns continued throughout the interwar years and beyond. Many physicians complained about colleagues who were not interested in obstetrics and seemed to suggest that obstetric work was somehow demeaning and of minor importance.[12] Within their professional world, physicians who delivered babies often did not believe that they had the respect of their medical peers.

One source of status anxiety was the tension existing between two views of childbirth, between the natural and the pathological. In the early decades of the century, those who espoused the former were at times depicted as contributing to the lesser status of obstetrics vis-à-vis surgical specialties.[13] Those emphasizing the pathological nature of childbirth were trying to raise the significance of obstetrics in the eyes of their colleagues, who deemed intervention a measure of a specialty's importance and a physician's skill. Childbirth as a natural physiological process did not mean an unproblematic process, but it did suggest to its adherents a process in which intervention would be infrequent. Thus, the difference between the two views of childbirth focused on the degree of intervention. Those who specialized in obstetrics instructed their students that the line between the physiological and pathological was unclear, thereby preparing them to be on the lookout for possible difficulties in childbirth. A perusal of examinations in obstetrics and gynaecology at medical faculties bears this out; the emphasis was on the abnormal in childbirth, not the normal. For example, in 1902 the senior obstetrics and gynaecology exam at Queen's University consisted of seven questions, all of which focused on what could go wrong in childbirth.[14] The pathological view could reach incredible heights of rhetoric – one physician referred to the pregnant uterus as an 'abdominal tumour.' While the word *tumour* does not necessarily imply malignancy (it means a mass or a lump), it does suggest a growth that should not exist or does not normally exist. It aligns the pregnant state with an inherently problematic condition. The same physician, however, assured his students that 'labor is a natural and a comparatively easy process, in the large majority of cases.'[15] Students received mixed messages.

Some physicians seemed to be aware of the peculiar stance they were taking. Women had been giving birth for millennia with little help from the medical profession. Why, in the modern period, could women no longer give birth on their own? To explain the shift, physicians acknowledged birth as a natural process in the abstract or in situations where the woman was influenced only by 'natural environments.' However, as the authors of a turn-of-the-century text pointed out,

The Indian squaw, in the early history of this country, gave birth to her child without delaying her companions when on the march, and was able at once to join them in their journey. To-day we have to deal with an entirely different being. Woman has inherited from her ancestors a physical organism so far removed from that belonging to the savage that what was once a physiological act, pure and simple, now verges on the pathological. Indeed, it requires the astuteness of the careful physician to recognize deviations from what should be normal and yet what is too frequently pathological.[16]

Such a view picked up on evolutionary theory and the importance of the environment. It also labelled cultures that still treated birth as physiological as 'savage.' Modern woman was civilized and thus in need of assistance.[17]

After the First World War, the image of birth as pathological gradually intensified. Because more births took place in hospitals; it was increasingly difficult to see birthing as natural. Sick people went to hospital; people in need of help went to hospital. The message of childbirth's dangers inundated the field. Dr C.B. Oliver of Chatham, Ontario, warned: 'The dangers that lurk along the pathway of the pregnant woman are legion. Always, she is travelling "close to the border-land of pathology" and she needs a guide familiar with every shallow and quicksand and portage along the way.' Birthing was a 'hazardous occupation' stemming from 'a disease of nine months' duration.'[18] Belief in a society that had progressed to the point where birthing was no longer natural continued to be the explanation. In 1924 a publication by the Ontario Department of Health noted: 'Our present-day knowledge of the process connected with childbirth makes it easy to understand how, since the early ages of the human race, with the beginnings of the struggle for existence, and the appearance and spread of disease, all interfering with the natural growth and development of the body, the function of childbearing ceased to be a normal function, as designed by its maker, and became one fraught with danger to both mother and child.'[19] Some within the profession worried that such views could lead to excessive interference. Recognizing this, Lennox Arthur, visiting obstetrician at St Boniface Hospital, in Manitoba, suggested that although physicians should consider birth pathological, they should treat it conservatively and with 'masterly inactivity.'[20] J.S. Fairbairn, in his 1924 text, distinguished obstetrics as a preventative specialty whose sole purpose was to preserve the physiological state, although he added that doing so took skill, dexterity, and experience and was deserving of esteem.[21]

Another cause for anxiety among some practitioners was the belief that they received inadequate training in midwifery. Some observers felt that medical schools did not stress the teaching of obstetrics enough because of the belief that childbirth was a normal physiological event. Anything deemed normal or natural did not need significant training. According to an early-twentieth-century writer in the *Canadian Journal of Medicine and Surgery*, 'both in teaching and in examinations, the study of obstetrics has been relegated to a position totally unworthy of its immense importance to the practitioner and to the national welfare.'[22] Some of the blame stemmed from the teachers themselves. As noted in chapter 1, physicians trained in an earlier era continued to practise long after new advances had overtaken some of what they had learned. Unless the physician kept up, he was destined to practise medicine in a way that seemed out of date to many new medical graduates. The same could be true of the teachers of these new graduates.

Some professors of obstetrics remained at their job for decades, not always moving with the times. William Gardner, the first professor of obstetrics and gynaecology at McGill University, had graduated in 1866 from McGill, and in 1873 he left the Department of Medical Jurisprudence to become head of the new Department of Gynaecology at Montreal General Hospital. In 1893 he went to the Royal Victoria Hospital as a gynaecologist and the next year became professor, remaining so until 1910. While his reputation was high, one historian has summarized his technique as 'very deliberate'; little seemed to phase him: 'He would interrupt the operation to retire for a cup of tea and a biscuit; when he came back his students would have left.'[23] His career suggests that there was a lack of training for specialization in the early years. It also indicates an approach to patient care that some would consider outdated by the time he retired.

Despite what some researchers have suggested, the call for improved education continued throughout the interwar period and beyond.[24] W.W. Chipman of McGill University insisted that training needed to be 'broad, practical, and sufficient, if we are to ensure a general improvement in our obstetric art.'[25] The *Manitoba Medical Bulletin* in 1929 contained an article by the provincial minister of health and public welfare, himself a physician, in which he pointed out that the time devoted to obstetric training was not sufficient and that the local university had admitted as much by increasing teaching hours in obstetrics from 119 in 1919 to 160 in 1929. Even when medical education and teaching in obstetrics improved, there was always a sense that training facilities could do better. As late as 1950, the chairman of the Committee on Maternal Welfare for the Canadian Medical Association acknowledged that there was a widely held perception that medical education in obstetrics was still bad.[26] And Canada was not alone. Some historians have suggested that in Britain the teaching of obstetrics had actually declined since the turn of the century.[27]

The major complaint made in Canada about the teaching of obstetrics throughout the first half of the twentieth century was that medical students did not get enough practical hands-on experience. In the early years, the viewing of births was relatively new. Not until 1906 were students admitted to the birthing rooms at the Burnside Lying-In Hospital.[28] While this was certainly an advance, it did not ensure that students were well prepared. H.L. Burris, recalling his own training, noted that fourth-year students had to attend six deliveries, but those six seldom prepared students for the complications of birthing.[29] Burris clearly felt that while attendance at births was a positive move, students needed a great deal more to prepare for the reality of childbirth in practice. Harold Atlee, looking back at his training in Halifax, shared the frustration felt by Burris: 'In practical obstetrics we were expected to witness only four deliveries. Having witnessed two of these at the Poor House, conducted under a blanket by a dear old Victorian obstetrician who felt that it was a mortal sin to expose a female perineum, I finally saw a baby being born only because Dr. Kenneth Mackenzie kindly allowed me to deliver two of his Grafton St. patients.'[30] The lack of practical experience was especially frightening for the new physician, who often had to deliver his first child in the presence of others who had more experience in seeing babies born.

The situation did improve. In the 1920s medical students at Dalhousie University were expected to deliver twenty babies and attend five difficult births. The University of Manitoba increased the required attendance at births from ten to twenty-five. In Britain the same movement was occurring. In the early 1930s the British Ministry of Health recommended two months' training in a maternity hospital and proposed that each medical student should personally deliver thirty patients. However, this still did not match the Swedish requirement of having medical students live and work for four months in a maternity hospital. Some Canadian medical schools tried to give students a feel for the reality of practice. At Dalhousie, for example, students attended three home births. While a few were uncomfortable with the conditions they found when they entered the homes of some patients – fleas, poverty, the necessity to place newspapers under the woman – the experience would have been invaluable for those destined for general practice.[31] Despite this, complaints that there was not enough practical education continued.[32] Such a situation was true of most professions; education cannot prepare students totally for what they have to face when they enter the real world. But the situation left some physicians in practice uncertain.

H.J.G. Geggie, who practised in the Wakefield area of Quebec from 1911 to mid-century, often wondered whether his diagnosis had been correct and whether his approach had been the best. He and others also questioned whether what medical students were taught had much application outside hospital practice.[33] In medicine, a gulf existed between theory, with its emphasis on book learning, and the actual practice of medicine – between the science of medicine and the art of medicine. Even though there was increased emphasis on longer and more practical education in obstetrics, there were many physicians such as Geggie who had been trained before the improvements occurred. Also, it is unclear how mandatory were some of the new requirements demanded of students. One physician, trained in the 1930s, recalled that she never witnessed a delivery until her internship. Another, trained during the Second World War, fainted when viewing his first childbirth; and because of the pressures of wartime training, he never had to see or attend another.[34]

One aspect in the development of obstetrics that influenced its teaching was the role played by gynaecology. As evidenced by the career of William Gardner, gynaecology and obstetrics, which once had been separate, became joined in the minds of physicians and administrators of medical faculties. Gardner held, professorships in both specialties at McGill, although it was not until after his retirement in 1910 that McGill formally joined the two. In 1912 the University of Toronto followed suit.[35] Outside the teaching institutions, physicians appointed to maternity hospitals were often cross-appointed as gynaecologists at general hospitals. The alignment of obstetrics with gynaecology meant that the increasing orientation of gynaecology toward surgery influenced the practice of obstetrics. B.P. Watson even argued that 'obstetrics is a branch of surgery.' In looking over the North American situation in 1914, he maintained that joining the two was a positive move. Separation between them 'tended to exaggerate the surgical aspect of gynaecology, often to the exclusion of non-operative and more conservative lines of treatment, and on the other ... deprived the obstetrician of opportunities of perfecting himself in operative technique, and today surgical intervention is more and more resorted to in obstetrics, as being in many instances the safest and most conservative line to adopt in the interests of mother and child.'[36] While the relationship between the two may have seemed natural to some, the result was a depiction of childbirth as a problematic occurrence often resulting in damage which, of necessity, the gynaecologist would address.[37]

In the interwar period and beyond, most physicians continued to accept the alliance between obstetrics and gynaecology.[38] It had long existed and appeared to be an obvious pairing. However, looking back from the vantage point of 1977, Harold Atlee wrote a condemning analysis of the field. He pointed out that while joining gynaecology and obstetrics seemed 'logical,' it was not. Underlying gynaecology was the premise of pathology; underlying obstetrics was the premise of physiology. The result for obstetrics had been disastrous. Physicians had increasingly seen birthing as problematic, with the consequence that intervention had increased. Too often physicians resorted to operative procedures.[39] The obstetrical/gynaecological association was, of course, not the only reason for increased intervention rates. Many times patients insisted that physicians 'do' something to ease the pain of childbirth. Evidence also exists that women who had experienced a complicated pregnancy sought the help of physicians for subsequent ones in the belief that physicians would be able to offset difficulties.[40] Nevertheless, Atlee had caught a significant shift in medicine – the dominance of surgery – which could not help but impinge on obstetrics.

Because of the close relationship between gynaecology and obstetrics, those who focused their attention on the latter felt at a disadvantage at times. They knew that surgical specialties garnered the attention and prestige of both the public and their medical colleagues; it was in the surgical aspects of medicine that the great advances were being made. Yet not all physicians who practised obstetrics were willing to defer to the surgeons. Joseph DeLee, one of North America's most famous obstetricians and surgeons, noted the respect that surgical specialities had, and in an effort to raise the prestige of obstetrics he argued, 'Even a normal confinement is worthy the dignity of the greatest surgeon' – a view endorsed by many in the field.[41]

In the interwar period, a backlash of sorts occurred as physicians responded to the surgical orientation of medicine. In 1932, J.N.E. Brown, a Toronto doctor, argued that 'the attendance on an obstetrical case, even normal, is just as important as upon an appendectomy; and that a proper handling of placenta praevia [when the placenta is in the lower part of the uterus and partially or entirely covers the internal os, which means that any expansion of the cervix could lead to tearing of the placenta and bleeding, and potentially could result in the death of both the mother and the foetus] or a face presentation is more difficult than a simple hysterectomy or gastro-enterostomy. Obstetrics is too often considered as of minor importance.' In 1942 Harold Atlee complained to the executive meeting of the Nova Scotia Medical Society that its recommended fee schedule for obstetrics underrated the skills necessary.[42] While not arguing that obstetrics was a surgical specialty, Brown and Atlee were making a case for its specialized nature. Other physicians were not as confident. An editorial in the 1929 *Canadian Medical Association Journal* advised that students be taught that childbirth was a normal process not requiring surgical intervention in most cases. When it did, however, it demanded more expertise than any undergraduate course could provide.[43] Obstetrical surgery should be left to the surgeons.

The surgical comparison accentuated the lack of prestige experienced by those delivering babies. Surgery connoted prestige. In a fascinating and revealing statement, Alton Goldbloom, one of Canada's most noted child specialists, talked about why he went into paediatrics and in doing so exposed his feelings about the status of surgery and what it demanded of a physician: 'A short physician cannot stand up to a tall patient, a short man as a surgeon could not possibly be a symbol of strength to a prospective victim – submitting to surgery connotes yielding, and who – man or woman, would yield to a tiny man. Obstetrics and Gynaecology is replete with symbolic yielding – but not to a tiny mite of a man.'[44] The quotation suggests not only the sexual aspect of obstetrics and gynaecology but also the prestige of surgery. Even in teaching, surgery held pride of place. Complaints about the teaching of obstetrics focused not only on the limited practical training provided but also on the fact that more time was spent learning surgery – the ratio was almost two to one. In England, Scotland, and Australia the ratio was similar, but in the United States the discrepancy was even greater, almost five to one.[45] Such teaching recognized and reinforced the increasing operative direction that obstetrics was taking.[46] Surgery had prestige, status, and dominance throughout the period under review because it, more than other aspects of medical care, was linked to laboratory science.[47] And more than any other branch of medicine, it could divorce itself from the patient in all her complexity and could concentrate on the body.

Another issue with which those involved with obstetrics had to deal was the rising importance of specialization in medicine. Family physicians especially might feel insecure. Even early in the century, those who taught and specialized in obstetrics argued that the family physician or the country doctor simply did not need – or was unable or, even worse, unwilling – to keep up with new advances. The medical press referred to specialists taking over.[48] While clearly an exaggeration, it is an indication of what the specialists hoped for and what the general practitioners feared. In 1913 DeLee fuelled such fears by connecting specialization in obstetrics with better care for patients and advancement for physicians. He reminded his student readers, 'The conduct of labor is not a simple matter, safely intrusted to every one.'[49] The assumption was that general practitioners could undertake normal deliveries but specialists should be called in if complications arose. Of course, this assumed that specialists would be both available and affordable, a situation that would not exist in most practices. Nonetheless, the push to specialization had begun – even though, in 1940, only Toronto General Hospital and Montreal's Royal Victoria Hospital had received the recognition of the American College of Surgeons for graduate training in obstetrics and gynaecology.[50]

As the files on childbirth patients became ever larger and more detailed in the interwar period, the apparent need for specialists was accentuated. Meanwhile, obstetricians stressed the broad scope of information with which they believed they needed to be familiar in order to give the best care to their patients. This included the 'cognate sciences of eugenics, sociology, public health, embryology [the science of the development of the individual during the embryonic stage], teratology [study of abnormal development and congenital deformations], endocrinology [study of internal secretions, particularly through the endocrine glands which regulate bodily activity], dietetics [science of diet and nutrition] etc.'[51] Clearly, only those who specialized in obstetrics would be able to absorb all this. The technology surrounding birth supported the need for specialists, as did major obstetrical procedures. Increasingly, specialists dominated the field or gave the appearance of doing so. In 1928 the American College of Surgeons set standards for accredited obstetric departments in hospitals which required

> a properly organized and equipped department of obstetrics, providing exclusive and adequate accommodation for mothers and the newborn ... segregation or isolation of infected mothers ... adequate clinical laboratory, x-ray and other facilities, under competent supervision ... adequate supervision by a chief and/or head of service or department, adequate and completed records, major obstetrical procedures to be performed only after consultations, the adoption of a standard for morbidity, minimum monthly review/analysis of obstetrics, and the opportunity for theoretical instruction and practical experience for student nurses.[52]

The significance of standards lay not in whether they were pervasive or even enforced, but rather the benchmark they established for good care. For physicians delivering children, whether at home, in small hospitals, or even in accredited teaching hospitals, the certainty that they and their actions were now under scrutiny must have reminded them that they were losing control over how they could practise medicine. A 1931 editorial in the *Canada Lancet and Practitioner* suggested that specialists visit local medical societies and lecture local physicians on how best to care for women in childbirth.[53] One can imagine how such a suggestion would have been received by the physicians on the front line of family care. But we must be careful not to exaggerate the rise of specialists in obstetrics. While they dominated the teaching fields and the medical literature, most babies delivered in Canada during this period were delivered by family practitioners, most of whom had not received any extra training in the field of obstetrics. Nevertheless, the professional climate was such that it could make these practitioners feel inadequate.

Obstetrical practice was important for family practitioners because it provided an entrée to treating the rest of the family, particularly after the turn of the century. If a physician provided good care to the parturient (about-to-give-birth) mother, the chances were that she would call on him when family members became ill. Obstetric work could form much of a general practitioner's case load.[54] By 1922, medical personnel cared for up to 50 per cent of birthing women in Canada.[55] Doctor-assisted birth was becoming the norm, and governments were introducing schemes that allowed women to be attended by physicians.[56] But the work of general practitioners was not easy. They faced a wide array of complications, which they had to deal with themselves. In 1931, looking back on almost fifty years of practice, Dr Robinson Cox from Upper Stewiacke, Nova Scotia, recalled that he had attended 1,550 cases of childbirth and 'had samples of about every known complication.' He had 'succeeded in all complications without help, except two, both cases of craniotomy [puncture of the skull and removal of its contents to decrease the size of the head to facilitate removal of a foetus].'[57] Family and rural practitioners were sensitive to the fact that they did not have access to the most up-to-date equipment for their patients. Some consoled themselves that the precision of technological birth was a bit exaggerated. Despite all the antenatal examinations, the resort to pelvimetry, and even x-rays, the relationship between the mother and child could not be totally known. 'Nature knows a thing or two not yet dreamed of by even the most experienced hospital physician.'[58]

The nature of obstetrical work itself was a problem. D.W. Cathell's turn-of-the-century guide to physicians described it in terms that would not be enticing to the ambitious physician:

Midwifery is a wearing and exhausting branch of medicine, – the hardest kind of hard work, – and in filth but little superior to the Nightman's; it seriously interferes with regular, healthy living, and is full of care and responsibility; and, although it does lead to other family practice, you will find, after some years, that the ordinary fees for attending cases of confinement are, on account of trouble, and anxiety while absent from them before or during labor, loss of time in waiting and consequent interference with the fulfilment of other duties and engagements, together with the nights of work, after days of toil, loss of sleep, risk of breaking down, etc., which they occasion, proportionately more meagre than in any other department of practice.[59]

Throughout the period, many others commented on the difficulty of obstetric work, the physical strength it demanded, the time it took, the anxiety it raised, the irregularity of the hours, and the need to be always on call. It was 'a young man's job.'[60] Not only was obstetrics difficult work, but for the just-graduated physician faced with childbirth, it could be awkward, terrifying, and embarrassing. Nonetheless, those committed to obstetrical practice were convinced of its significance. In the words of one, 'It involved the fundamentals of life itself.' When Marion Hilliard wrote about the first time she saw a baby being born, she remembered feeling that 'this is what life is all about.' Even at the end of her career, in the 1950s, she could still say, 'I never fail to be moved to my soul at the drama of birth.'[61]

Closely linked to the wear and tear of obstetric practice was the perception by those engaged in it that they were not particularly well remunerated. In 1910 A. Edmond Burrows of Harriston, Ontario, warned readers of the *Canada Lancet* that physicians had to take care and protect their status, and part of this protection was demanding suitable fees for obstetric work. In the early years of the century, physicians charged about $5 for an ordinary childbirth case and $10 to $15 if there were complications, such as sepsis (bacterial contamination) or use of instruments. In the interwar period the fee increased to about $25, although this could vary from place to place. In Vancouver in 1921, fees were estimated at $35 for a normal delivery, $35 if a miscarriage occurred, $50 if the physician had to deal with a haemorrhage, and $45 for use of forceps. Yet at the same time in rural Saskatchewan, under a maternity benefits scheme, doctors received only $15 for attending needy mothers, and that only if the physician earned less than $1,500 a year. By 1932, fees in some parts of Canada could be as high as $50 for a normal delivery. During the Depression, such fees were impossibly high for many people. Even with the economic recovery, rates remained stable; in 1945, $35 for a normal delivery was a figure that had some acceptance, although there were some physicians in the country who were still charging only $15.[62]

Whatever the fee and whatever it represented, many physicians complained to one another that it was not sufficient. Referring to the 1920s, one Toronto physician remarked: 'We, in this part of the country, average $30.00 for pre-natal care, delivery and post-natal care; for a medical man to take the blood pressure, examine urine every two, three and four weeks; spend a couple of hours at a delivery during, perhaps, busy office hours, that amount is not enough, and the average medical man will not do it.'[63] When patients complained, the defensive response was that the fees being charged were not excessive for the work provided.[64] The public did not understand that many physicians treated poor patients free, and at times made up for it either by charging their wealthier patients more or by absorbing the loss themselves.

Another financial worry for those working in obstetrics was the possibility of a malpractice suit. The medical superintendent of the Montreal Maternity Hospital warned in 1906: 'It is not at all uncommon for women about the time of confinement to consult scientific books from which they obtain an idea of the physician's responsibility for infection, and suits for malpractice are not unknown when infection occurred.' Similarly, J.S. Fairbairn's 1924 text *Gynaecology with Obstetrics* pointed out that the public was becoming aware of the need for careful examinations during pregnancy and thus resented 'any unexpected complications and their consequences in labour.'[65]

Nor did competition from others offering assistance to parturient women offset the practitioners' sense of insecurity. Male physicians had to deal with increasing numbers of women physicians. The numbers certainly would not have warranted concern, but what they represented did. A 1928 editorial in the *Canada Lancet and Practitioner* stated it bluntly: 'Given equal training, the woman obstetrician has an advantage over one of the male sex in her greater patience and her sex-sympathy, both of which may be drawn upon heavily in a protracted case.' Others even went so far as to suggest that women physicians might eventually take over the field of obstetrics.[66] But this was going to take some time, given their limited numbers.

At a conceptual level, nurses were not competitors since their role was to be the helpers of physicians. In reality, however, they often found themselves in situations where they did deliver children. Some who no longer nursed professionally used their training to help their community in an ad hoc manner. Public health nurses found that it was not always possible to call in a physician. Red Cross nurses often practised when there were no medical practitioners close by. Of special note was the work of the Victorian Order of Nurses. Created by the National Council of Women to celebrate Queen Victoria's Jubilee in 1897, the VON was originally intended to aid women in childbirth. However, opposition from physicians ensured that the VON's mandate was reconfigured so that VON nurses would only assist medical practitioners in helping women in childbirth. This was easier said than done. Often VON nurses worked in areas where few physicians practised and thus acted as midwives through necessity. In addition, a woman who did not want the services of a physician or perhaps could not pay for one sometimes delayed calling the VON nurse to her bedside so that when the nurse arrived she had to deliver the child.[67] In 1925 the VON raised the issue at its annual meeting. The question asked was, 'Is a V.O. Nurse to Answer a Confinement Call Before the Doctor Arrives?' The answer was yes.[68]

Maternity homes run by women with some training hired trained nurses to help them in their work. Miss Bessy Cook, who had trained at and graduated from St Paul's Hospital, Saskatoon, took up a post at the maternity home in Shaunavon, Saskatchewan, run by Mrs Ross, who herself was a practical nurse. While most of the maternity homes in Saskatchewan called on physicians, it was not always possible to do so. Lola Boyd of Lafleche acknowledged that in her nursing years she had 'brought a number of children into the world unassisted by a doctor not because [she] wanted to, but because [she] was caught.' She added, 'I'm proud to say I never in my nursing career had a case of infection in childbirth.'[69] Even hospital nurses were not exempt from going beyond the helpmate role if the physician did not arrive in time. As Kathryn McPherson noted when commenting on the Winnipeg General Hospital of the 1920s and 1930s, 'Enemas were commonly given to parturient women as a natural method to induce labour, but this often had more rapid effects than predicted.'[70]

In 1943 the University of Alberta set up an 'Advanced Obstetrics Course for District Nurses,' which it hoped would improve maternity care in isolated districts.[71] But more needed to be done. In 1950 Helen G. McArthur, the national director of nursing services for the Canadian Red Cross Society, wrote an article for the *Canadian Journal of Public Health* summarizing the situation:

I would like to mention, in passing, the question of nurse midwifery. In 1945, the Dominion Council of Health passed a resolution acknowledging that, in certain areas in Canada, doctors are not available for attendance on obstetrical cases and recognizing the value of public health nurses with training in obstetrics for attendance on such cases. The Council endorsed the principle of employing qualified graduate nurses from accredited teaching centres to attend such obstetrical cases. The Canadian Medical Association in October, 1945, and the Canadian Nurses Association in December, 1946, passed similar resolutions.[72]

As the above quotation reveals, the medical profession was supportive of childbirth care being provided to women even if the providers were not doctors. This was a significant about-face for the medical profession, which had long opposed the use of any but medical practitioners in childbirth. However, the above endorsement was not what they viewed as the ideal situation; it was simply the best that was possible when medical practitioners were not available.

Although midwives were never very numerous, particularly in the twentieth century, they still existed, working in isolated areas and among certain ethnic groups. While the reality of midwives did not really pose a problem for physicians, the idea of them did. They represented an alternative to medical care. Articles appeared in the medical press about how well midwives worked in other countries, how well trained they were, and how under them maternal mortality rates were better than those in Canada.[73] Physicians could mount arguments to explain the differences between obstetric practice in Canada and elsewhere that could account for the differences in mortality rates; but the bottom line was that good midwife practice appeared safer than the general medical care provided to women in Canada.

Practitioners delivering children in the first half of the twentieth century had much to contend with. As in other aspects of medicine, they tried to focus on the certainties of the scientific approach. They gathered increasing amounts of information on their patients, which provided them with a sense of 'knowing.' They were encouraged by what they believed to be the promise of scientific obstetrics – the eventual ability to meet the problems of childbirth. Nevertheless, they appeared anxious, and when their professional lives are examined, several causes of that anxiety emerge. There was a division among them over whether childbirth was natural or pathological, although the actual division was not so clear-cut. Childbirth was natural, at least in the abstract, but ... That 'but' and the emphasis individual physicians placed on it determined how problematic each considered childbirth to be. In addition, many felt that their medical education had been deficient, that their colleagues, especially those in gynaecology, did not appreciate what they faced when delivering a child, that their patients were unwilling to pay them their due, and – the final injury – that those not as well trained as themselves, such as nurses and midwives, at times usurped their role. Despite these pressures, the literature on childbirth has tended to see these practitioners as individuals with power, status, and prestige. From the perspective of the patient, this may have been the case, but the practitioner himself could see his position with a less positive eye.

The historiography on childbirth has understandably focused on how practitioners practised their art. However, the broader context in which the individual doctor worked may have affected the nature of that art. Did the status of surgery and surgeons within medicine and the alignment of obstetrics with gynaecology influence the direction of obstetrics? Did the insecurity which many physicians felt about their own obstetric training encourage them to cling to maxims longer than they otherwise might have? Physicians could comfort themselves that they had science on their side and that science would eventually win out. In the meantime, they had to cope with the reality that although they were becoming the dominant players in childbirth, others were available – not to challenge them but to hold out a different alternative or possibility. Midwives were the most significant of these.

CHAPTER THREE

Midwives Did Not Disappear

I delivered several babies in emergencies when there was no doctor around. Then knowing that, Dr. Gerald Smith ... came to me one Sunday morning during breakfast and asked if he could speak to me privately. In the living room he asked me if I would help him out with his maternity patients ... But I told him I had eight children of my own, that the teacher stayed with us and that I liked to provide meals for people travelling by train from St. Brendans (Free of charge of course) so that I was kept quite busy. Also, whenever the priest was in our part of the parish he stayed with us ... and he said 'Well you do your best for me and I'll do my best for you.' So that's how it all started.

Irene Farwell Bradley, midwife[1]

The literature on the history of midwives is vast. Historians have questioned why midwives declined in number in North America, whereas in other Western countries they were able to survive and indeed flourish.[2] The reasons for the decline are multifaceted, but most early feminist analyses focused on the medical profession's hostility to midwives, because of its vested interests (professional and financial) in controlling childbirth. In much of this literature, there is a sense of something lost with the decline of midwifery – the loss of a caring concern for women in birth and a loss to women in general, as physicians (most of whom were men) took over what had traditionally been a female-dominated sphere.[3] The response of physician historians to this view has understandably been less accepting and has focused more on what benefits the medical profession had to offer women.[4] In recent years, the historiography has gone beyond the doctors-versus-women dichotomy, integrating other factors into the explanation, although there remain remnants of the original antagonism.[5] In Canada, historians have noted that midwives had significantly declined in number and popularity by the end of the nineteenth century. Nevertheless, pockets of them still worked within immigrant communities, in isolated areas, in maternity homes on the prairies, and among the poor and the First Nations.

Newfoundland was a region where midwives dominated – a result of the isolation of many of its inhabitants in coastal communities and the lack of physicians outside the major centres. In Newfoundland, midwives were members of mainstream life and society rather than members of racial minorities, the poor, or immigrant groups, as they were in the United States. Consequently, in the first half of the twentieth century they maintained their status and position and were not the focus of any concerted effort to eliminate them.[6] Indeed, as the above quotation reveals, some physicians supported midwifery. The multiplicity of locales and types of midwives reminds us that there is no one history of midwives; there are numerous histories, many of which still need to be written.[7] But wherever midwives existed and in whatever guise, they represented an alternative to the medical model of care (more in theory than reality), and thus it is useful to examine them as a foil in evaluating physician-directed childbirth. Consequently, this chapter does not critique the work of midwives so much as serve as a reminder that alternative ways of birthing did exist.

In examining who midwives were, how they cared for women in childbirth, and how that care changed over time, several themes emerge. First is the need to accept that the term *midwife* had different meanings for different people; midwives varied in their training and in what they offered women. Second is the culturally based nature of midwife care, reflected in European and aboriginal-based societies. Third is the evolution of midwife practice to mirror that of medical practitioners more closely and the willingness of many midwives to accept this evolution as positive. Last is the physicians' response to midwives. Physicians were aware of their work, whether in Canada or elsewhere, and while in general they were opposed to the use of midwives in Canada, the opposition was never uniform and often was more complex than is suggested by much of the early feminist literature.[8]

The difficulty in studying midwives is that there exists no accepted definition of what a midwife was. The conventional view is that a midwife was a woman who was not a physician but helped another woman in childbirth. A woman with no experience who went to the aid of a neighbour in labour might acquire the reputation of being a midwife in her community. A woman who apprenticed with a midwife and then delivered babies in her community on a regular basis was a midwife. Similarly, women who took some kind of formal training (of various lengths) in midwifery were midwives. But did a midwife have to be a woman? One woman midwife who practised in western Canada mentioned that her father delivered most of the women in the area in which they lived. Trained by midwives in the United States before moving to Canada, he also depended for guidance on a book given to him by the local doctor. As late as 1940, an article in the *Canadian Doctor* referred to a letter received from a farmer in the Parry Sound district, who wanted to know 'if there was any place in Toronto where he could take midwifery training as he had been bringing the babies into the world for all the families around him for some time, and he would like to prove [*sic*] himself.'[9] Despite the examples of these two men, the vast majority of midwives were women. But their training and status within their own communities varied considerably, as did what they offered women. As C. Lesley Biggs has recently argued, their survival in the twentieth century 'suggests the trajectories for the decline of midwifery took place at different times for varied groups of women within Canada.' Too often the decline of midwifery has focused on a specific kind of midwife (the neighbour midwife), ignoring the survival of many other types.[10]

It is unclear how many midwives practised in Canada. In 1913 the *Canadian Journal of Medicine and Surgery* reported that in Prescott and Russell counties in Ontario, between 10 and 20 per cent of children's births were not registered. These births most likely represented the ones delivered by midwives or neighbouring women. This is certainly far less than the 50 per cent of births attended by midwives in the United States at approximately the same time. The large percentage in the United States was explained mainly by the significant percentage of the population who were black or immigrant and whose access to medical care was limited.[11] By 1930, however, only 15 per cent of births in the United States were attended by midwives.[12] In Winnipeg, midwives attended 18 per cent of births in 1917, 5 per cent in 1925, and only 0.1 per cent in 1945. Before 1939, some estimates were that 40 per cent of home births (which represented the majority of births) were unattended by medical professionals. In 1943 national figures suggested that 20,000 women gave birth without the benefit of medical attendance (leaving the question open as to whether these women had received other help); in 1947 the figure was 16,000. But official figures could not catch everyone, particularly First Nations and Inuit women. A conservative estimate in 1966 was that two-thirds of Inuit births took place outside hospitals or nursing stations and were thus not attended medically.[13] Neither did the figures include Newfoundland, which was outside Confederation until 1949. But sources on Newfoundland midwives are incredibly rich, and therefore these women are included as a significant focus of this chapter.

Midwives were often older women, though if they apprenticed with a midwife they began quite young. Such an apprenticeship might not have involved much book learning, and critics have suggested that it did not give the women expertise in problematic births, but it was rich in hands-on experience.[14] The tradition had a long history, and most Canadian medical practitioners had themselves trained under an apprenticeship system until the middle of the nineteenth century. Other midwives learned as they went. Even though her mother was a midwife, Annie Fizzard from Grand le Pierre, Newfoundland, had never observed her.

'Larn' it all on me own,' was her response to a question of training.[15] Still others knew what to do because helping women in labour was part of what they knew as women. As one Inuk woman recalled, 'Back then, the women had the knowledge to take care of a woman in labor ... We were informed by our elders on what to do and what not to do.'[16]

Some midwives had taken formal training. Retired nurses often served their communities, and some women with partial nurse training did the same. A Saskatchewan government listing of maternity homes indicated that almost 32 per cent of the operators were graduate nurses, whereas the rest depended on practical experience.[17] Olive Bishop from Pass Island on the southern coast of Newfoundland had partial training. Born in 1896, she graduated from high school at the age of seventeen, went to college for two years and then to nursing school, but had to leave after six months because of ill health. When she returned home, people came to her for medical aid. Once her health improved, she began teaching school and did so for four years until difficulties with her hands made her quit. At that point she began nursing when and where she could, and gradually built up a reputation along Hermitage Bay. She eventually took a three months' midwife course in St John's, and in 1939 the Board of Health formally recognized her as a district nurse – after nineteen years of service, much of it unpaid.[18]

The case of Olive Bishop reveals that even when they had had extensive apprenticeship, midwives often took advantage of formal training when it was available. This was especially the case in Newfoundland, where the state supported midwifery training. In 1919 Newfoundland established the Outport Nursing Committee to bring nurse-midwives to the district nursing services provided to outport settlements. In the mid-1920s the Newfoundland Outport Nursing and Industrial Association (NONIA), a voluntary organization that received government approval and some financial assistance, took over the work of this committee. Between 1925 and 1934 NONIA was able to provide nurse-midwives, often from Britain, to many of the isolated settlements.[19] In 1936 An Act to Govern the Practice of Midwifery provided for formal licences to be issued to trained midwives. Training under this Act varied from three weeks to three months, the difference perhaps reflecting the variable experience of many of the women taking the course. Although most women who attended were from the St John's area, attempts were made to train outport women. For example, the government instructed Myra Bennett, a trained nurse from Britain who had been working in Daniel's Harbour since 1921, to give six local women a six months' training session. In addition, officials from the Department of Health and Welfare, under which the Midwifery Act was regulated, travelled around Newfoundland examining women who were already working as midwives in order to provide them with official certification. By 1938, 143 communities were covered by the Midwifery Act in twenty-three nursing districts. Training emphasized the benefit of science and the limits of a midwife's experience and expertise. The women were taught: 'If the after-birth or hand presented you should call a physician immediately.' They could deal with a breech presentation, but in no circumstances were they to enter the birth canal, a prohibition that severely circumscribed their ability to respond to complications (as it was intended to do).[20] The training stressed the women's assistant role to a physician, but the reality of many Newfoundland communities in which these midwives lived meant that restrictions on their actions were seldom enforced.

While Newfoundland was the region most organized in terms of midwifery training, other parts of Canada made some attempts. In 1919 Alberta permitted 'any nurse who has taken a course in obstetrics, and has obtained the consent of the minister [to] practice mid-wifery in any designated part of the province, where ... the services of a physician are not available.' When physicians were available, a nurse-midwife would not be sanctioned. In 1924 B.E. Harris, a public health nurse from Oshawa, wrote a critical assessment of 'practical nurses' in which she stated that these community women were well meaning but really did not have the expertise to be safe helpers. She noted, 'We are considering now the holding of a class for Practical Women, teaching them the rudiments of asepsis, the proper care of a maternity case.'[21] Both Quebec and Nova Scotia permitted midwives to practise and also provided training, though few women took advantage of this opportunity.

The Salvation Army maternity hospitals offered training over eighteen months, with lectures in anatomy, physiology, obstetrics, gynaecology, paediatrics, materia medica, and bacteriology, along with practical supervision by graduate nurses. This training was available in Winnipeg, London, Toronto, Ottawa, Saint John, Halifax, and Sydney, with a total of fifty women training as maternity nurses. Most of the trained women eventually worked for the Salvation Army, though almost 50 per cent returned to their own communities. In Nova Scotia and Quebec, there was little to stop them from practising as independent practitioners of midwifery.[22] However, midwifery was not well paying, support from physicians was limited, and midwife training had emphasized the midwives' role as physician helpers. Nowhere in Canada did midwives receive the formal recognition of the state to the degree that they did in Britain under its Midwives' Act of 1902.[23]

There were various types of midwives in twentieth-century Canada because of the various needs. Some pregnant women preferred to be assisted in childbirth by another woman or had no other option, either because of lack of money or because of physical isolation. In 1906 the National Council of Women (NCW) reported on various towns and cities in Ontario and the situation in which poor women found themselves during childbirth. Even in areas long settled, problems existed. The NCW report stated that Kingston women were well served by two hospitals with forty physicians and trained nurses, but the women of Ingersoll and Lindsay were not so fortunate and, as a result, did not receive adequate care. In 1918 the VON reported that 5,000 out of 13,000 births in Nova Scotia went unattended by a physician. Western Canada, especially, could not meet the needs of women; there were not enough trained nurses, and the small hospitals being proposed would not be large enough to cope with the demands of maternity care.[24] In 1917 the federal government investigated rural Ukrainian districts in the prairie provinces and discovered that only one woman in eighty-five had had either a physician or a midwife attend them in childbirth. The NCW in the same year worried that in sparsely settled areas women often left their beds too soon after birth in order to take care of their families. Even worse, the hard life these women led might cause 'conditions' that could lead to morbidity of the mother and/or child or death. On the prairies, one response was the development of maternity/nursing homes. In Saskatchewan in 1926, forty-eight were being inspected. By 1941 there were 151.[25] Sophia Anstey recalled that in her community of North Summerford, Newfoundland, she was the only midwife within twelve miles, and until 1924 the nearest hospital was 125 miles away.[26] Women living beyond medical help were well aware of their situation. One recalled, 'Never until my dying day shall I forget the agony of knowing that if anything went wrong I hadn't a chance.'[27]

Rhoda Maud Piercey, from Winterton, Trinity Bay, Newfoundland, who had wanted to be a nurse, described how she became involved in midwifery: 'One day, a neighbour asked me if I would assist the doctor with the delivery of her baby. I was so surprised that anyone would ask for my help, that I was reluctant to say yes, but out of pity for the family, I agreed to do my best. These people were poor and could not afford the fees for a professional nurse. The Doctor was new to the province just having arrived here from his home in England, and he much needed assistance.'[28] Although reluctant, Piercey had a sense of where her duty lay and also a sense of her own worth in recognizing that both the woman and the physician needed her. The case was successful and word spread that the community had a midwife. The sense of community obligation was strong among midwives. Annie Andre became a midwife at the age of thirty-nine because the women in her village did not have anyone to go to whom they trusted. Consequently, Mrs Andre took it upon herself to contact Grace Hospital in St John's, and in 1949 she took a midwife course, leaving her children in the care of her mother and leaving 'her husband to care for himself.'[29]

For some women, midwifery was a way of remaining independent. In 1918 Lillian Moody was twenty-one and married to a cook on a ship sailing out of St John's. Planning eventually to move to her husband's family in England, Lillian found herself widowed with two children and a third on the way. After the birth of this child, her physician, Cluny MacPherson, suggested that she become a midwife to help provide her family with an income, and he encouraged her to take a midwifery course. She did so in the winter of 1921 at the Midwives' Club in St John's, which had been set up by the Child Welfare Association. Her situation was not unusual. The teacher at the Midwives' Club noted that most of the St John's women taking the course were widows, though she believed that this was not the case for those from outside the city.[30] In Saskatchewan, most of the maternity home operators were widowed women with families to support.[31] Yet, for most midwives, the payment was negligible. Sophia Anstey, who began practising midwifery at the age of thirty-eight in 1895 (and over a forty-six-year period delivered more than three hundred babies), was hardly ever paid, though she was sometimes given a meal; and she recalled that if a family was richer than the norm, she might receive fifty cents, especially if the case required her to stay over. Not all midwives could afford to be so generous and some did receive significant payment, but most worked for nothing and indeed saw payment as the exception rather than the rule.[32]

Some midwives had relatively small practices. During her career, Mme Hubert in rural Quebec delivered sixty-seven babies. Diddy Day in Quidi Vidi village, Newfoundland, in the early decades of the century delivered forty-four babies, seven with a physician and thirty-seven on her own. By contrast, others had both extensive and long practices. Annie Fizzard in the decades after 1916 delivered close to 350 children. Jane Ann Emberley delivered more than 323, not including cases where a physician was present. In more than fifty years of midwifery, Mrs Susan Eveleigh delivered 1,534 children, an extraordinary feat given that she had nine children of her own.[33] Certainly, the numbers some midwives delivered easily exceeded those of many physicians' practices.

What kind of care did midwives provide? Like that of physicians, it could vary from person to person. In general, midwives provided little formal prenatal care. A woman would approach a midwife to arrange for her services, and until the woman went into labour little explicit contact occurred. Yet, as part of the local community, the midwife would see the woman and caution her if she was doing something that the midwife thought was a danger to her own or her baby's well-being. Midwives did not view hard physical work as a problem for pregnant women, but many recalled advising them not to reach above their heads, for they believed that this would pull on the umbilical cord and strangle the baby. Some suggested that pregnant women wash their legs with soap and water and then grease them to overcome discomfort during pregnancy. Some counselled couples to engage in sexual intercourse in the last week of pregnancy to assist in the birth – advice physicians viewed with disapproval because it could increase the chance of infection or induce early labour.[34] By the 1930s, many midwives in Newfoundland began to visit daily in the two weeks before delivery, giving advice and checking on the progress of the pregnancy to determine when the child would be born. In her practice from the late 1930s into the 1950s, Mrs Freda Guinchard of Daniel's Harbour was even known to have women visit her during the early months of their pregnancy, and as the date of delivery drew near she would 'stay and look after the mother.'[35]

Generally, it was only when a woman knew she was going into labour that she sent for the midwife. Most midwife-directed births took place in the home of the woman, although some midwives had the women come to them.[36] In the home, the bedroom was the most usual room in which to deliver, but the kitchen or parlour might be used depending on which was warmer and most convenient. Among Finnish Canadians, women often gave birth in a sauna. It was a peaceful and quiet place; it could be heated to a comfortable temperature, and there was always water available.[37]

Helping to deliver a child in the woman's home was not as easy as it sounds. For the midwife, it meant time away from her own home and family. In Newfoundland and other isolated parts of Canada, transportation was difficult at best and in winter could be next to impossible. Jane Ann Emberley remembered that she 'had to travel through snow, get over fences, go [by] boat and everything else.' She recalled one case in particular: 'There was too much snow and I couldn't get through and Din and this other man had to get on each side of me and haul me through the snow. One on each side and they dragging me. Nobody knows how they done it! Another time Joey John took me over to Broom Cove in the punt and I had to walk back by land. I had to do that nine times.'[38] (Broom Cove was three or four miles from her home.) Mrs George Poole, who worked on the coast of Labrador from the mid-1920s to the late 1960s, had vivid recollections of winter transportation problems. Often she had to travel by dogsled for distances up to ten miles and received frost burns as a result. Nor did discomfort necessarily end with arrival at a family home. Sleeping arrangements might be minimal, the house cold, and food scarce. Some midwives returned home with lice. In addition, since midwives tended to work well into old age, they had their own infirmities with which to contend.[39]

In Newfoundland the traditional position for the actual birth was for the woman to kneel on the floor and rest her arms on a chair. This position allowed the woman to push and the midwife to reach up and assist the baby. If the woman was in difficulty, the midwife might encourage her to lie on the bed. Even when there was no difficulty, some women delivered in bed; a cloth or belt, on which they could pull during contractions, might be attached to the foot of the bed.[40] Myra Bennett, the British midwife working in Daniel's Harbour, found that the beds were deep boxes on legs, which meant that the mattress was surrounded by a 'board fence' too difficult to deal with. The first thing she did on seeing one was to knock the sides off.[41] Over time, more women gave birth in bed. One study of Newfoundland midwives traced the shift to the interwar years, a consequence of the increased medical training more midwives were receiving and also the increased contact with medical professionals. Clara McGrath recalled: 'Before 1935 I born the babies like this. I'd put a quilt or banket on the floor. The woman would kneel by a chair and drop the baby into the blanket. After I had my [public health] training I had them use the bed.' In other communities, however, the shift predated medical influence. Some felt that being on the floor 'Indian style' was no longer appropriate, that the bed was more comfortable.[42]

The reference to 'Indian style' was accurate only in part. The Kwakwa Ka'wakw (Kwakiutl) of the West Coast dug a pit and lined it with soft cedar bark so that the child could safely drop into it. During the birth, one of two midwives held on to the woman.[43] An Inuk woman described the custom of her people: 'Some woman gave birth while sitting up, sometimes they were helped physically during the actual delivering of a baby. I have never seen this process of midwifery myself before. But I have heard that a midwife would position her behind the woman's back in order to keep the woman's back who is in labour straight. Sometimes when the woman in labour was kneeling down, she would keep her hands on her thighs in order to give balance.' The Inuit believed that if the woman became too comfortable, the delivery would be slow, so the position often changed during labour.[44] While specific customs varied from culture to culture and from community to community, seldom did First Nations and Inuit women have their children lying down. As one Métis woman dismissively put it, such a custom was a 'disgustingly dirty habit.'[45]

The cultural specificity of birthing practices was also reflected in who was present at the birth. The southern Kwakwa Ka'wakw excluded husbands from the birthing room. Nevertheless, the husband did have a role to play. While his wife was in labour, he had to walk from house to house, entering through the rear door and leaving through the front.[46] In Western culture, men usually did not enter the bed chamber, nor did they have a ceremonial role, but they often assisted by keeping the fire going in the kitchen so that water could be boiled or by bringing water when necessary or going for help if it was needed. Otherwise, most stayed out of the way. As one woman recalled, 'My husband wouldn't come near the house at all only to stir up the fire. He spent most of the time out in the stable standing in the shutter door.'[47] Some midwives believed that the presence of the father in the house was bad luck. Others did not even seem to consider the idea of a man helping. Rhoda Maud Piercey of Trinity Bay, Newfoundland, told of a case in the 1930s when, knowing that the baby was going to come quickly, she sent the husband to get a neighbouring woman to help her. She never considered letting the father help. 'It was unheard of that the father should be in the room when his child was being born.'[48]

But midwives did often call on others, such as a neighbour, the mother of the woman in labour, or possibly a woman they were training. A. Lapthorn Smith of Bishop's University in Quebec recalled one of his cases in 1902 when on entering the home of the patient he faced six old women waiting to pass judgment on what he was about to do.[49] For some midwives, having a witness to their work was important. Susan Eveleigh believed it to be a legal requirement until the local doctor told her it wasn't necessary. After that she delivered babies on her own. As midwives increased their contact with medical personnel, they tended to work alone as a way of offsetting the dangers of infection.[50] But although infection rates dropped, there was a corresponding decline in the sharing of childbirth culture among the community of women.

The equipment that midwives brought with them could vary, and generally it increased over time. Nevertheless, in all periods it was minimal compared with that carried by physicians. In the early part of the century, midwives often had the following: an enema bag, rubber gloves, a lubricant, scissors, and fine muslin. Some claimed not to have taken anything; one said she had attended women 'with just a crucifix in my pocket.'[51] H.J.G. Geggie recollected that Mme Hubert in his rural Quebec practice carried 'the burnt rag for the cord; the great scissors to cut the tongue-tie; the large teaspoon of thick castor oil to "cut the phlegm" in the baby's throat ... Beaver's kidneys in gin was always ready for the after-pains ... [and] wheat grains "to settle the childbed."' Some also brought 'medicinal drops' for the baby's eyes (to protect against infection) and sewing cotton with which to tie the umbilical cord.[52] One Scandinavian midwife working in the 1920s in the Rainy River area of western Ontario never used eye drops and had no equipment, but she claimed to have her 'tricks' for difficult cases.[53] Those who worked with or were advised by physicians had access to more aids. Some doctors provided midwives with ergot (a rye fungus that can cause cramping and abdominal contractions), while giving them very careful instructions on how to administer it.[54]

Just as in other aspects of birthing, culture played an important part in what equipment was available. In northern Native communities, a mother – who might be her own midwife – would gather moss and make a bag out of it; she would also make cord from twisted fibres or sinew to tie off the umbilical cord. A moss pad, perhaps covered by fabric, would be made to place under her at the time of the birth, and she would have a pole ready to use as a crossbar support to lean against.[55] Native people were not particularly impressed by modern scientific ways. Dr Mary Percy Jackson told the story of her work with Métis women in the late 1940s. She had just saved a mother in childbirth, and this had impressed the old women of the community. But she noted: 'My gown, mask and gloves are accepted as a harmless eccentricity; they know that all that is really required is a pair of scissors and a piece of string.'[56]

One of the medical complaints about untrained midwives was their lack of attention to antisepsis. Yet each culture had its own way of ensuring cleanliness. Among the Finns, taking saunas was part of their emphasis on cleanliness, and the fact that birth often occurred in a sauna connected it with that concern. The heat of the sauna provided comfort, and apparently the carbon in the smoked saunas prevented the growth of bacteria.[57] A study of early Newfoundland midwifery found that midwives were quite familiar with the concept of antisepsis. Some carried Jayes Fluid and carbolic with them; others applied scorched muslin to the child's navel area and to the mother's vagina. Midwives also used soap and hot water liberally, and some used peroxide. Many made sure that they had boiled all their utensils and sealed them in glass jars before the time came to attend a labour.[58] Jane Ann Emberley made a point of noting that she never 'carried the same apron from one patient to another.'[59] As time passed, midwives adopted more scientific ways of sterilizing, especially the use of previously prepared sterile pads. But this did not necessarily ensure that sterilization was any better. Some physicians understood this. When Nurse Banfill was working with the Native people of the Pacific Coast in the 1940s and 1950s, she was given good advice:

> Dr. Provost advised me to stand by for abnormal maternity cases, but warned me against interfering with Indian deliveries. They seemed immune to their own germs, but readily picked up germs introduced by other races. He insisted that a normal delivery by an Indian midwife was usually without infection. Many times Indian mothers had been infected when delivered by a white person. The mother, or midwife, bites off the cord. Nature provides certain types of moss and reeds, which seem to be germ proof, and the only anti-septic measures needed. Used as a cord dressing, no more infections were encountered than when sterile gauze dressings were applied.[60]

Provost's advice to Banfill raises the issue of intervention. Historians who have been critical of midwives suggest that midwife intervention could be extreme, whereas historians sympathetic to midwives stress the non-interventionist aspects of their work compared with the custom of medical practitioners.[61] It is important to go beyond this simplistic dichotomy to examine the customs many midwives followed and to appreciate their diversity. Seldom did midwives shave the genital region, although some who had more formal training did. Nor did midwives perform episiotomies. However, some midwives brought enema bags with them because of concern that constipation might cause discomfort in delivery or impede delivery – and also that by creating intestinal contractions, it might speed deliver. For the same reasons some used purgatives, although other midwives resorted to these only in cases of long or overdue labour.[62]

Writing about Olive Bishop, who was a midwife nurse on the south coast of Newfoundland, Joyce Murphy pointed out the demands placed on Bishop: 'She dealt with normal and abnormal deliveries. Everything from twin births and breech births, to corded babies and premature infants. She had antepartum and postpartum hemorrhages, toxemias (eclampsia [convulsions and coma] and pre-eclampsia), placenta previas, as well as numerous abortions and miscarriages.'[63] Midwives dealt with such complications in a variety of ways. For incorrect presentations, some midwives turned the baby externally, whereas others greased their arms and physically tried to shift the baby in the womb.[64] To offset bleeding, Mrs Annie LeMoine from Port-au-Port had the woman drink the juice of boiled blackberry or blackcurrant roots beforehand. Others simply tied a green string around the waist of a woman who was haemorrhaging.[65] While not aggravating the situation, this would of course have done nothing to stem the blood flow, but it may have calmed the woman by seeing something done. At times, doctors working with midwives taught them how to intervene. For severe haemorrhages, one Newfoundland physician advised midwives to tip the woman back in a chair until she was almost upside down and then pack towels between her legs until the physician arrived.[66] Complications of birth could occur anywhere, and the women attending simply did the best they could, as did physicians. At times the best could be very good indeed. One study of the Canadian North confirmed the kinds of situation that Native women might have to face. One elder stayed with a woman for two days until she could remove a retained placenta and control the bleeding. The women of Fort Rea told the story of a woman who 'suffered a prolapse [falling down] uterus a month or so after the birth of her child and was nursed by the older women in camp who used hot compresses and massage until the condition corrected itself.'[67]

Most midwives accepted pain as a normal accompaniment of birthing. It was 'God-given.'[68] John W.S. McCullough, Ontario's chief medical officer, argued that women preferred to have physicians attend them because only trained individuals could provide anaesthesia.[69] Legally, trained individuals did not include midwives. Consequently, midwives could not give anaesthesia, but they tried to alleviate pain in other ways. Some advised the mother to wear the hat of the baby's father or to place an axe under the bed to ease the pain of childbirth.[70] While such folk customs may not have worked in a physiological way, they would have comforted the woman in labour that she had done something to help herself. Other midwives provided medicinal teas. For example, Mary Margaret Drover, who practised midwifery in Island Cove, Newfoundland, in the 1920s, gave her patients a tea made from ginger wine and strained juniper.[71] The aim was not the elimination of pain but its alleviation. Unfortunately, this was not enough for some women in labour, and there was little more that a midwife could do. Mrs Maritta House, who worked in Trinity Bay in the late 1930s, remembered that she had threatened 'to shove the blanket down [the] throat' of a screaming woman unless the woman quietened down and stopped reacting to her pain so excessively.[72]

Because pain alleviation was limited in midwife-directed births, some midwives were very sensitive to prolonged labour. To encourage a faster birth, some stretched the vagina. In Newfoundland, although midwives would not deliberately break the amniotic sac as a matter of course, some might do so to shorten a very long labour.[73] One physician told of the death of a woman in childbirth which he blamed on a midwife who had obtained ergot from a druggist because the birth was not progressing rapidly enough. As already noted, other midwives used ergot given to them by physicians and did so very carefully, appreciating that it should be 'administered strictly.'[74] In Native communities, women attending the mother might squeeze her in an effort to make the delivery progress. Or they might wrap a blanket around her as tightly as possible, with two women pulling it.[75] In Dr Wilfred Bigelow's rural Manitoba practice, in 1908, a midwife introduced him to a new technique. He had gone to an isolated farmhouse, where he was met by an old midwife who told him that the woman had been in labour for over a day and that the birth was not progressing. The midwife thought that the woman should be 'quilled.' Not knowing what this was, Bigelow proceeded with the examination, checking the uterus, which felt hard, showing little evidence of progress occurring. Meanwhile, the midwife kept suggesting quilling. Curious about what this was, Bigelow eventually told the midwife to proceed.

> She immediately got up from her chair and pulled down the wing of a goose which was hanging on a nail behind the stove. She got a nice long goose quill ... and cleaned the inside of the quill, cutting off both ends. She went to the cupboard and dipped one end of the quill into a small package of cayenne pepper. I wondered what the devil was coming next, so I followed her into the bedroom. She took the quill and inserted it into the nostril of the patient, then gave it one big blow, and away went the cayenne pepper into the poor woman's nasal cavity. I knew what was liable to happen. She began to sneeze immediately. With the sneezing the midwife said, 'Doc you'd better get ready.' By the time I had taken a look at things, the perineum was bulging and with another few sneezes, the baby was born.[76]

Circumstances and results habitually determined whether intervention had been necessary and whether it was benign. Dr Samuel Peikoff told of going to the home of a Manitoba woman and meeting the midwife, Rosie, who informed him that she had been there working for sixty-two hours and the baby still had not come. He listened for a foetal heartbeat but heard nothing. He then decided to do a pelvic examination: 'I walked over to Mary's bed and pulled the blanket down to her knees. She lay in a pool of blood and what I thought was greasy meconium from ruptured membranes. But it was thick and black over the pubis and perineum. I was puzzled. Since the midwife had been reputed to have twenty-five years experience, I asked her: "What is that dirty brown stuff? It looks like axle grease."' The 'brown stuff' was fresh cow manure which Rosie had used to 'grease' the child (who was successfully born). Although upset at what she had done, Dr Peikoff recognized that Rosie was exhausted and that 'this was not the time nor the place for a confrontation.' Knowing that midwives could be jealous of physicians, he felt he had to tread carefully.[77] What is fascinating about Peikoff's telling of this incident is his ability to empathize with the midwife despite his horror at what she had done.

Once a child was born, the immediate task at hand was dealing with the afterbirth. In the 1923 *Canadian Mother's Book* (1923), Dr Helen MacMurchy suggested that women who found themselves acting as midwife should use a clenched fist to massage the mother's abdomen, both to prevent haemorrhage and to help expel the placenta by getting the uterus to contract.[78] Midwives themselves did not discuss this much, though some hospital patients reported that their midwives had used considerable force to expel the afterbirth. One midwife described having the woman blow into the neck of a bottle to cause contractions and deliver the afterbirth. She had learned this from a physician. To help with the afterpains, others brewed various teas, for example, from the boughs of the juniper bush. The tea, they believed, would cleanse the body of 'corruption' and rid it of any remaining placenta.[79]

What to do with the afterbirth was a matter of concern to midwives. One study of Newfoundland midwifery described midwives rolling the afterbirth in salt, wrapping it in newspaper, and then burning it in the oven. Some believed that if they did not take the right steps, the woman might 'dry up' or even bleed to death. Even those who did not follow such beliefs were concerned about the way in which the afterbirth was cared for. One midwife made sure that she placed it in a chamber pot, away from the sight of the husband. She then burned it in the kitchen stove. When people no longer used chamber pots, she wrapped the afterbirth in newspaper before burning it. Others threw it into the privy.[80]

Among the Inuit and First Nations people, there were taboos connected with the afterbirth in order to protect the mother and child, and the whole community. On Coronation Gulf and Victoria Island early in the century it was the custom to hang the afterbirth high in a tree. Similarly, Angela Sydney of the Tagis and Tlingit people remembered her community doing this when the baby was a boy. The afterbirth was left in the tree to be eaten by the 'camp robber,' the Canadian jay, in the belief that this would ensure that the boy became a good hunter. If the baby was a girl, the people placed the afterbirth in a gopher den. Among the southern Kwakwa Ka'wakw, treatment of the afterbirth was gender specific as well. The midwife would carefully wrap it in cedar bark and bury it in a location dictated by the sex of the child.[81]

After the third stage of labour, the midwife had time to focus on the mother and her baby. Chores included suturing perineal tears, washing both mother and child, changing the bed, and putting clean clothes on the mother and baby. One midwife remembered a family so poor that she ripped her own petticoat to make diapers. Some baptized the child if they thought it was not going to live. Binding the mother was also something that midwives did. There were two types of binding. If the mother was not going to nurse – perhaps because her child had been stillborn or her own health would not allow it – binding the breasts would dry the milk. The other type of binding was that around the woman's abdomen. Tightened each day for nine days after the birth, it helped encourage the stomach to return to its usual shape and contributed to the woman's comfort.[82]

During the postnatal care period, midwives insisted that the new mother be on a restricted diet of tea and toast, avoiding fats such as butter. Dr H.J.G. Geggie recalled that in rural Quebec in the early part of the century, midwives forbade women in labour to drink cold water. They heated the water or cut it with gin. In Newfoundland, when friends visited the new mother, they ate a piece of dark fruit cake, called a Groaning Cake, which the new mother had made.[83]

The postnatal period was the time when midwives were particularly useful. They would visit daily for nine or ten days after the birth and help cook meals and wash clothes. Sometimes these visits were twice daily, in the morning and in the afternoon or evening.[84] One settler on the prairies in the early twentieth century recalled: 'I was only married a year, and my first girl was born in the house, but we had a nurse. Mostly all the coloured people there in Amber Valley had this same midwife. She went north of us too, to the white people. She'd stay right in your house until nine days even, and cook and do the wash. Everybody just loved her.'[85] Depending on the circumstances, the midwife might stay longer than nine days. If the birth had been premature, she might stay until she could be sure that both mother and baby could manage. As well, neighbours would help. Even in the 1930s this kind of pattern continued. One midwife told of staying with the mother for nine days and then visiting twice a day for two weeks to 'dress the babies [sic] belly button.' Others tried to stay with the mother for two days, providing the subsequent care through visits. However, prolonged stays were not always possible, especially when other women needed the midwife's services.[86] Nurse-midwives tried to follow the same procedure. Margaret Giovannini remembered that during the 1940s she visited twice a day for the first three days after birth and then once a day until the tenth day as long as things were progressing well.[87]

The length of time a woman stayed in bed also varied. Dr Geggie recalled that many women were out of bed on the third day after the birth but went back again on the ninth day. This seemed to coincide with many midwives' belief about the importance of the number nine in some aspects of birthing. (Geggie also noted that Mme Hubert advised women not to put their hands above their heads and not to comb their hair for ten days or wash it for six weeks).[88] Other women seemed to stay in bed for the full nine days of the midwife's visits in order to offset the possibility of haemorrhage. Over the years, some midwives began to let mothers get up earlier. One midwife recalled that when she first practised in the 1920s she kept the women in bed for the traditional nine days, but by the end of her practice, after increased contact with the medical profession, she kept them in bed for only three.[89] Recalling her experience in the 1920s, one woman summarized much of the midwife care provided:

The treatment we got after the baby was born was something else. You got tea with bread and butter the first day. Then no more for three days, dry toast I lived on for three days. They wouldn't even give ya a drinka cold water. You were not allowed to sit up in bed. Your weren't allowed to comb your hair, nor put yer hands in cold water. The windows were not allowed to be opened. I don't know what way it was, but you had to go along with it. The midwife had the responsibility of you and the baby, she was afraid you'd hemorrhage. They would let you up the fifth day just to sit in the chair. The tenth day, mother was coming downstairs and that was a big day. The blanket was put on the rockin chair. And my husband would say don't open the doors mother is getting up today. Then when ya got up, ya couldn't walk, ya were practically starved to death.[90]

Keeping women in bed for so long and the special consideration given them was not always healthy, but removing them from their normal routine did focus the attention of their families on the seriousness and importance of what the women had gone through. It was also in keeping with wider medical practice. In these various ways midwives could both psychologically comfort and give practical aid to the new mother. Once up, the woman might rest for another week or even longer, though the pattern varied depending on the needs of the family. The rest period in bed and afterwards was possible only because of the work of the midwives and the willingness of women neighbours to help.

Even when women began to go to hospital to give birth, the work of midwives did not end. Rhoda Maud Piercey, for example, often accompanied the mother to the hospital and then visited the mother after she came home if her dressings needed to be changed because of infected breasts or if she was worried about the condition of the baby's cord.[91] Having a baby was a significant event, and the customs surrounding it, combined with the attention of the midwives, celebrated that fact. Some communities did not expect women to go out into society until 'churched.' Anglicans and Roman Catholics in Newfoundland followed this tradition, which was both a thanksgiving for the safe delivery of the child and a 'purification' of the woman.[92] Until 'churched,' a woman was not to put her hands in flour or make bread, or even cut it.[93] The final sign that the woman was ready to resume her usual life was the resumption of sexual relations with her husband – six weeks after the birth.[94]

Midwives took incredible pride in the success of their work. In the first forty years of this century, Sophia Anstey did not lose one of the more than three hundred babies she delivered. Many of the midwives interviewed or who left records made similar claims.[95] Losing a child was hard. Annie Fizzard recalled that of the close to three hundred and fifty cases she helped deliver, she had only one still birth – and she 'cried when dat' came into the world.'[96] Having had children of their own, midwives knew how difficult losing a baby was, and perhaps for this reason they were reluctant to give up on them. As Rhoda Maud Piercey stated, 'Never once ... in any of my many births did I ever feel the urge to give up. I always had faith and hope in what I was doing. I thank God that I never lost a baby.'[97] At times physicians, too, recognized that the work of the midwives was successful more often than not. Dr Geggie recalled of Mme Hubert: 'Never was an obstetrician more meticulous in her regimen, never was a paediatrician so careful of details. Her patients came through very serious illnesses, all of them with the happiest results. Nor did she let you forget that she'd had sixty-seven babies in her time, never lost one, nor mother either. The rest of us could not say as much.'[98]

For both midwives and physicians, particularly if they were not Catholic, the survival of the mother was more important than that of the child. Midwives prided themselves on keeping their mothers alive, and some doctors were struck by the low maternal mortality rate among mothers who did not have access to medical care.[99] But occasionally death occurred. Mrs Susan Eveleigh remembered one woman in the 1920s who had been told by her physician that she would have difficulty giving birth. He advised her to go to the hospital. She refused. The doctor then advised Eveleigh not to attend the woman if she was called. But Eveleigh felt she had no alternative: 'Somebody had to do it.'[100] Many women were intensely grateful for the work midwives did. Typical was the experience of a woman from the Alberta prairies:

I had a doctor. I never had anyone to stay with me after my baby was born, but I had a doctor, and I had a nurse. She was a Nurse who had come from the old country where she'd been trained in nursing and midwifery. If I hadn't had her when my youngest son was born I would have been dead. We had a doctor who wouldn't take any notice of what she said, even though she had good training in the old country ... She must have been about 55 then. She saved my life, because the doctor told my husband he couldn't save me. I was really sick but she did the trick, she knew what to do.[101]

In a similar vein a Newfoundland woman observed: 'The midwives were great women, they never lost heart, never gave up and wouldn't let you give up either ... They knew just what to say. They were as brave as lions you know, they never got upset and wouldn't let you get upset either.'[102]

A sense of a female community emerges out of the descriptions of midwife care. Yet as time passed, many women clearly saw midwife births as part of an older order, born of necessity, although some mourned their passing.[103] But many midwives did not. Some thought that perhaps the 'cottage hospital' scheme was best; there the midwife could work in a controlled environment and have a sense of professionalism and autonomy.[104] Nor did they miss the hard and sometimes stressful nature of their work.[105] Many felt that the shift to 'doctor-attended hospital' birth signified progress and modernization. Others, however, had a more positive view of the past and took pride in their personal touch and low mortality figures. Clara Tarrant made it clear that something had been lost in the transition to hospital birth: 'It's not the same thing now. No, no. Not the same at all. The mother is gone and when she comes back, brings the baby in and lays it down. No ... I think there's a bit of something gone there ... Something missing ... The feeling is gone out of it.'[106] Midwifery lasted longest in cohesive communities that were isolated from the pressures of modern industrialized society as a result of geographic or cultural separation.[107]

As noted in chapter 1, some practitioners were concerned about the lack of feeling in medicine. However, few thought that midwifery was the answer in childbirth. Indeed, throughout the first half of the twentieth century, doctors as a professional group ensured that it would not be. Some, while against midwifery, saw no reason to oppose it overtly, for they were confident that the superiority of medical training would win the day. Others made a point of distinguishing between two types of midwives, the dividing line being training. Others were much more accepting, acknowledging the need for midwives and grateful for the assistance they provided to physicians.

The turn-of-the-century Baltimore physician D.W. Cathell, author of a widely read advice manual for physicians, told them that when a midwife sought their help in a difficult case, they should cooperate; in doing so, they would illustrate the 'practical superiority of qualified physicians over the unskilled midwife' and thus raise the status of physicians among the public. Of course, his advice begged the question of the comparison with skilled midwives. In 1902 an editorial in the *Canadian Medical Record* seemed to endorse the *trained* midwife in order to encourage the elimination of what the editor saw as women 'whose natural intelligence and education is such that it is impossible to bring them to the required level.' The training envisioned was formal, culminating in a set examination. Dr Edmund E. King, vice-president of the Ontario Medical Council and a member of the Academy of Medicine, told the Ontario Medical Commission that many trained women were needed in the crowded cities of the day. Rather than a short midwifery course, however, he thought that the system as it existed in Britain was the best option.[108] Training that was both formal and experiential, where the boundaries between practitioners and midwives were clear, would thus legitimize and exalt the formal training physicians were already receiving.

Not all agreed. Adam Wright, who was professor of obstetrics at the University of Toronto and obstetrician and gynaecologist to Toronto General Hospital, made clear the advantages provided by physicians: 'The importance of exact and correct knowledge of normal labor with all its preventive possibilities is perhaps better appreciated on this continent than in older countries, because a kind of Providence has thus far mercifully preserved us from the licensed midwife.' Note the use of the words 'exact' and 'correct' with respect to knowledge. In Wright's eyes, doctors had access to scientific knowledge that was better than or could be a supplement to experiential knowledge. Wright privileged book learning – up to four years of study in subjects such as anatomy, physiology, and pathology. Only this kind of study would allow the physician to discern abnormality early enough for preventive measures to be taken.[109] American physicians made similar arguments, separating themselves from the situation in Europe, where midwives received formal training.[110]

Physicians took for granted the superiority of medical science over midwifery experience. In all probability, most physicians came into contact with midwives only when these women had not been able to help their patients. The successful births managed by midwives, whether trained or not, went unnoticed or were deemed unworthy of comment. Certainly, the only time hospital records mentioned midwives was in cases where a previous labour had gone wrong. Mrs Ann Powell, age thirty-eight, entered Victoria General Hospital, Halifax, on 25 October 1900 suffering from prolapse of the uterus. Her case record stated that when her second child was born, the midwife had pulled on the cord to remove the afterbirth and as a consequence had pulled the womb down as well. It took a doctor's skill to help the woman recover, but after her third child was born the problem reappeared. A similar case was that of Mrs Mary Mott, age thirty-seven, who entered the hospital in 1905 and had been delivered by a midwife when she was seventeen. Her file noted: 'Patient says that the midwife used considerable force in pulling away the afterbirth. Patient was very sick and lost a great deal of blood.' Once again a physician had helped the woman in her immediate recovery, but since then Mrs Mott had been experiencing bearing-down pains.[111]

In St John's, Newfoundland, where in the second decade of the century midwives cared for up to 50 per cent of women in childbirth, it was the midwife who decided whether and when a physician was needed. This scenario gives an interesting twist to the traditional medical view of the midwife who, through her incompetence, is forced to admit her failure and call in a physician. In the view of at least some physicians, the midwife was not necessarily admitting the superiority of a practitioner when she called him in; rather, she was exerting agency (even if in doing so she was admitting her need for assistance) and determining the physician's participation. Patients in St John's often engaged both a midwife and a physician, though the midwife and patient understood that if the birth was normal they would not call the doctor. Whether the physician was under the same understanding is not clear. If not, it would explain why some were rather perturbed; being called in only for problem births limited their clientele and thus their income.[112] A similar situation existed in the maternity hospitals in Saskatchewan, where the matron in charge determined not whether a doctor would be present (he usually was) but when.[113]

Not all physicians found working with untrained midwives problematic, particularly in the early years of the century when there was more contact between midwives and doctors. Wilfred Abram Bigelow recalled going to the bed of a woman in childbirth in his Hartney, Manitoba, practice. When he arrived, two midwives were present. They were wonderful women, he said: 'We called them "gamps," but it would take a lot of nurses these days to do what those women could do in their practical way.' In 1916 an article in the *Canadian Practitioner and Review* noted that there were good midwives and bad ones, just as there were good and bad physicians. It also observed – probably not to the pleasure of its medical readers – that midwives were nurse and doctor rolled into one and could provide the services of both at a much lower cost than physicians. While not willing to endorse such women, Dr Helen MacMurchy, in 1911, suggested licensing and training midwives in order to help reduce maternal mortality among women who had no access to physicians.[114] But this clearly was not her preference. Even in Newfoundland where midwives were common, one historian has determined that physicians 'tolerated' midwives because they saved the doctor time and allowed him to continue the rest of his practice rather than overseeing lengthy labours. But physicians still preferred that they should be present for the actual delivery, if possible.[115] Thus, midwives were to work to the advantage of the physician, without cost to him.

Seldom did physicians or anyone else compare the care given by physicians with that provided by midwives, trained or untrained. When such comparisons were made, physicians did not welcome them. In 1919 Dr M. Seymour, medical officer of health for the Province of Saskatchewan, reported to the Saskatchewan Medical Association on a study he had done comparing maternal mortality rates for the 50 per cent of women in the province who gave birth without the assistance of either a physician or a nurse, with the other 50 per cent. The former experienced a 'much lower' mortality rate, he noted. 'I was very strongly taken to task by some of the members for even compiling these figures,' he said, but explained: 'I thought the proper place to give these figures was to a meeting of medical men. I was taking care that they were not being published.' Research in England for an earlier period also linked a decline in maternal mortality with the increased number and skill of midwives, rather than with the improved skill of physicians.[116] Most physicians did not want to address the issue and, when forced to, simply refused to engage in serious discussion.

Little changed in the interwar period. The arguments had become pro forma. Doctors easily rejected the use of midwives because they focused on the untrained ones. In 1931 Dr W.B. Hendry from the Burnside Lying-In Clinic called them 'unkempt, gin-soaked harridans, unfit for the work they were supposed to do and a menace to the health of any women they might attend.'[117] The negative way in which physicians portrayed midwives suggested a class bias, and the occasional reference to foreigners suggested an ethnic one as well. The focus on untrained midwives, of course, begged the meaning of the term *trained*. Historian Cynthia Comacchio has argued that the midwife issue was so contentious and central to the autonomy and authority of physicians that most medical practitioners simply could not face the issue head on.[118] Perhaps that is why they most often assumed that midwives were untrained.

The medical profession had won the battle over midwives and

in many respects did not have to engage in polemics. Compared with the number of physicians practising, there were few midwives. As subsequent chapters will show, the Canadian solution to the needs of pregnant women was to provide medical not midwifery assistance. Midwives were in no position to protest their weakening position. They had little contact with one another and had few influential champions. There was little, then, for physicians to oppose actively. They simply kept an eye open in case anyone raised the issue of strengthening the midwife role in Canada. In 1929 J.R. Goodall, clinical professor of obstetrics and gynaecology at McGill University, reflected the rather distanced tone of the discussion:

> This argument [for midwives] has to be met frankly and my answer applies only to Canada. Let other countries find their appropriate solution. We have committed ourselves for generations to the policy of physician-accoucheurs. We cannot turn back now even if we should wish to. Our policy has been an evolution, slow, and cumulative. The physician-accoucheur has come to stay. That is the positive answer. The negative side is that we have practically no midwives, nor have we a class of women who would be willing, in large numbers, to undertake this type of work. It would mean years of training to make them efficient. Lastly, our public (except those recent imports from the Near East) are not favourably disposed to midwives, and the public have the say as to who may or may not attend them in labour. What an indictment of our training in obstetrics to admit that a midwife, with poor schooling and short medical training, is a more effective obstetrical agent than is a graduate in medicine![119]

Goodall's statement illustrates the way in which the medical profession dealt with the challenge of midwives. Instead of looking at the experience of other countries, which suggested that midwives could lessen maternal mortality and meet the needs of women,[120] Goodall circumvented the issue by stating that midwives were fine for other countries but not for Canada. He did not deny the experience of other countries but fell back on the specificity of the Canadian context in order to justify opposition to midwives. The situation was just what it ought to be – no midwives. He ignored the historical reality that the current situation was a function of many variables, one of which was the hostility of many within his profession to midwifery. His reference to the lack of public support was also somewhat disingenuous, since several major women's organizations, such as the National Council of Women and the Women's Grain Growers, had come out in support of midwives.[121] Ignoring such support, Goodall maintained that it came only from 'recent imports,' with the implication that these were hardly worth recognizing. In the last sentence, however, the emotional underpinning of the opposition emerged. The status and prestige of physicians would be in jeopardy if Canadians considered midwives as capable as physicians in the childbirth room. If that occurred, how could physicians continue to demand the respect they felt was their due as a result of their extensive schooling?

As Goodall's diatribe suggests, Canadian physicians were well aware of the work of midwives elsewhere. Articles written by British doctors appeared in the Canadian medical press on a regular basis. In a 1928 *Canadian Medical Association Journal*, for example, Dr James Young of the Edinburgh Royal Maternity and Simpson Memorial Hospital, reported on the low contagion rate among patients cared for by midwives. He also noted that obstetrical intervention was not high among midwives, whereas physicians often felt pressured by the time constraints or other aspects of their practice into intervening unnecessarily.[122] Yet articles such as Young's did not stimulate debate about the pros and cons of midwifery. As members of a professional group, medical practitioners continued to reject it as not being applicable to the Canadian situation. They recognized that some women in Canada did not receive the care they deserved, but midwifery was not the answer.

John McCullough of the Ontario Department of Public Health acknowledged that there was a need for nurses – less expensive ones than the trained nurses already working in Canada – who could 'take the place of the incompetent and not always "too clean" handy women upon whom the rural doctor is obliged to depend.' McCullough was even willing to grant that in normal cases of childbirth a midwife was equal to a physician. 'But,' he said, 'she has to meet any condition that may arise and in a complicated case is obliged to call in a doctor. Most women nowadays demand an anaesthetic; it must always be in skilled hands and is an element of more or less danger. First-class results are almost always achieved in the private wards of the hospital with competent nurses and specialists ... In simple cases the home with a competent physician is cheaper and better.' So while giving some recognition to the midwife, McCullogh wanted to explain that most women in Canada would not want one. And he was clear about what was needed: 'The motto of the pregnant woman should be: "Constant supervision of doctor or clinic during the entire pregnancy." It is chiefly through the observance of this motto, and not by the substitution of midwife for doctor, that the maternal mortality will be reduced.'[123]

Others also picked up on the use of nurses to offset the midwife threat. Some accepted the notion that 'high-class obstetrical nurses' could oversee the first stage of labour – until a physician arrived on the scene.[124] In the early 1930s, the Committee on Maternal Welfare of the Canadian Medical Association raised the issue of midwives and sought opinions from members of the association. It found that the Nova Scotia branch was hostile to the use of midwives but supported having trained nurses for rural areas.[125] A 1935 review of *Midwifery for Nurses* in the *Canadian Medical Association Journal* also emphasized a limited role for nurses. Noting that the book implied that nurses could make a vaginal examination, the reviewer argued that this might 'be recognized in Great Britain under a midwifery system, but is not considered good practice in this country.' In Canada, nurses could be kept in their place both by being trained to defer to physicians and by limiting the obstetric training they received.[126] Emphasized by Goodall, McCullough, and the above reviewer was training; it was the dividing line. The only training good enough was medical training. Anything less might be sufficient for a helpmate role but for little more. Nevertheless, the midwifery sys-

tems of other countries continued to be impressive in their results. In 1932 Goodall noted what most physicians and nurses
did not want to hear – that physicians and nurses could be an
actual danger to their patients. They transferred septic material
from their non-obstetrical patients to their obstetrical patients,
with the result that their maternal mortality rates were much
higher than those of women cared for by midwives.[127] However,
Goodall's assertion did not signal a change of heart from his
earlier rejection of midwives in the 1920s. Then he had directed
his opposition at untrained women, whereas now he was advocating the use of trained midwives within a health care system in
which the lines of responsibility were clear.

One of the few vocal supporters of midwifery was Harold
Atlee. The interesting thing about his stance is not his emphasis
on training – he assumed a very formal midwifery training system – but his raising of the gender issue. He discussed the fact
that in the past women had controlled birthing, and he told
nurses that it might not be a bad thing for women to take it back.
He also argued that women were more patient and less interventionist than men and that the low mortality rate of European
midwifery systems suggested to him that nurse-midwives should
be considered.[128] But although Atlee spoke out so supportively,
there was little else he could do. He recalled a midwife in eastern
Canada who had been pressured by local physicians to quit her
practice:

> She had a place where she took the better class of unmarried
> women ... and she delivered them. But the profession ganged up
> on her – every step she made was watched like a hawk ... They
> thought they were losing money. The midwives would take money
> away from them. And then, of course, there was the all-abiding
> anti-feminism. How can a woman deliver a baby, sort of thing ...
> They tried to hit her for malpractice but they could not do it. She
> gave up – she was the last one.[129]

Atlee raised two important issues: the antifeminism of some
physicians and the financial reality of practice. Physician oppo-

nents of midwifery seldom mentioned the former specifically, but it was reflected in their concern about women within the profession. They did, however, worry publicly about the financial issue. Some even argued that governments must get more involved in financing health care to parturient women in order to help eliminate the need for midwives.[130]

Some physicians who supported midwifery did so if the midwives cared only for certain groups of women. Dr J.H. Duncan from Manyberries, Alberta, referring to the fact that poorer women could afford only a 'part-time nurse or neighbour woman' in attendance, asked, 'Why complain? Their score is generally fair.'[131] Dr E.L. Gainer from British Columbia was quite willing to recognize that minority cultures in Canada, such as the Japanese, used midwives. But behind his sanguine attitude was his belief that 'all our own people have a doctor and someone to help them.'[132] Physicians were also accepting of midwives who helped them. Dr William Victor Johnston, writing about practising in the 1920s, stated: 'I learned in my practice that nurses were the doctor's best friends – both practical and registered nurses, including midwives.'[133] In Newfoundland, physicians were often very supportive. One gave Mrs Susan Eveleigh advice about postnatal care and what to charge for her work. The latter was perhaps a bit optimistic, since he advised $15 dollars. As Mrs Eveleigh pointed out, 'Some poor people could not afford to give me money. So I born most of my babies free of charge. If they had money to give me, they would give it to me.'[134] Many Newfoundland women became midwives because physicians had encouraged them to do so, but these women worked mostly in isolated areas and thus did not take patients away from physicians.[135]

Midwifery was never a major focus of medical practice. Physicians took the decision not to encourage the development of a midwifery system before the turn of the century, and the twentieth-century discussion simply occurred in response to the lack of care being provided to women living in isolated areas and partly in response to the high maternal mortality rates. What the discussion did do, however, was to encourage the medical profession to face both issues and to place pressure on various governments to respond. Once maternal mortality rates began to decline significantly in the early 1940s, the issue became less urgent. Nevertheless, even in the 1940s occasional voices supporting midwives raised the issue of poor obstetric training in Canada and low maternal mortality rates in countries with midwives.[136] Yet opponents still refused to engage in direct debate. Dr Ernest Couture, author of *The Canadian Mother and Child* – a federal booklet that was widely distributed throughout the country – felt that the 1940 edition should include a description of birth that would be helpful for a neighbour woman if she found herself in a situation where there was no medical attendant. For this, he came under some criticism. Charlotte Whitton, the outspoken head of the Canadian Council on Child Welfare, worried that such a chapter might be 'used by practical nurses and midwives to increase independence of the medical profession amongst certain ranks of the population, particularly among those of foreign birth.'[137] Medical attendants at birth was the Canadian way, and immigrants had to learn this.

In the first half of the twentieth century, midwife-directed birth was significant for the alternative model it offered to physician-directed birth. But its oppositional position should not be exaggerated. Midwives varied greatly. Some were neighbour women who helped deliver babies occasionally, whereas others were community-designated as a result of apprenticeship or formal types of training, and a few were men. The practice of many mirrored that of physician-directed births. Some sought out medically based education; some shifted the position of the women in labour to emulate that demanded by physicians; and most easily adopted different ways of maintaining cleanliness. Over time, they limited the number of people in the delivery room and increased the amount of equipment they carried with them. They intervened to shorten labour and kept women in bed after birth for the same amount of time as physicians did. Many were comfortable working alongside physicians and willingly took direction and advice from them. The culture of the midwives and their communities played an important role in determining the equipment used, the people present, the position of the birthing woman, and disposal of the afterbirth. Midwives existed because there was a need for them and because so many women felt the obligation to respond to that need. Certainly, the limited remuneration they received does not suggest a strong economic motivation. They took pride in the high percentage of safe deliveries and the postnatal care they provided. But this pride did not prevent many from being grateful to see the end of their practice; their work was physically hard and emotionally draining. In addition, many believed that medical births had much to offer.

Many doctors were not as opposed to midwifery as some historians have suggested. For those willing to discuss the use of midwives, training was the central concern. Midwives who were trained were more acceptable than those who were not. The best training was medical training, and the best midwife was a helpmate to the physician. Opponents of midwifery tended to focus on the failures of midwives and resented situations where midwives were the gatekeepers to obstetric practice. But by the interwar years, the opposition had become simply a matter of form; midwives no longer posed a serious threat even in doctors' minds. Doctors believed in their training and felt that they, not midwives, could offer the best possible care to Canadian women. Although for centuries childbirth had been the prerogative of women, some physicians were convinced that it was only when men became involved that advances were made. After all, the 'science of obstetrics [owed] its existence to men.'[138] Science was what doctors had to offer, and in the modern world it was superior to any kind of experiential wisdom offered by midwives. Nowhere did physicians apply this belief more than in the prenatal care they offered women.

CHAPTER FOUR

The Expanding World of Prenatal Care

This woman is going to have a baby. Hopes for that baby fill her heart. Life, for her has taken on an added importance, and her whole existence glows with a new resolve and a new purpose. Will her hopes be fulfilled? Will things turn out as she dreams they will? That, to a great extent, depends on her. Ninety-eight out of every 100 births are safe and normal – if the proper care is taken during pregnancy. And the most important step toward proper care is to consult the doctor as soon as you suspect a baby is coming, and to keep in touch with him.

Parke, Davis, and Co., advertisement, 1937[1]

The medical community in the first fifty years of the twentieth century assumed responsibility for prenatal care, a significant departure from the previous century, when a woman generally did not see a physician until she went into labour. Doctors believed that their formal knowledge and experience would enable them to become aware of problems early and do something about them before they got out of hand. Using their knowledge, they were able to define the limits of discussion on pregnancy and prenatal care, and thus determine the outcome of the discussion – prenatal medical care was necessary for *all* women. But what did that care entail? This chapter first looks at the care provided in Aboriginal communities – their concern with the type and extent of activity engaged in by the pregnant women, their food customs, and their beliefs surrounding the determination of the child's sex. Taken together, they emphasize the degree to which every society has its own traditions regarding birthing. In this respect, prenatal care in itself is more than 'an exemplar and a facilitator of the wider social control of women,' as some have argued.[2] It is a reflection of culture. Certainly, Canadians of European extraction had their own ways of dealing with pregnancy outside the medical model. Many of them were ambivalent about pregnancy and looked to other women for advice. Unlike Aboriginal women, they focused on sex prediction, not sex determination. But like Aboriginal women, they developed food customs, some of which were closely linked to their belief in maternal impressions, a belief that provided them with both agency and responsibility. Increasingly, however, Canadian women accepted the medical view of pregnancy.

The medical view in the first half of the twentieth century encompassed more of women's experiences than before. While some physicians worried about fertility rates and felt the need to express their concern, more focused on issues revolving around the nature of conception, how the sex of the child was determined, and the general significance of the prenatal period. But these discussions were somewhat abstract in nature. Physicians' real involvement with their patients began with the diagnosis of pregnancy, a process fraught with significance and uncertainty. Having diagnosed a patient as pregnant, the care and treatment provided was shaped by the medical perception of pregnancy as a time of danger. As the Parke, Davis advertisement quoted above indicates, the medical literature told physicians (and women) to have their patients see them on a regular basis so that the physicians could monitor changes in the pregnancy. Further, they were to provide advice on what activities the women should follow, the clothing they should wear, and the food they should eat. In addition, the literature stressed its general hostility to the persistent belief in maternal impressions, although ironically the medical view was more a shift in focus than a refutation of the concept. Underlying the medical care provided to women was the anxiety of doctors about pregnancy's complications, three of which – miscarriage, vomiting of pregnancy, and eclampsia –

are the focus of this chapter in an effort to understand how the dangers of some women became the potential dangers of all and how dealing with those complications could be incredibly frustrating for many physicians and at times a source of division among them.

The involvement of physicians with pregnancy and prenatal care signalled a significant shift in attitude. Because doctors attended patients, the pregnant woman who saw one took on the patient role with its 'illness expectation.' Pregnancy, became aligned to illness – the physician looked for the *symptoms* of pregnancy, *diagnosed* pregnancy, and compared the pregnant state of the woman with her normal (non-pregnant) state.[3] But physicians had an urge to divide pregnancy into various components and stages, which they could then measure in order to determine what changes were healthy and what were not. In doing so, they defined what was natural and unnatural. *Natural* necessitated significant prenatal supervision and measurement to assure the physician that the pregnancy was indeed healthy. *Unnatural* necessitated prenatal intervention. The need for prenatal care became an unquestioning belief in the interwar period. But belief in it narrowed the range of acceptable variations among pregnant women; healthy, pregnant bodies (rather than persons) were to behave in a similar fashion. The corollary was that physicians agreed on acceptable responses, and diversity among responses was circumscribed. While neither women's bodies nor the responses of physicians could ever approach the ideal, medical literature continually put forward guidelines as a reminder of what the ideal was. These guidelines encompassed the taboos and customs of science.

The medical view of pregnancy was not the only one. Peoples not exposed to Western medicine had their own rules and customs, though in fact the focus of many was similar to those of the West. A concern of both traditions was the amount of activity that women should engage in leading up to the actual birth. For most First Nations people, the demands of survival had traditionally meant that reduced workloads were not possible – and perhaps not necessary, given their belief that birth was a natural event. Many peoples of the North believed that a lazy woman would have a slow and difficult birth and give birth to a lazy child.[4] An Inuk woman told how she had worked until she went into labour, using her protruding abdomen as a support for the ice she took from the lake.[5] Another northern woman recalled: 'When we're pregnant, we're always chopping wood – chopping, chopping, chopping! That way we'll have an easier labour.'[6] Nonetheless, they did take extra care. Concerned about miscarriages, the Inuit advised women in the first stage of pregnancy not to stretch skins.[7]

Other customs were more ceremonial in nature. The people of Cumberland Sound believed that if a woman wore the teeth of a wolf, no harm would come to the child. Women tied their front hair at the sides with rings of thread so that the umbilical cord would not strangle the child they carried. Kitty Smith, a Yukon elder of Tlingit, Tagish, and Athapaskan heritage, recalled: 'When they have a baby, they put a belt on the lady's stomach. When you're going to have your first baby, you get up in the morning. You rub some kind of feathers – rub your stomach and then blow in the air. Then that baby is going to be easy born.'[8] Food taboos were common, though eating restrictions varied from people to people. Some Inuit believed that if a pregnant woman ate seal kidneys, the womb would be too dark for the child. Others believed that a pregnant woman should not eat a caribou shot through the heart, a seal that died underwater without having come up to breathe at least once, or a walrus whose intestines had been cut.[9] These customs and taboos were to ensure the well-being of the mother and the child. Others cast a wider net and sought to protect the family and community. Vilhjalmur Stefansson reported that among the Nunatama of the Arctic, pregnant women did not relieve themselves inside their homes. Nor could they be on the ice during whaling, since it was bad luck for the hunt if they (as well as menstruating women) urinated on the ice.[10] While these various strictures limited the actions of the woman, they were a recognition of her control, within limits, over what was happening to herself and her community; the limits defined the culture of communities and peoples, and the strictures became comforting guideposts to a safe birth.

Many Native communities had strong beliefs about sex determination. These revolved around three themes: the fragility of the male sex, the lack of sex 'fixedness,' and the connection between a hard birth and the birth of a female child. Many in the North believed that if a woman pushed hard and her labour was short, a boy would be born; if the labour was long, a girl. Maleness was fragile and could easily be turned into femaleness. For instance, when a boy was born, the midwife would make sure that she protected his penis so that it would not disappear. And after a hard and long labour, during which a boy might have changed into a girl, the mother sucked on the umbilical cord to make the penis return and thus make the baby into a boy again.[11] While such beliefs focused on the birth process, others took their cue from the pregnancy itself. Some Inuit believed that a woman carried a girl child higher than a boy and that her abdomen was rounder.[12]

The situation was not all that different for women in European-based society. They had their own customs about what to do and what not to do as a way of lessening uncertainty and placing power in the hands of people (often the pregnant woman herself), rather than leaving it to fate. Women talked to one another and took strength from the traditions that were part of their culture. Among them was an ambivalence about pregnancy. Many Canadians referred to it as an 'interesting condition,' as 'being in the family way, confined, indisposed, sick, having a cake in the oven, or knocked up.' They seldom used the word *pregnant*.[13] In the early decades under study and even after, pregnant women were not always comfortable about being in public. In 1912 Francis Marion Beynon, in her *Grain Growers' Guide* column, railed against 'the false modesty which demands that the expectant mother shall hide herself away by daylight.' Yet the attitude persisted. As Mrs Adelaide Plumptre noted in the 1928 National Council of Women's *Yearbook*, 'Pregnancy – especially in Anglo-Saxon communities – is wont to be regarded as a condition to be concealed – either as a sacred or a guilty secret – as long as possible.'[14]

Women seldom wrote about their experience of pregnancy. One who did was Lucy Maud Montgomery. When expecting her first child in 1912, she confessed that although she was 'mentally and emotionally uplifted by it,' physically she didn't 'seem to be taking to it so kindly.' The fact that Montgomery was thirty-seven years old may help explain her weariness; that she was not experiencing a happy marriage would also be a factor in her sense of unease. As her time drew near, she was disturbed by more than the physical discomfort, fatigue, and even fear of childbirth pain. She worried that she would give birth to a 'monstrosity,' to a child who had special needs, or that she would not be able to love her child. She also faced the possibility of her own death. All of the above might be considered first-birth anxieties, but she had the same anxieties during her second pregnancy, in 1914. Indeed, she was more anxious, because she knew that she had been fortunate in that the first birth had gone so well. Unfortunately, her fears were well founded. She gave birth to a still-born son, a tragedy she would never forget and would forever mourn.[15]

Some pregnant women took comfort from reading advice manuals. One recalled her pregnancy for the readers of the *Grain Growers' Guide* in 1914. Throughout she ate sparingly, she said, chewed on slippery elm to drive off hunger pangs, and drank copious amounts of flax tea.[16] Older women offered younger women advice and the wisdom of their experience. At times the advice could be frightening. For example, some Newfoundland women remembered being told that keeping a jewel around their necks would ward off evil spirits and that the pain of birth was a result of the devil trying to wrest control of the child.[17] As well as striking fear in a woman's heart, this type of advice made pregnancy and birth an epic struggle between good and evil.

The support structure provided by older women was significant. But as we shall see, doctors saw it as a threat and urged women to look only to their medical adviser. Doctors were not the only ones who rejected it. Women who considered themselves modern thought it a mistake for a mother to give her daughter advice 'based on her own experience of twenty or thirty years ago – regardless of the progress made in medical thought and practice in the last quarter century.'[18] This attitude denied women's experience and culture, and paved the way for increasing dependence on medical professionals. It also left some women unprepared for what was going to happen. Nevertheless, others found comfort in believing that by following medical advice they were doing all they could to ensure the health of themselves and their unborn child.[19]

Unlike the Inuit, Western society did not focus on the birth process either as a predictor or a determining factor of sex. Neither did it believe in the changeability of sex. It did, however, take some interest in predicting the sex of the child before birth. For some, trying to guess the sex was an innocent pastime, engaged in as a way of preparing for the birth; for others, it reflected the desire to have a specific-sex child. Alice Stockham in her 1916 advice guide to women put forward the theory that the partner 'whose mental forces ... are most active and vigorous' at the time of conception determines the sex of the child.[20] Like the Inuit, some thought that the shape of the woman's abdomen during pregnancy was an indication of the child's sex. If the woman 'stuck out in front' she would give birth to a boy, whereas if she 'stuck out behind' a girl would be born. It was also thought that pregnant women carried a boy higher than a girl and more to the right. Such beliefs had a long history and have lasted to the present day. Another sign was the appearance of the mother's face. A clear face indicated a boy, whereas a freckled or cloudy face, a girl. And unlike the Inuit, many believed that boys resulted in harder labour than girls.[21]

Food customs were also part of pregnancy in mainstream society. Dr H.J.G. Geggie recalled that in his rural Quebec practice in the early years of the century, women would carefully eat 'nine hand-picked grains of whole, unground wheat' in the late stages of pregnancy to ensure an easy delivery.[22] For the 'modern' woman, popular magazines were replete with advertisements of women claiming the wonders of various substances taken during pregnancy. In the interwar period, Irma Avery heard of a diet for pregnant women that was said to increase the child's IQ by ten points.[23] In making choices about their diet, women were able to do something for themselves, to feel part of what was happening, and to feel that they controlled or at least directed it somewhat.

Agency could also be found in the belief that a woman's experience, thoughts, and feelings (maternal impressions) could have physical, moral, and intellectual repercussions on the child she carried. Of most concern were the harmful effects of maternal impressions that placed blame on the mother. The physical marking of a child, always deemed negative and unwanted, was a particular focus. In 1936 the author of an article in the *Dalhousie Medical Journal* described one such folk belief in Newfoundland: 'If a pregnant woman has a great desire for a particular food and at the same time touches her baby a birth mark will appear on the child in the same place.' Midwives also believed in the harmful power of not satisfying a pregnant woman's food cravings. A mother's fear was said to have a similar effect.[24]

While we might smile on hearing of such beliefs, common sense informed them. Certainly, Canadians in all parts of the country were familiar with the concept of heredity – they only had to look at their own children. Making a connection between the actions and experiences of the mother during pregnancy and the resulting characteristics of the child differed only in suggesting that physical traits were not fixed at conception. In the early decades of the century, and to a lesser extent later, such beliefs were common. In addition, many Canadians, both lay and medical, had long believed that heredity was significant in determining mental and moral characteristics as well. Physicians working with the insane always questioned patients about a family history of insanity. Members of the Woman's Christian Temperance Union argued that the intemperate habits of parents could be visited on their children in a variety of ways. The Government of Canada, through its immigration laws, acted as if certain people were more fit than others. It feared that if the unfit (morally, physically, or mentally) were allowed into the country, they would propagate their own kind. Canadians believed in the power of heredity, and maternal impressions were part of their understanding of how it worked.

The ability to 'mark' a child endowed the pregnant woman

with power. In the case of food cravings, family, friends, and the woman herself needed to placate her needs, otherwise the child would suffer. This belief had the benefit of ensuring that a woman had enough food at a time when her nutritional needs were increasing. The power of pregnant women to mark their children was fearsome because it was uncontrolled and unpredictable. It could be the consequence of fright, an accident, or forgetting the need for vigilance. It seemed to reflect the general societal attitude that women were more emotional than men, less able to act in a rational way. Alice Stockham advised that husband and friends must become the woman's 'guardian. She must be held in check.' Others agreed and warned of the need to keep certain news from her.[25] Women who did not control themselves or were not controlled would suffer the consequences through the dire effects on their children.

Belief in the power of maternal impressions provided community control over spheres otherwise seemingly influenced by chance. For example, people clearly saw markings on a child as problematic. Attributing them to a woman's experiences during pregnancy provided the community with an explanation that kept a potentially frightening aspect of life at bay. In 1934 a woman wrote to Ontario's chief inspector of health, John McCullough, concerning a story about an expectant mother frightened by a mouse whose child was subsequently born with a mark resembling a mouse. McCullough dismissed this as sheer coincidence.[26] But most people wanted more than this as an explanation and continued to make a connection between events that McCullough saw as coincidence. Ilka D. Dickman, a nurse in Newfoundland in the late 1930s and early 1940s, recounted the case of a baby who was born deformed and eventually died: 'In the house of the newborn, there is the mother crying in her bed; the father, sitting next to the dying baby, deeply shaken; the grandfather, utterly upset; all of them worrying themselves to death not because of the misfortune itself, but rather on account of the unknown sin they must have committed, to which this deformed child is ascribed.'[27] The desire to ensure the well-being of the child and the inability to do so led the family to accept responsibility for what had happened to it. People strove to maintain or exert control. In the October 1929 *Chatelaine*, an advertisement entitled 'World's Most Beautiful Child' depicted a healthy child whose mother testified, 'I took Virol myself before baby was born.' The moral: 'Give *your* child the same chance.'[28] Advertisers knew that most mothers wanted their children to be healthy and beautiful and would be willing to do almost anything to guarantee this. Is the taking of Virol any different from satisfying cravings and avoiding fright? Both acknowledged the intimate relationship between the woman and her unborn child.

But women's agency had limits. As the medicalization of pregnancy increased, there was less opportunity for women's networks to function. It became more problematic to believe the tales of food taboos when faced with scientific opposition. However, even within the scientific modality, room for agency existed. Many women internalized the push to medicalize prenatal care and, having done so, demanded it. No longer did some feel it was a matter of choice; it was a necessity. After all, physicians told them so. It was incumbent on the government to ensure that such care was possible for all women, and it was the duty of physicians not to refuse a case simply because a woman might lack the means to pay. If it was a matter of life and death, as many physicians argued, then surely the Hippocratic oath would mean that commercial wants should not hold sway. Middle-class women, especially professional women, could insist that poorer women did not know what was good for them and could exert their own agency in trying to 'reform' the situation of such women.[29] The acceptance of the medical paradigm was part of the culture of Western society. It is to that paradigm we will now turn.

Physicians' interest in pregnancy began even before a woman became pregnant. For most of the years under review, the fertility rate of Canadians declined, a phenomenon of which Canadians and Canadian physicians were well aware. In a 1935 issue of the *Canadian Doctor*, E.L. Chicanot lamented the decline and raised a particular concern for physicians: 'While the average citizen may be inclined to ask "where is the population of the future to come from?" the doctor could scarcely be blamed for querying "Where are we to get our patients?"'[30] Not even the famed high birth rate of French Canada was immune. Only in the 1940s did the tide begin to shift.

Observers speculated on the causes of the declining birth rate. The editor of the *Canadian Journal of Medicine and Surgery* in 1905 suggested that people in previous generations had probably been made of 'sterner stuff' than those in the present, but he pointed out that domestic help had been a lot cheaper in the past, as had the nursing help needed before and after childbirth. Many modern couples did not feel that they could cope with a family and the demands that went with it – though it was really the women, he said, who made this decision. Not that he blamed them; he called them 'good' but 'desperate' women and concluded that, with respect to Ontario: 'moralists may deplore, statisticians may regret, and publicists fuss over the race suicide ... but the married women, the strictest of logicians in matters pertaining to the family, have settled the birth-rate of Ontario and it is going to be small.'[31] Perhaps women needed encouragement. Six years later, the editor told his readers of the financial assistance given to couples in New Zealand, which seemed to be having a positive influence on the birth rate. He did not think it would work in Canada, however; it smacked too much of 'pauperism.'[32] While legislative solutions were interesting to contemplate, some physicians looked to causes closer to their own area of expertise. Frederick Fenton, associate in obstetrics at the University of Toronto, suggested that women were avoiding childbirth because they feared its pain. If physicians could reassure women and offer them 'even a moderate degree of relief,' that might 'do much to eliminate "race suicide."'[33]

Physicians in the interwar period similarly speculated on the causes of the declining birth rate. The author of one physiology textbook pointed out that poor nutrition lowered fertility, as did hard physical labour by women. The age of the women was also a factor. Less analytical was Harold Atlee, who focused on what he saw – the pain, disability, and even death that women faced as a consequence of pregnancy and childbirth. No wonder that some opted not to have children! At least one woman commentator agreed. She reported that the introduction of caudal anaesthesia would take away the pain of childbirth and thus encourage a woman to have more children than she might otherwise do. Less sympathetic was H.S. Wasman who, in the November 1947 *University of Toronto Journal*, picked up on the concerns of the time regarding women rejecting their prescribed role: 'Some women, after giving birth, feel as though they have done their bit for the rest of their lives. They never "get their strength back" because they never could assume much responsibility. By means of invalidism they avoid further pregnancies, marital responsibilities and are able to live a thoroughly self-centred life, controlling their environment by illness.'[34]

While some physicians might speculate on the reasons for the declining birth rate and on what they could do to stop the spiral, the real interest was in conception. Physicians were fascinated by the physiological nature of conception, believing that if they understood it they could better advise their patients on the timing of sexual relations to ensure conception or to protect against it. Understanding it would also help protect the health of the child and maintain the health of the mother.

In the early years of the century, there was much discussion of when the most fertile time in a woman's monthly cycle occurred. This was a continuation of the late-nineteenth-century debate and did not change significantly until the interwar period, when an accurate understanding of the monthly cycle revealed that most physicians in the earlier period had been wrong. What was particularly intriguing about the discussion was the role that sperm was believed to play. Adam Wright of Toronto General Hospital diplomatically recognized the active role of both the father and the mother; while acknowledging the 'vibratory' motion of the sperm, he recognized that they were 'sucked up by the uterus.' Others were much more willing to give primacy to the father. William Maddock Bayliss, in his 1915 *Principles of General Physiology*, made a point of telling his readers that the female cell was basically stationary, and the male cell 'sought' it out. He acknowledged that the child grew from the fertilized female cell but insisted that the male cell 'set into activity the dormant powers of segmentation and growth of the female cell.' He concluded: 'It is easy thus to lose sight of the fact that the male cell also brings with it the capacities of the organism from which it has arisen.' J. Clifton Edgar in 1907 had posited that the 'shelf life' of the spermatozoa was seventeen days in the vagina – lying in wait, so to speak, to fertilize the ovum. Others were similarly in awe of the abilities of the spermatozoa to survive. E.C. Dudley in his 1908 text explained that the actual place of connection between sperm and ovum was in the Fallopian tube at the abdominal end; to get there, the 'persistent and virile' sperm went through an incredible ordeal of several days' journey 'traversing the long distance; they have been observed at the abdominal end of the tube as late as five weeks after the last sexual intercourse.' Most medical estimates of sperm life, however, varied from seven days to three weeks.[35] By the 1940s, the reality check was in. Unlike that of 'lower' animals, the potency of human sperm lasted only about thirty hours. The same was true for the ovum.[36] With new understanding about the limited life of the sperm and ovum, physicians deemed that the fertile period for women coincided with ovulation. So this became the period on which medical attention focused for the purposes of birth control and fertility treatment.

Nonetheless, concern about which partner played a more significant role in conception continued. A 1940 text gave what appeared to be a straightforward description of conception: 'Under favorable circumstances the penetration of the ovum by the male cell or spermatozoon may take place, which process is called *fertilization* or *conception*.' Such descriptions, and earlier ones, focused on the male being active and the female being less so. In explaining the fertilization of the egg, a 1948 text postulated that 'the unfertilized ovum in some unknown way exerts an attractive force upon the spermatozoon,' which by the 'lashing movements of its tail' reaches the egg and 'penetrates' it.[37] This description rendered the attractive force of the egg vague, whereas it vividly portrayed the 'lashing' movements of the sperm. While some physicians might lament that men did not get enough credit for their role in procreation, the gendered nature of the descriptions of conception went a long way to offset this perceived deficiency.[38] These descriptions reflected the gendered divisions of society at the time. Canadians tended to view men as more active than women, particularly in sexual matters.

But what encouraged conception? Was sexual arousal in women an aid? In the early decades of the century some denied that it was, arguing, 'Many women are always passive in coitus, and all women are entirely passive in conception.'[39] This view placed the sexual initiative in the male domain rather than the female. Most physicians, however, seemed to feel that orgasm would make conception more likely, though it was not necessary.[40] Sexual arousal on the part of women remained an issue of contention. The authors of texts in the interwar period repeated the widespread belief among women that arousal was necessary for conception. The physician authors themselves remained cagey. They denied that it was a necessary factor but often admitted that it didn't hurt and could help. In 1935 one argued that orgasm would allow the sperm to enter the cervix before it was 'injured by the acidity of the normal vaginal secretion.' Indeed, he went so far as to suggest that 'excitation without relief leads to chronic pelvic congestion' and eventually produces 'degenerative changes in the ovaries.' He was thus positing the idea that orgasm was perhaps not necessary for conception but that without it the chances could drastically decrease not only for that sexual encounter but for future ones as well.[41] The discussion of arousal being necessary for conception was part of a broader societal-legal debate in cases of rape that resulted in pregnancy. For many, the pregnancy proved that the woman had enjoyed the rape – otherwise how could she have become pregnant?

Closely linked to conception was the issue of sex determination, but physicians' interest was less in predicting the sex of the child and more in understanding how sex determination actually worked. One turn-of-the-century theory, which had a long tradition, was that older or riper ova, if fertilized, would result in males. James S. Freeborn from Magnetawan, Ontario, apparently subscribed to a version of this belief. He speculated that a determining factor was the timing of conception in the menstrual cycle – girls being conceived early in the cycle and boys later. Thus boys were conceived from older ova. Freeborn argued that knowledge of this was important: 'Nature has not always balanced the sexes in individual families and I consider it our duty to suggest the remedy – regulate the family and you regulate the nation.'[42] While old theories continued to hold sway, some physicians were attempting to persuade their colleagues to give some of them up. The 1906 text edited by Thomas Clifford Allbutt, W.S. Playfair, and ThomasWatts Eden dismissed the belief that the sex of the child was determined by which ovary produced the egg. Their text assured readers that despite the reemergence of this theory, in fact if surgery removed one ovary and tube from a woman, she was quite as likely to give birth to either a boy or a girl.[43] Few were aware of the role that the sperm played in determining sex.

Physicians in the interwar period and after had a much better understanding of the role of the sperm in sex determination. As a consequence, they discarded many of the old theories. But interest in sex determination, while less urgent, still existed. Some felt that the acidity of the vagina played a role. In a 1932 issue of the *Canadian Nurse*, William J. Stevens, the attending obstetrician at the Ottawa Civic Hospital, argued that 'sex determination is impossible to modify,' but he noted that 'some advocate [the use of] bicarbonate of soda douches [to] produce males and lactic acid douches to produce girls,' though he was sceptical of their efficacy.[44]

While contemplation of the beginning of life at conception and sex determination remained abstract, there was a more practical approach to the prenatal period that followed. Here, physicians felt they had something to offer. In the early decades of the century, they tried to educate Canadians and one another on the importance to society of childbearing women. Peter Bryce, the chief medical officer of immigration in 1914, described how a Spartan mother, 'when asked how it was that the women of Lacedemon rule the men, replied: "Because we grow men."'[45] Bryce reminded men that if it were not for women, they would not exist. Woman herself was not significant, but what she was able to accomplish was. Such women needed care. Of special concern was the woman facing her first pregnancy. W.P. Manton, writing in the 1906 *Canadian Practitioner and Review*, asked:

> What can such a woman know of the dangers which may threaten from indiscretions in diet, from inadequate bodily protection, from excessive or unwonted exercise, or from the thousand and one daily indulgences and habits which she has hitherto practiced without thought or evil consequence? And is it not eminently within the province and duty of the physician to guide her in the manner of loving, to instruct regarding personal hygiene, to alleviate as far as possible the annoyances and minor ailments to which she is liable, and to direct her in the matter of even the smallest detail preparatory to the final event – labor?[46]

Direction of the pregnant woman in 'the smallest detail' was, of course, wishful thinking. In the early decades of the century, most women did not see a physician during pregnancy, and most physicians did not have the time to supervise them to the extent being suggested. Nonetheless, Manton's advice reflects how some in the field thought physicians should handle the prenatal period.

In the interwar years, pressure placed on various levels of government to ensure that women received care attested to the increasing importance given to the prenatal period. The National Council of Women, the United Farm Women of Ontario, and the Trades and Labor Congress all thought that governments should provide more assistance. The hearings of the British Columbia Royal Commission on Health Insurance and Maternity Benefits, in 1919–21, raised the concept of providing benefits for women so that they could afford obstetric care. Other jurisdictions also expressed interest. Dr J.E. Hett of Kitchener even called for the establishment of a Ministry of Motherhood.[47] As the focus on maternal mortality in the interwar period became a major issue for the medical profession, many physicians could see how state benefits or subsidies for prenatal care could benefit women (and also themselves, by enabling more women to afford such care).[48] While most women easily survived pregnancy and birth, there was no guarantee that any individual woman would. Even an apparently healthy woman could have some condition that might complicate events. As for an unhealthy woman, the situation was problematic. But as an author in the August 1926 *Canadian Child* maintained, 'In civilized communities ... skilled and kindly doctors step in and save these weak mothers, and their babies.'[49]

Maternal mortality rates were high, but what role did prenatal care or lack of it play in this? Rural women received less care than urban women, yet their maternal mortality rates were not as high. The main killer of women in childbirth was puerperal septicaemia, which good prenatal care could not prevent, though it could prevent some complications of pregnancy. Interwar studies of maternal mortality reveal that it was non-medical factors, such as poor nutrition, poverty, and overwork, that created many of the problems that affected women. Yet the focus on medical care and intervention during pregnancy implied that medical care could overcome almost any problem. Over and over again, physicians stressed the importance of prenatal care and the need for both the public and their colleagues to understand its importance. Some argued that prenatal care had become 'one of the most efficient forms of preventive medicine.'[50] Probably wishful thinking, such a statement served the purpose of presenting prenatal care as a given. Any physician who did not practise it was out of step. It was wishful thinking also for the many women who could not afford a physician's care throughout the nine months of pregnancy. Even in the 1940s, when the economy was booming, prenatal exams had not yet become the norm. Mrs William Dietrich, who entered the Kitchener-Waterloo Hospital on 2 January 1943 and gave birth to a stillborn child as a result of a prolapse of the umbilical cord, had only had prenatal care since her seventh month.[51] Certainly, when governments gave financial help to women who could not afford prenatal care, it was not generous enough to meet the levels of care that physicians thought necessary. In 1946 the Ontario government provided to any expectant woman one free prenatal exam from the physician of her choice.[52] By the mid-1940s, however, physicians were suggesting a regular regimen of exams.

The first issue of pregnancy faced by both women and physicians was diagnosis. Some women suspected pregnancy and went to the physician to have it confirmed. Others did not bother and saw the physician only when they were well along in their pregnancy. For physicians, the diagnosis of pregnancy was important since it placed their reputation on the line; all textbooks stressed this and gave detailed descriptions of the various signs of pregnancy, coupled with warnings that its diagnosis was seldom foolproof. In the interwar period a specific test for pregnancy existed, which led to great excitement among physicians in Canada and elsewhere in the Western world. Nevertheless, in all the discussions, commentators made explicit separation between the medical signs on which doctors could depend and the subjective symptoms as related by the woman on which physicians could not depend.

In 1900 William Gardner explained to his readers in the *Montreal Medical Journal* the importance of making a diagnosis of pregnancy, the way to do so, and the difficulties involved. He pointed out that a patient would not forgive misdiagnosis. Adam Wright agreed. He noted in his 1908 text that the physician 'will get little credit for making a correct diagnosis, while, on the other hand, he will be seriously blamed for a mistaken diagnosis. It is very important in certain instances that no mistake be made, especially where the reputation of the patient is at stake.'[53]

A definitive diagnosis of pregnancy was not easy. Medical literature warned physicians not to base the diagnosis on what a woman told them. Gardner was very clear about the danger of the 'designing' woman who came to the physician denying her pregnancy in the hope that a physical intervention would result in a miscarriage. Another physician reported a cautionary tale: 'I was once caught napping and overcredulous in trusting to the statements of a supposedly respectable and innocent young unmarried woman. After a hasty and superficial examination a diagnosis of ovarian cyst was made. To my chagrin, on opening the abdomen, a five months' pregnant uterus revealed the true

nature of the tumor.' Lapthorn Smith, professor of clinical gynaecology at Bishop's University, told of women who denied the
possibility of being pregnant because 'they were widows or that
their husbands had promised not to impregnate them or because
they were wearing a little piece of sponge which of course was
lost in the vaginal vault; or they were using a syringe after
intercourse.' Others mentioned that menopausal 'neurotic' women
might exhibit all the signs of pregnancy.[54] The moral of all these
warnings was that since a physician could not distinguish a
'designing' from an 'innocent' woman, or a 'neurotic' from a
'non-neurotic' woman, he had to view all women with suspicion
in order to protect his own reputation. But women did not need
to be designing to deny or be unaware of pregnancy. Mrs Sally
Torrence was admitted on 21 May 1900 to the Victoria General
Hospital, Halifax, complaining of the stoppage of menstruation
and an abdominal tumour. She had had a previous tumour,
which under medical treatment had disappeared, but she feared
it was back again. Her patient record stated that she was examined and found to be pregnant.[55] Given Mrs Torrence's medical
history, that pregnancy did not occur to her was understandable.
For other women, the lack of sex education and the unwillingness of many to talk about their bodies meant that they did not
always know the symptoms of pregnancy.

Physicians had to take great care and base their diagnoses on
'careful investigation of history, symptoms and physical signs,
negative and positive.' Gardner instructed his students: 'If, with
empty bladder and rectum, and everything else favourable in the
position of the patient, you cannot easily define the uterine body,
so distinctly firm in the nulliparous condition, then suspect pregnancy.'[56] But the word 'suspect' reveals that diagnosis was not
straightforward. J. Bland-Sutton and Arthur E. Giles in their 1906
text went through all the signs of pregnancy from the least to
most sure: among them amenorrhoea, morning sickness, fullness
of breasts with the presence of milk, pigmentation of the mam-
mary areolae, soft tumour in the hypogastrium (the lowest middle abdominal region), movement of the foetus, softness of the
cervix, and the foetal heartbeat.[57] To help distinguish between

characteristics of pregnancy, David Berry Hart in his 1912 text separated the *signs* of pregnancy from the *symptoms*. The former referred to what a physician could see or test for, the latter what the patient experienced and related. The distinction between the two was applied to all diseases. For Hart, sign was more significant than symptom.[58] The diagnosis was between the physician and the woman's body; of less interest was the woman's experience of her body.

The theme of uncertainty regarding diagnosis did not disappear. Wilma Hallman remembered going to a physician in the interwar period to have her pregnancy confirmed, but even her physician did not realize until much later that she was pregnant with triplets. Hallman's mother, however, was convinced that she was carrying more than one child, for multiple births ran in the family.[59] J.S. Fairbairn in his 1924 text echoed the teachings of the earlier period. In the first weeks of pregnancy positive diagnosis was impossible. As the pregnancy progressed, signs and symptoms increased so that diagnosis became more certain. But only at mid-term, when foetal movements and heartbeat could be detected, was the diagnosis positive. The problem with this medical reality, according to Fairbairn, was that the public did not accept it. They seemed to feel that diagnosis of pregnancy was straightforward and should be given early on. Fairbairn warned his medical readers that the public would not forgive errors in diagnosis and would regard such errors as carelessness on the part of the physician.[60] The medical literature had plenty of tales of mistakes, such as gynaecologists opening an abdomen in order to remove a tumour and finding a foetus instead. Mrs Lillian Cowper, age thirty-two, was admitted to the Victoria General Hospital, Halifax, on 12 October 1930, complaining of pain in the lower left abdomen, dysmenorrhoea (painful menstruation), menorrhagia (excessive menstruation), frequency of micturition (urination) – all symptoms that she had had since previous surgery. The case record reported: 'Pt draped in lithotomy position [patient lying on her back with legs flexed against the thighs and thighs flexed against the abdomen] and examine p.v. [per vagina] to determine if pregnant. No evidence of pregnancy on this p.v.

exam ... Abdomen opened by incision surrounding old scar ... & uterus found large adherent by a strong band of adhesions from right upper edge of fundus ... wall ... found to be pregnant. Abdomen closed in layers without disturbing uterus.'[61]

There was need for a better way of diagnosing pregnancy and of diagnosing it earlier in the pregnancy. A 1930 editorial in the *Canadian Medical Association Journal* told of the Zondek-Aschheim reaction, whereby a hormone in the urine of pregnant women 'when injected into immature female mice, produced effects closely resembling those caused by the implantation of pituitary tissue.'[62] This test allowed for earlier diagnosis, and advocates claimed that it gave correct results in more than 98 per cent of cases. However, since the test necessitated the use of a laboratory where female mice were always at hand and trained personnel available, it was expensive.[63] Nevertheless, the excitement surrounding this test was high. Other tests followed. In 1933 an article in the *McGill Undergraduate Journal* described five different tests based on hormone reactions. Physicians felt they were entering a new period in which certainty of early diagnosis was possible, though some did worry that the test took up too much laboratory time simply to let a patient know that she was pregnant before a clinical diagnosis was possible.[64]

The existence of these tests did not do away with clinical diagnosis. Physicians still relied on their skill in distinguishing between the symptoms and signs of pregnancy. Some even questioned the kind of accuracy that the hormone tests gave. Harold Atlee, for instance, did not believe the claimed 98 per cent accuracy rate. He argued that the laboratories at his disposal were only 75 per cent accurate and at times produced false positives and negatives, a situation not good enough for him.[65] But it was getting to be good enough for most physicians and some women. One physician wrote about cases of imaginary pregnancy when most of the symptoms of pregnancy were present but the signs were not. When the physician told these patients that they were not pregnant, the women refused to believe him. But they would believe a laboratory test.[66] Belief in a laboratory test was an extraordinary expression of faith in science. The women believed these tests more than the experience of their bodies.

The physicians' view of pregnancy conditioned the care they provided to pregnant women. They tended to compare the pregnant body with the non-pregnant body, assuming the latter to be the norm. Thus, they often considered that experiences usual for pregnant women were problematic. Early in the century some physicians referred to pregnancy as a 'morbid condition' verging on the 'pathological.' Not willing to go that far, others argued that pregnancy was a healthy state 'within certain limits,' and they believed that most women actually improved in health, as if the body was preparing itself with extra energy for the 'coming ordeal.' With the help of physicians, women could maintain their physiological normalcy.[67] A 1919 *Health Bulletin* entitled 'Save the Babies,' distributed by the Alberta board of health, assured readers that 'motherhood should cause no fear or trouble. Giving birth to a baby is natural and normal.' Yet in the next sentence it told women to 'engage the best doctor, they could afford and to place themselves under his care' as soon as they knew they were pregnant.[68] At a time when most people were under a doctor's care only for the most serious ailments, such a directive underlined the fearsome possibilities of pregnancy. Writers of medical literature warned medical students and practitioners about the 'perversions of taste, smell, etc.' that occurred, the neuralgia of face and teeth, the alteration in respiration. Physicians could not ignore that pregnancy placed strains on the body, and they cautioned one another to be vigilant, especially with women they deemed too young or too old to be pregnant. Certainly, they could not depend on the women themselves, whom they usually regarded as being ignorant about most things concerning their pregnancy.[69]

Physicians also saw pregnancy as a time of added emotional stress. No doubt, some considered the changes brought about to be bordering on the neurotic. They depicted women as losing control of themselves. Pregnancy 'exaggerate[d] any previous defect or susceptible point in the patient's mental ... organization.' Time and again, descriptions of the mental or emotional state of pregnant women stressed its abnormality – the 'exalted nerve tensions,' 'nervous instability,' 'mental affections,' 'neuroses,' 'psychical disturbances,' 'irritability,' – or stated that the

woman became 'fretful,' 'peevish,' and 'unreasonable.' Furthermore, in extreme situations, the emotional upset of pregnancy
could lead to melancholy, mania, and psychosis. Pregnant women,
physicians argued, could not be reliable witnesses; the acuteness
of their perception had altered, so their interpretations tended to
be false. Women were not 'responsible' for what was happening
to them, and they should be 'humoured and shielded' so that
they did not experience stress.[70] In such a scenario, the physician
played a key role. As a 1915 editorial in the *Canadian Journal of
Medicine and Surgery* made clear, a pregnant woman needed guidance and advice: 'Her husband or parents can get no better
adviser than a thoughtful, earnest physician.'[71]

Even as late as the 1940s, although many physicians recognized that most pregnant women did not have emotional difficulties, at the same time they could warn that pregnancy placed
added strain on their 'psychic makeup,' leading to personality
changes and problems such as irritability, despondency (happy
and cheerful pregnant women were a minority), moroseness,
excitability, hysteria, and psychosis in rare cases.[72] But few went
as far as some had in the earlier period in questioning women's
competence. Nonetheless, a 1947 article in the *University of Toronto Medical Journal* raised its spectre:

> DeLee noted that in olden times pregnant women were consid-
> ered mentally irresponsible because of their increased suggestibil-
> ity. Today they are not considered reliable as witnesses for as one
> author expresses what he thinks is the case, 'their perception is
> less acute, their reasoning deficient, and their interpretation false.'
> Yet rather than a certain dullness of intellect associated with preg-
> nancy, it would seem more likely that the woman's thought and
> feeling is concentrated on the approaching birth and its conse-
> quences, and that this focus is responsible for the relatively greater
> indifference to the environment seen at this time.

While the article did not agree with DeLee on the reasons for
women not being reliable witnesses, it gave credence to his
conclusion – that pregnant women were less dependable, less

competent than other adults – albeit in a way that was sympathetic to women.[73] Some women themselves shared the view that women were 'not normal' during pregnancy.[74]

Because of their great concern about maternal mortality during the interwar years, physicians could not help but see pregnancy and childbirth as inherently problematic. W.W. Chipman, a Montreal physician, quoted the sentiment expressed in an earlier period that 'the most common tumour in the lower abdomen, in the adult woman, is a pregnant uterus.' For James Robert Goodall, clinical professor of obstetrics and gynaecology at McGill, 'Every pregnant woman is a toxic woman and ... she possesses great potentiality for developing pathological states.' As late as 1946, when Mrs George Cunningham went to Montreal General Hospital, her case record described her as suffering from amenorrhoea – that is, she was pregnant.[75] Physicians were torn between telling one another that pregnancy was normal and preparing themselves for the difficulties that ensued with some pregnancies. They viewed women as high or low risk, but almost never did they see a woman as no risk. Was there not danger in this attitude? Herbert M. Little, assistant professor of obstetrics at McGill University in 1924, thought so. Women received the message that pregnancy was a sickness and acted accordingly.[76]

As well as encouraging women to see them on a regular basis during the prenatal period, physicians advised one another about the kind of care they should provide. Of particular concern in the early years was estimating the size of the pelvis. If the pelvis was too small, the child would have trouble being born, and both the physician and the mother needed to be prepared. Doctors were to examine the breasts and nipples, to inquire about vaginal discharge, and to check the woman's blood pressure. An article in 1909 pointed out that no physician would deny the importance of at least one pelvic examination during pregnancy but that 'many practitioners shrink from recommending it on account of the suspicion and reluctance with which the suggestion is still only too often regarded.'[77] Recognizing this problem, Henry Jellett, the author of *Manual of Midwifery* (1910), suggested the use of abdominal palpation, which in his opinion compared well with a vaginal examination, which could expose the patient to danger, discomfort, and at times pain.[78]

Some physicians and teachers were much more ambitious regarding good prenatal care, advising monthly urine testing for the first six months of pregnancy, twice or more in the seventh month, and weekly in the eighth and ninth months. Most wanted women to see them as early as possible in their pregnancy. Not only did they think that specific medical care was necessary, such as urinalysis and pelvic measurement, but they also thought they needed to give women advice on a wide range of issues. Noteworthy is the all-encompassing nature of their advice, ranging from diet, clothing, exercise, and bathing to care of breasts.[79] Pregnancy was such a drastic change in a woman's being that all the normal rules and habits of living might not apply and could be dangerous. Physicians believed they needed to warn and advise women; they could offset problems before they occurred but could only do so if the patient let them.[80] All this advice created a benchmark for ideal care, which was next to impossible to achieve: either the woman would not cooperate or the busy family physician could not devote the time needed.

Increasingly, more women had opportunity for prenatal care. Metropolitan Life set up a visiting-nurse program in Montreal and Halifax as early as 1910 and later expanded it to other Canadian cities. The nurses visited policy holders, and much of their work involved prenatal care. At the peak of the program, a woman could receive up to eleven prenatal visits.[81] The Victorian Order of Nurses (VON) did yeoman service providing prenatal care. Some hospitals set up prenatal clinics for the community. While W.B. Hendry, a Toronto physician, noted that the care provided by the Burnside Lying-In Hospital's clinic could 'just as easily be carried out in private practice,' he was afraid that 'the busy practitioner ... lulled to a sense of false security by long series of successful deliveries, relaxes his vigilance.' Between 1910 and 1920 the maternal mortality rate of women who had attended the Burnside clinics on a regular basis was less than one-quarter of that for women who were semi-private patients in the hospital. For Hendry, the difference was an indictment of private practice prenatal care.[82]

Despite the encouragement of women to see a physician, one lecturer in obstetrics at McGill University estimated in 1911 that 80 per cent of women approached their first labour without having had a preliminary examination.[83] For many women, either their living conditions or their financial situation made it difficult. Some viewed the whole process as natural, not necessitating professional help. Also, there was a plethora of popular advice literature for women if they needed reassurance. Physicians, of course, did not consider such literature a substitute for a doctor's care. More acceptable were government publications, largely because they advised the pregnant woman to place herself under the care of a physician or, if that was impossible, to go to a hospital clinic or dispensary.

The surveillance of women throughout their pregnancies increased over time. The emphasis during the interwar period on reducing the maternal mortality rate meant that physicians and others intensified their encouragement of women to seek prenatal care. Nonetheless, many women still did not consult physicians to the degree that physicians wished. The sugested number of visits kept increasing and was beyond the ability of most women. To physicians, it was obvious that the need was there. Physicians could not wait for women to tell them if they were experiencing difficulties; instead, they had to be 'on the *qui vive* for all those abnormal deviations which may and do occur so often during pregnancy and the puerperium.'[84] But this required frequent visits. One physician suggested in 1924 that a visit every month until the fifth month was suitable; after that, the woman should see her physician every three weeks to the seventh month and then every two weeks until labour began. Others felt that weekly visits were necessary during the last six weeks. In either case, it was more frequent than that recommended in England. During the visits the importance of taking urine samples and blood pressure was stressed, though how often varied from physician to physician. Some physicians warned their colleagues that prenatal care included not only urinalysis and taking blood pressure but measurement of the pelvis, cervical smears, blood count, temperature, weight, position and rate of foetal heart, the removal of infected teeth and tonsils, and so on.[85]

The lure of measurement was strong. Many physicians saw it as something certain in which they could have confidence. The need or desire for certainty stemmed from the minority of problematic childbirth cases. To lessen these, all women needed to undergo monitoring. If not taming the natural, monitoring would at least keep track of it. The normalization or standardization of care that resulted from monitoring was important. For many women it ensured a safer delivery; for all women it constrained choice; and for the individual physician, it meant that responsibility was shared with the wider fraternity of physicians.

Prenatal care emphasized the 'patient' role of women, who were now encouraged to go to doctors even when they were not ill. Pregnancy became medicalized. This did not just affect the relationship between a pregnant woman and her physician, it created that relationship. The advice givers assumed that women would implement their advice; but at the same time, the insistence on frequent doctor's visits suggested that women needed to be monitored to ensure that they did so. With the number of tests and examinations deemed necessary, there was the danger that the physician might focus on them and ignore the emotional needs of the patient. One physician warned his colleagues: 'The attitude of the physician during history-taking and especially during the making of the physical examination should be one of tact and such as to inspire confidence in his care, ability, and integrity.'[86] Going to see a physician during pregnancy was the first time some women had visited a physician. For Dorothy Atkinson it was the first time she underwent an internal examination. She recalled that her physician did not explain to her what it involved and she did not question him: 'In those days I thought that doctors were gods more or less and you just lay back and let them do it.'[87] Women under the prenatal care of a physician had probably never gone to one so frequently. This could not help but deliver the message that they were somehow fragile, in need of care, and sick. The ideal patient did as she was told. Physicians advised one another and their patients that the pregnant woman was to assume very little without checking with her doctor. He was to direct the kind of housework she did, her way of living, and her leisure-time activities, as well as her diet, sexual activity, and the amount of sleep she was to get. Physicians exhorted women to cooperate with their physicians.[88] The fear, of course, was that women would not. English doctors shared this fear. In the early 1930s, two reports on maternal mortality and morbidity in England suggested that 17 per cent of avoidable deaths in pregnancy and childbirth were the result of patient negligence.[89]

Prenatal clinics, classes, and services expanded considerably during the interwar years. The Metropolitan Life scheme that had begun before the war continued. In 1932 there were prenatal visits to 2,200 expectant women in Montreal alone.[90] The VON estimated that in 1929 its nurses made 42,196 visits nationwide. To ensure that physicians were on side with this program, VON nurses urged women to seek out physician care.[91] Hospitals continued to provide prenatal clinics designed for working class women. But clinics had mixed success. At the Dalhousie Obstetrical Clinic, women averaged 2.5 visits.[92] Prenatal classes were being introduced in some areas by the 1940s. Unlike the clinics, they attracted predominantly middle-class women, who were demanding information and wanted to participate more in the birth of their children.[93] The value of prenatal care had become a truism, providing physicians and prospective mothers with the certainty that they were doing all they could and the best they could.

As services expanded, they exposed the needs of women who had been ignored for years. The 1922 report of the VON described how some of its prenatal work began. In Winnipeg that year, a Ukrainian woman had come seeking help, so the VON had started a prenatal class in the Ukrainian district 'with a view of interesting the mothers in medical and nursing care.' The report went on in a tone dismissive of Ukrainian culture and its non-scientific ways: 'Most of these mothers are the victims of midwifery instruction and have gone no farther and are now paying the debt of ignorance.' The VON nurses separated themselves from the Ukrainian women on the basis of ethnicity and class, feeling that part of their job was to imbue them with

'Canadian ideals' as represented by scientific medical care. At the same time, they had some semblance of gender solidarity in seeing the women 'down trodden by their men' even if they connected this not to gender but to the foreignness of the culture.[94]

The theme of these years was consistent: pregnant women should see a physician. Physicians tended to make what Janice Raymond refers to as eschatological statements – ones that suggested dire consequences if women did not follow their advice and a rosy future if they did.[95] Dr Helen MacMurchy told women, 'There is always something the Doctor can do to make you better. That is what a Doctor is for.' Prenatal care could prevent maternal mortality.[96] Assuming that care was available, women were to take advantage of it and to follow the physician's advice. But not all physicians could or would provide the care their colleagues advocated. In 1927 Elizabeth Smellie, chief superintendent of the VON, condemned some for neither providing a urinalysis nor encouraging patients to return on a regular basis. W.B. Hendry noted in 1934: 'There are still a few doctors in this country who do not recognize the necessity of pre-natal care; these men should not be practicing obstetrics. There are others who practice it only in a casual way.'[97] But not all were able to give the ideal care, because they lacked facilities and time.

The federal, most provincial, and many local governments issued advice literature to pregnant women. All stressed the importance of medical care. Organizations such as the Canadian Red Cross, the VON, and private companies such as Metropolitan Life distributed pamphlets on both prenatal and postnatal care.[98] Popular literature for pregnant women was also available. Some read Dr Spock. Betty McKenzie read *Childbirth without Fear* by Grantly Dick Read.[99] The latter earned the ire of some Canadian practitioners. One complained in 1946 about Read's insistence on 'detailed explanation of the physiology of birth and the leisurely development of a confidential relationship between patient and physician.' Many physicians simply did not have time to develop such relationships. Others, influenced by Read's attitude, adopted the idea that the monthly visits with women should be a sharing of information, though they advised women to write down the answers to their questions 'to prevent [them] asking the same questions too many times.'[100] After all, the physician's time should not be wasted. Even when popular books did not challenge conventional wisdom, some doctors worried that they could lead to misinterpretation and needless worry on the part of women.[101] Advice literature gave women more options from which to choose, and almost all encouraged dependence on 'experts.'

Despite the concern about prenatal care, many women were still unable or refused to take advantage of it. In St John's, Newfoundland, the first prenatal clinic opened in 1927 but closed quickly because of lack of attendance. Even in 1957 most women in the city did not visit a physician until they were midway through their pregnancy.[102] Outside Newfoundland, the situation was a bit brighter from the physician's perspective. Toronto physician J.N.E. Brown reported in 1932 that progress was being made but that much still needed to be done. Of the women under the supervision of VON nurses during the mid-thirties, 26 per cent had contacted their physician before their fourth month and another 26 per cent did so before the end of their sixth month. Another 16 per cent contacted their doctor by the end of the ninth month, and 6 per cent contacted him after they went into labour. (For 17 per cent, time of contact was unknown.) This meant at least 22 per cent left consultation until relatively late in their pregnancy. In rural areas the situation was not as promising. Some rural physicians commented that patients often did not come at all until they were in some crisis or were about to go into labour. In Manitoba in 1939–40, hospitalization records revealed that of 10,600 patients only 2,636 received 'adequate prenatal care,' which consisted of five or more physician visits; 48 per cent had partial care (one to four visits), and 29 per cent had no care at all. Anglo-Saxon women had twice the rate of adequate care as non-Anglo-Saxon women. Since non-Anglos were 55 per cent of the patients, the differential was problematic. Physicians also worried that unmarried women, because of shame and social ostracism, did not seek prenatal care.[103] Clearly, many patients failed to live up to the expectations of the ideal prenatal regimen.

Nonetheless, more women were taking advantage of the services offered, especially with the economic upswing after the Second World War. Between 1947 and 1953 the percentage of women in Ontario receiving prenatal examinations rose from 39.4 to 66.5 per cent.[104] By 1949 Dr Ernest Couture, chief of the federal Division of Maternal and Child Welfare, depicted a utopia of prenatal care that he felt existed:

> Today, all Canadian mothers without exception, can obtain the benefit of proper guidance during and after pregnancy, if they are willing to seek it. If at all possible, they should remain throughout these months under the constant supervision of a medical man. To the honour of the medical profession it must be said that most doctors are willing to render such services even though their only reward be the satisfaction of accomplishing something for the well-being of mothers. Where a doctor's services are not available because of distance, the mother should have the advice and help which a nurse can give, and usually a nurse's services are within the reach of every mother.[105]

The ideal was care from conception to at least six weeks after delivery.[106]

Physicians criticized women who refused to utilize medical services. It was a rejection of science and thus illogical and irresponsible. William Victor Johnston recalled that in his country practice in the 1920s, one of the most fearful aspects of childbirth was pre-eclamptic convulsions, which were largely preventable through monthly urine testing for albumin (a protein which if detected in urine indicates malfunction of the kidneys). Yet 'despite efforts to popularize the idea of monthly check-ups, it took years to educate women to the importance of this program.' Some felt that women were so reticent about being pregnant that they delayed going to see a physician. Some women simply did not want or apparently did not feel they needed the assistance of nurses or physicians.[107] A report on the Gaspé area said that nurses were 'stunned' to find that their help was not wanted because they represented 'new-fangled ideas,' which the local women found foreign.[108] But how fair was it to blame women? Geraldine Mitchell remembered seeing a physician on a regular basis for her first pregnancy but not for her second, simply because with a young child to care for she didn't have the time. In one northern Ontario community women had difficulty getting prenatal care because the men were reluctant to spend money on prenatal programs or have women see physicians on their own.[109] The medical and social ideology of the time was based on individualism, which as Cynthia Comacchio has argued, weakened society's ability to appreciate underlying structural problems such as, in this case, the isolation of women within the family.[110]

If prenatal care was increasing over the years, prenatal advice was doing so even more. Unlike more traditional cultures, Western society tended to be wary of physical activity during pregnancy. Pregnant women were to avoid violent exercise in particular. Thus in the early years of the century, railway travel, carriage driving, motoring, cycling, and horseback riding were suspect, as were long journeys. Dancing was problematic, though one commentator felt that family square dancing was acceptable. Joseph B. DeLee advised against golf, sea bathing, and tennis.[111] A 1901 text prohibited 'lifting, and all violent muscular strain and overwork.' In addition, 'crowded and ill-ventilated rooms should be shunned.'[112] Of course, the physicians proffering such advice made few suggestions about how a woman was to follow it and still run a household. Instead, they emphasized that during pregnancy women needed to be 'treated with an extra degree of consideration and indulgence' in order to reduce the pressure of work on them.[113] Physicians directed their advice at the middle-class women who were their patients. On occasion, however, they recognized working-class realities. Jennie Gray, a Toronto physician, noted that pregnant women who had to wash and scrub for a living were at risk. A 1910 text advised women to avoid certain pollutants and contaminants, such as carbonic acid gas, carbon monoxide gas, and work that brought them into contact with lead, mercury, and phosphorous. Unfortunately, most women working with such poisons could not afford to leave their jobs.[114] Even when pregnant, many women continued to put in long and physically hard-working days, whether at home, in factories, or in primary industries. The reality of these women's lives gave the lie to the practicality of physicians' advice, though not the validity of it.

Not all activity was prohibited. Women needed exercise, and physicians recommended daily walking, simple gymnastics, and sea bathing in certain circumstances. The class bias of much of the medical advice emerged again in the physicians' encouragement of women to continue their normal lives, including theatre going and concerts.[115] A 1915 editorial in the *Canadian Journal of Medicine and Surgery*, contrary to DeLee's advice, suggested that golf was good. Recognizing that most women did not play golf, the editorial assured them that the exercise they received doing their housework was perhaps even better, and that the 'only limitation on these duties [was] that of no reaching up, or climbing ungainly distances.' Women were not to work as hard as they usually did and they were to ensure that they received at least nine hours' sleep at night, in addition to a rest in the afternoon.[116] If a woman did overdo things, her child would pay the price.

Physicians deemed bathing helpful to women. They believed it relieved strain on the kidneys and kept the vaginal canal clean. However, the water had to be warm, not hot, and the bathtub not too full. Hot baths, they warned, could disturb the pelvic blood vessels and result in miscarriage, and some feared that a full tub-bath in the latter part of pregnancy could cause infection.[117] Of course, the problem for many women was that they did not have access to water, so could not bathe on a regular basis; in that case, a sponge bath would do. But as one nurse noted in a rather superior way, 'It is always very gratifying to give a thoroughly good scrubbing to such a patient who comes to the hospital to be delivered.'[118] Part of the hygienic regimen was keeping the bowels free. Physicians generally believed that women were more constipated than men, partly because of the problem of relieving themselves when facilities were awkward to use. Pregnancy compounded the problem. One turn-of-the-century text even suggested taking a laxative 'each night or every other night on retiring.' Concerns about regularity and bathing persisted well into the interwar period.[119]

The concern about other activities of pregnant women also persisted. As with conventional wisdom, medical wisdom advised women not to lift or reach up for fear of wrapping the umbilical cord around the baby's neck.[120] In the home, women might be able to work around such prohibitions, but without help it would be difficult. H.J.G. Geggie recognized this. Responding to the death of a mother and the miscarriage of another, he focused on the lack of household help that both women had experienced and considered such help necessary for a 'complete [prenatal] program.'[121] Paid work, outside the home, would require a different response. In 1931 John W.S. McCullough of the Ontario Department of Public Health argued for maternity benefits to allow women to have at least two to three months free of excessive work. A writer in 1936 stated insisted that clerical work was fine but that industrial work should be given up for the last month. Dr Marion Hilliard did not have problems with women working up to about the seventh month of their pregnancy as long as they managed to get some extra rest. Ideally, she said, they should not work during the first three months, though they could return to work for the next three; but she realized that this was not feasible given the structure of the working world.[122]

Physicians continued to place limits on pregnant women. One Toronto physician worried that too many younger women acted as if nothing was happening – 'attending parties, keeping late hours, riding too much in autos, playing bridge excessively and otherwise keeping up a life of excitement and strain.'[123] Some repeated the prohibitions of the earlier period. Dr T.R. Nichols from Stratford, Ontario, in his *Instructions for Expectant Mothers and the Care of Infants* (1932), warned:

> In the latter months the amount of exercise taken should be gradually diminished. Avoid much climbing of stairs, the use of the sewing machine and heavy housework. Violent exercise such as horseback riding, playing tennis, motoring, swimming, etc., may

induce miscarriage and should be avoided. DON'T FORGET THAT
RIDING OVER ROUGH ROADS IN AN AUTOMOBILE MAY ALSO BRING ON
MISCARRIAGE. DRIVE VERY CAREFULLY AND SLOWLY.[124]

While such warnings focused on the latter stage of pregnancy,
they had the tendency of suggesting that they should be followed throughout the full pregnancy, especially when coupled
with directions to avoid exertion around the time of normal
menstruation. In 1949 Dr Ernest Couture, author of *The Canadian
Mother and Child*, the federal government's major advice pam-
phlet, made it clear that he did not approve of pregnant women
attending hockey and football games because of the excitement
of the games and the exposure to cold. He acknowledged that the
increased comfort of automobiles and the better condition of
roads meant that many physicians were not as concerned about
travelling as they had been, but he said that long trips were still
problematic.[125]

Other physicians were not so limiting. Indeed, in the years
following the First World War, physicians seemed more willing
to have women be active. They still had concerns about the early
and late months of the pregnancy and deemed long journeys a
problem, but they encouraged golf, dancing, swimming, walking, and travelling, in moderation.[126] Experience often played a
role in what a physician did or did not endorse. Harold Atlee
discouraged long automobile drives because two of his patients
who had had healthy pregnancies had miscarried after long trips.
While he realized that most women (and their unborn children)
could survive 'violent forms of exertion' during pregnancy, he
did not see the point of taking the risk. Thus, he standardized the
advice, applying it to all women. But he said that apart from
avoiding long car rides, violent exercise, and swimming, pregnant women should change their routine as little as possible.[127]
Others agreed, arguing that as long as a woman increased her
rest and sleep, very little was beyond her. One physician used the
example of a rather extraordinary woman to prove his point. She
was a patient of his who had come to him in the early months of

pregnancy: 'At the same time, [she was] carrying on with her profession of a circus bare back rider. With the pursuit of scientific data, and the accompaniment of a small boy, as excuses, I went to see the circus and watched this lady do back-flips, front-somersaults and cartwheels on and off the horse and over the circus ring without apparent trouble, and this had been a bi-daily procedure for several months.'[128] While clearly exceptional, the woman demonstrated to her physician what was possible.

One activity about which many physicians had concern during the early decades of the century was the frequency and timing of sexual intercourse during pregnancy. While most did not see the possibility of prohibiting it, they did feel that sexual excess could lead to miscarriage, as could sexual intercourse in the early and late months of the pregnancy and at what would have been the usual menstrual period.[129] There was an uncomfortableness with the idea of sexuality during pregnancy. One text pointed out that 'even uncivilized nations have condemned the privilege of sexual intercourse' during pregnancy; another said that 'if the analogy of the lower animals and of many savage races is to be followed, coitus should be entirely forbidden.' Still others felt or perhaps hoped that 'the usual marital relations [were] distasteful to most women at this time.'[130] Class at times entered the discussion. Joseph B. DeLee referred to those among the 'lowest classes' who engaged in sexual intercourse even in the final weeks of pregnancy. He also condemned 'certain midwives' who believed that intercourse would encourage labour pains.[131]

Physicians in the interwar period seemed less concerned about sexual intercourse in itself, but they continued to worry about its dangers early and late in pregnancy – miscarriage and infection, respectively – and when the usual monthly periods would have occurred.[132] But the moral overtones of the previous decades had lessened considerably. Harold Atlee in his inimitable way caught the shift in attitude: 'We have now given up the preposterous belief that two healthy and loving young people will sleep for weeks in the same bed without moving towards the middle. There seems no clear evidence that this does any harm, but a considerable amount that its deprivation does no good, since not all sex-starved husbands are content to lower their libido by merely taking cold baths.'[133]

Of less interest to physicians was the clothing pregnant women wore. Indeed, they expressed more concern about the clothing of non-pregnant women, perhaps feeling that the realities of pregnancy led women to dress in a pragmatic way. The major issue was to ensure that clothing was not tight.[134] Some advocated the use of abdominal support. One physician in New Aberdeen, Nova Scotia, supported the use of the binder in his practice between 1904 and 1924, believing that it strengthened the muscles and helped shorten labour in women with 'pendulous abdomens.' Certainly, many women seemed to find the binder a comfort. One woman in the interwar period remembered wearing a support that hung from the shoulders and supported the belly with straps around the buttocks, which she claimed prevented stretch marks and back pain.[135]

Physicians deemed the diet of pregnant women more important. In the early decades, some believed that diet could control the size of the child. One diet advocated 'allowing the woman during the last three months of her pregnancy, wasted and boiled meats, without sauces, fish, green vegetables, salads, cheese, butter if desired, and a very small quantity of bread. Water, soups, potatoes, the farinaceous foods and beer, are proscribed, and sugar is to be replaced by saccharin.'[136] Most medical men were not this specific in their advice, but generally they encouraged the consumption of fruit and vegetables and a limited amount of meat. In addition, they advised drinking water and discouraged alcohol consumption and excessive drinking of tea and coffee.[137] Seldom did they discuss the reasons for recommending certain food over others.

Proper nutrition could offset some of the problems of pregnancy. In the interwar period and after, doctors seemed focused on weight gain. An editorial in the *Canada Lancet and National Hygiene* of 1924 blamed too nutritious a diet for the birth of large children who in delivery caused their mothers significant pain.[138] As a result, some physicians tried to monitor their patients' weight.

Dorothy Atkinson remembered her physician placing her on a special diet to ensure that she did not put on too much weight. Irma Avery recalled that her doctor had been 'disgusted' about her weight gain, though he did not advise her how to stop it – that was up to her.[139] While other physicians denied that diet determined the size of the child, they still thought that devising a normal weight gain model would be beneficial, even though they were not able to make definite predictions about what weight gains were or were not problematic.[140]

Food nutrition increasingly became part of medical care. The Depression, in particular, raised awareness of pregnant women not meeting the dietary standards being set.[141] In 1940 P.J. Darns of the Royal Victoria Hospital's Montreal Maternity Hospital reported a case of a woman, twenty-eight years of age, who had had two pregnancies and, in the thirty-fifth week of her third, developed ulcers of the vulva. When doctors discovered that her economic circumstances were poor and that she was unable to buy proper food, they prescribed large doses of vitamins A and B; the ulcers healed. After Joan Carr experienced a miscarriage, her physician during a subsequent pregnancy placed her on vitamin E. Advertisements in medical journals often referred to the increased nutritional needs of women during pregnancy.[142] The Canadian Dietary Standard recommended 2,000 calories a day for a woman doing no manual labour, 2,400 for a woman doing housework or something similar, 2,400 for a pregnant woman doing no manual work, and 2,800 for a pregnant woman doing housework. The only woman who needed more was a nursing mother, who required 3,000 calories a day.[143] Proper nutrition could lower the complications of pregnancy and childbirth, lower miscarriage rates, and improve the chances that the new mother would be able to nurse her child.[144] Unfortunately, the nutrition deemed necessary was not accessible to all. Many women in poor circumstances put the nutritional needs of their husband and children above their own. A Mennonite woman remembered that during the 1930s her mother always gave the children 'first access to milk, with no consideration given to the unborn child she was carrying.'[145] Despite the recognition that nutrition was significant, few programs existed in Canada to ensure that poor women received the dietary supplements they needed.[146] And unlike Britain during the Second World War, Canada did not implement a milk and vitamin supplement program for pregnant women, in spite of rationing.[147]

Plain and easily digestible food was best. Milk and cocoa were fine, as was weak tea and water. Indeed, physicians felt the latter was necessary. For many, alcohol remained anathema.[148] Often physicians assumed that women should know why a certain food was being prohibited and therefore offered no explanation for the prohibition. Either that, or they thought that women should simply accept their advice without questioning. In his 1932 advice manual, T.R. Nichols suggested that women avoid fresh bread. He added: 'Animal foods, such as eggs, fish, beef, chicken, and lamb may be taken only once each day. Avoid such meats as pork and veal.' Bland foods were best especially in the latter stages of pregnancy: 'Soups, eggs, cooked cereals with milk, all *stale* breads, an abundance of vegetables, both *raw* and cooked.'[149] Yet times did change and with them advice. In his 1942 manual, Dr Percy Ryberg suggested that while smoking and drinking were not good for the unborn child, if the woman found it too difficult to cut them out totally, she should at least reduce them. Jane Rutherford remembered that there was no prohibition on smoking or drinking during her pregnancy; she felt that women simply knew enough to cut back. After moving from Toronto to western Canada, Betsy Lawrence recalled smoking and having the occasional drink throughout her pregnancy, and no one said anything to her about it, not even her physician.[150] Not all physicians were so accommodating. One Halifax physician reported that pregnant women should not smoke at all because studies revealed that it could affect the child's heart.[151]

The discussions of diet during pregnancy became more scientific over time, couched in terms that suggested the rigour of investigation and technical understanding. The advice turned away from prohibiting specific food and instead focused on what ingredient in certain food was necessary or harmful. By the mid-1940s, physicians felt they had a better understanding of nutrition. As one observer said, 'The pre-natal diet is close to rating as an exact science.'[152] But it was a culturally informed science. In the November 1945 issue of the *Canadian Medical Association Journal* a Vancouver physician and other health professionals discussed the changing view of nutrition:

> The training of students only a few years ago was that, at the appearance of increased blood pressure, oedema, or proteinuria, meat, fish, eggs and other protein producing foods were eliminated. Today, as a profession, we are more cognizant of the vital role of protein in the diet, and especially in the diet of our pregnancy cases ... We occidents derive our protein for ourselves and our unborn progeny from the protein of animals rather than from that of the cereal grains. We are a taller and better proportioned people than our oriental neighbours, perhaps chiefly because of the animal protein in our diet.[153]

Not only was the importance of protein stressed but its source was aligned with a sense of occidental racial superiority.

The advice physicians gave to pregnant women clearly went beyond the measurable. Their desire to oversee pregnancy was strongly reflected in their response to maternal impressions. At best they were ambivalent; at worse, hostile. This had not always been the case. At the turn of the century, there was no great gap between what the laity and physicians believed. A 1901 medical text told its student readers: 'It is an interesting question to what extent the unborn child is affected by the mental condition of the mother. There is no doubt that her mental state may be the cause of modifications in the physical, the intellectual, and the moral characteristics of her offspring. The mental hygiene of the mother is, therefore, important.'[154] And although J. Clinton Edgar in his 1907 text was not prepared to engage in a discussion about maternal impressions, he admitted their possibility and stated that it would do no harm to treat women as if such influences existed. Jennie Gray was particularly concerned about the moral marking of a child; a child whose parents were not sexually continent during the pregnancy would be more prone to commit self-abuse. In this case, Gray acknowledged the influence of both parents, but in other statements she made it clear that the mother was the chief architect of her child – physically, mentally, and spiritually.[155] Society and the individuals who lived in it were all interconnected, and given that mother and child were especially so, the one obviously influenced the other.

For many physicians as well as other Canadians, belief in the influence of the mother on her unborn child was part of the broader belief in heredity and the overwhelming conviction that 'like begets like' – the underlying premise of concern about the feeble-minded, the insane, the morally depraved, the criminal, and the physically weak. If only society could control who pro-created, social problems would be reduced. These beliefs had their culmination in the eugenics movement of the interwar period, when heredity gave the science of eugenics credibility and helped explain the transference of physical and moral de-fects from one generation to another.[156] These beliefs did not always focus on the mother, but her close relationship with the foetus made her influence particularly suspect. The age-old be-lief in maternal impressions, in part, made eugenic beliefs plausi-ble and acceptable.

While some physicians in the early decades of the century certainly seemed to share their patients' belief in maternal im-pressions, others referred to them as superstitions. They urged one another to 'dispel the woman's anxiety' and assure her that there was 'just ground and stronger ground for the belief that such impressions do not affect the foetus.'[157] Assurances, how-ever, were not enough, and some tried to give an explanation for what caused physical markings on a child. Winfield Scott Hall in his 1913 manual, *Sexual Knowledge*, argued that they were the result of some disruption in the nourishment of the foetus, caused by 'fright or accident, or fits of temper.' Ironically, while he saw his explanation as disproving the power of maternal impres-sions, he actually explained how they worked. Nor was Hall consistent in his apparent rejection of them. In the same book he argued that at the time of conception the mother should have a mental attitude 'of joy and willingness, so as to impress the child with nobleness of character.'[158] While her attitude may not have physically marked the child, morally it did.

The renowned American obstetrician Joseph B. DeLee exhibited similar inconsistency. In his 1913 text he raised the possibility of emotions being not only nervous in action but also chemical. If the latter, toxins produced could pass from the mother through the placenta to the child. Despite such conjectures, he belittled the woman who believed that by reading good literature and listening to good music she could positively affect her child through her emotions.[159] He rejected the idea of maternal impressions as superstitions when held by untrained and non-scientific individuals, yet he seemed willing to accept them when presented by researchers in a scientific manner. Physicians such as DeLee separated themselves from their patients and stressed physicians' modernity and scientific outlook. Any seeming connection between the thoughts of the mother and the deformity of a child was simply coincidence. Yet what DeLee and other physicians were doing was wrapping maternal impressions in scientific language. They offered more specific and complex paths for investigation but made the same causal link between mother and child. The medicalization of the link, however, kept the pregnant woman at a distance. While her biochemistry might explain the impact of maternal impressions, only physicians could understand it.

One reason why some physicians were reluctant to entertain the notion of maternal impressions stemmed from their perception of the relationship between the foetus and its mother. Physicians in the early years of the century saw the foetus as differentiated from the mother by the end of the second month of gestation. They believed that at that point the woman usually was not even aware of her pregnancy and 'frights and emotions would therefore, play a very unimportant role.'[160] The logic here is interesting. It suggests that because the woman does not know she is pregnant, her emotions cannot affect her child. The argument seems to be that for maternal impressions to work, the woman has to be aware of the possible relationship between these impressions and the child she carries. Without the awareness of the latter, the former are irrelevant. And they can never be relevant, since when the woman is aware of the connection, the foetus has already become separate from her.

In the interwar period, medical personnel were even more dismissive of maternal impressions. A 1928 *Chatelaine* article referred to the persistence of the 'old wives tales.' The author, a nurse, argued that they were part of a bygone, prescientific era and that 'scientific research' had disproved them. A 1925 editorial in the *Canada Lancet and Practitioner* claimed, '"Maternal impressions" is a bogey.'[161] Nonetheless, they could not so easily be rejected. William J. Stevens, attending obstetrician at Ottawa Civic Hospital, made clear that such impressions were not possible since 'there is no nervous or circulatory connection between mother and child' and without either one there is no communication between the two. It is unclear what he believed the function of the placenta was, and his confusion became more explicit when he admitted that 'profound mental emotion occasionally causes abortion or premature labour.'[162] Physicians seemed to be searching for explanations that would not incorporate something as vague as maternal impressions. Almost anything would do, even the season of birth, except power residing with the pregnant woman.[163] Scientific explanation became the neutral, objective force that took influence and power from the mother. As Toronto physician W.A. Dafoe noted, the child was already fixed in its physical and mental abilities by the sex cells of the parents long before it took the form of a child. Thus, he appealed to what physicians were learning about chromosomes. He viewed the child as a 'parasite living off its parent' and was not willing to concede that there was a relationship between the parasite and its host (the mother).[164] He was describing a situation in which he posited a disconnection between the mother and child. Whatever relationship existed between the two was a scientifically mediated one.

The attempts to find cause and explanation beyond maternal impressions were in essence a reconfiguring of impressions. In 1948 an article in the *Canadian Journal of Public Health* maintained:

It is true there is still much to be learned about the effect of the emotional state of the pregnant woman upon the child. However, enough is now known to prove that both physical and mental characteristics of the child depend to some degree upon experiences in the prenatal period. It is also known that such symptoms as nausea and vomiting, bleeding, and even spontaneous abortion may be caused by the emotional state of the woman. Even more definite is the knowledge that the emotional state of the pregnant women influences her attitudes to the child. Many a child was rejected before his birth and continued to be because the mother could not accept her pregnancy.[165]

Physicians wanted to assure women that they could not physically mark their children. At the same time, they insisted that women act in a way that would ensure the birth of a healthy child; in doing so, many came very close to endorsing a form of maternal impressions. What all could agree on was that a healthy mother made for a healthy baby. The push for comprehensive prenatal care that occurred in the interwar period and afterwards was testimony to that. Physicians had found what satisfied their need for explanation. Their focus on the physiological nature of the connection between mother and foetus (even if sparked by emotion) placed causation and solution in the medical arena.

Even with the best of care, pregnancy was not free of complications. The rest of this chapter will examine three of these – miscarriage, vomiting of pregnancy, and eclampsia – as examples of the way in which physicians approached their patients and medical issues. Miscarriage was frequent. In 1915 physicians estimated that 16 per cent of all pregnancies resulted in miscarriage, or that they occurred at a rate of one to five live births. A 1940 text calculated that about one-third of all pregnancies resulted in a miscarriage. Others felt the rate was closer to 10 per cent.[166] Over time, physicians were able to offset some of the conditions that led to miscarriage, but it remained a potential threat to all women. It was an experience that most never forgot. Florence Edenshaw Davidson, a Haida woman, remembered that in the early years of the century she had a miscarriage after four months of pregnancy. For her, the fact that the baby was not fully developed did not matter. 'I cried real hard,' she said, 'just like I lost a big baby.'[167]

The causes of miscarriage were many. Some physicians focused on sex during pregnancy as problematic, especially at the beginning or during the time of the usual menstrual cycle. Others blamed too strenuous activity. In the interwar period, doctors gave more emphasis to diet.[168] But whether the cause was thought to be sexual congress, physical exertion, or diet, doctors seemed to be telling women that many miscarriages were the result of women not taking sufficient precautions. Whatever the cause, classifying them provided physicians with a sense of certainty, of knowing more than they perhaps did. Early in the century, J.J. Ross, a demonstrator in anatomy at McGill, described a classificatory system that linked causes specifically to the father, mother, or foetus. The causes could be predisposing or exciting. 'Exciting causes [linked to the mother] act quietly, or more directly on the uterus or ovum, e.g., blows, falls, contusions, lifting, sea bathing, stretching of arms and running of a sewing machine. Many of these causes are not active save in connection with some constitutional predisposition.' Among causes linked to the father were syphilis, youth, old age, feebleness, and debauchery. Predisposing factors revolving around the mother were multitudinous: syphilis, tuberculosis, heart disease, malnourishment, kidney disease, poisons, vomiting or continual coughing, fright and anxiety, hot baths, and so on, as well as anything that could result in a uterine contraction.[169] Why this physician and others deemed some causes exciting and others predisposing was not always clear, but the accumulation of causes over time was evident. If a physician thought he could pinpoint the cause of a patient's miscarriage, then he added that cause to the list. Yet physicians seldom prioritized causes.

An exception to this was venereal disease (VD). In the early years of the century, race and gender played a role in physicians' perceptions of VD. W.G. Cosbie, reporting on the obstetrical and gynaecological service at Toronto General Hospital stated that Wassermann tests done on 1,674 mothers at delivery showed a 4.3 per cent positive reaction. Cosbie noted that the results were in keeping with clinics elsewhere, 'allowing always for the presence of a negro population in certain of them.'[170] Physicians were convinced that syphilis was often caused by, in the euphemistic words of David Berry Hart, 'the mischief in the husband.' Showing an early-twentieth-century sensibility to the double standard, Hart explained to his readers how a physician should discern whether syphilis was a possibility: 'Inquiries ... must be made from the husband as to a special phase in his bachelor life; but nothing must be said to his wife, and if she asks any explanation of the unfortunate terminations of her pregnancies she can be told that the after-birth is in her case diseased. This answer includes the truth, and the real reason is a professional secret. Usually she pushes her inquiries no further, and if she does, the medical man can give her no information.'[171] Thus, Hart was suggesting that information be withheld from the patient because of the privileged nature of the physician's conversation with her husband. Hart clearly did not feel that a woman had the right to know what was causing her miscarriages. That she might blame herself was not something he considered.

Most physicians in the interwar period did not worry themselves with the race or gendered nature of VD contraction. They accepted it as a problem that all could potentially face. Gerald H. Pearson of the Ottawa Social Hygiene Council stressed that every woman early in her pregnancy should be examined for syphilis, which 'lurks unseen in many homes from the highest to the lowest.'[172] James Goodwin, a Toronto physician, believed that the consequences of syphilis in pregnancy demanded 'unfailing prenatal watchfulness.' These words reveal Goodwin's confidence in his own profession. The routine Wassermann would catch the disease before it had time to wreak havoc on the foetus and it would allow treatment of the mother with Salvarsan, which he argued would increase her chances of giving birth to a living child. Although he acknowledged that the incidence of syphilis was low in obstetrical patients, he concluded, 'It will be kept low only by reason of our individual efforts.'[173] In seeing all women at risk, all women became suspect.

Herbert M. Little of McGill worried about this very issue. He argued that in the urgency of dealing with syphilis, too many prenatal clinics had instituted Wassermann tests as a matter of course and frightened patients away. He questioned whether a Wassermann was even accurate in pregnant women and challenged using the test on patients where syphilis was not even suspected.[174] The two sides of the issue were difficult to reconcile. Little's view placed trust in women and assumed that physicians knew who their patients were and who the husbands were; Pearson's and Goodwin's view treated everyone the same – but as guilty until proven innocent. However, the 'guilty until proven innocent' attitude might save a woman's life and that of her unborn child, especially if the woman had been infected with syphilis unknowingly. Given the double sexual standard of the day, this was quite possible.

The long list of causes of miscarriages created the image of a woman at risk from almost any aspect of life. It could also lead to more intervention. A 1932 text advised its readers to perform a monthly vaginal examination to help in offsetting 'a symptomless oncoming abortion or miscarriage.'[175] Ignored was the possibility that such an examination could itself become the cause of miscarriage. With the increasing interest in hormones in the 1930s, some suggested administering various mixtures to habitual aborters. In 1947 in the United States, the Food and Drug Administration approved diethylstilbestrol (DES), a synthetic estrogen, to prevent miscarriage, despite animal studies that suggested it was carcinogenic. The next year an article in the *Alberta Medical Bulletin* endorsed it. Even in the early 1950s, when a study indicated its use was not efficacious, the manufacturers continued to advertise DES for routine use in all pregnancies.[176]

A more common complication of pregnancy was morning sickness. J. Clifton Edgar in his 1907 text had a very pragmatic suggestion: the woman should eat an early breakfast, after which she could sleep for an hour or so before getting up.[177] Of course, some women would not have been able to follow such a regimen, but it placed control in the woman's hands. In the interwar years, doctors did not seem particularly concerned – they saw morning sickness as common and almost physiologically normal. They encouraged women to rest more, to refrain from sexual relations, to eat more and smaller meals, to drink more fluids, and to make sure that their bowels were regular.[178] But morning sickness could become serious when continuous – it could result in the loss of the child and the death of the mother. In the early years of the century, doctors could do little for it. In the interwar period, however, a debate arose about the nature of the vomiting of pregnancy, which determined the medical response to it.

The Canadian physician who wrote most on this subject was Harold Atlee. In 1925 he described his way of dealing with it:

I have been using the suggestive method of treatment for all cases of vomiting of pregnancy, including the pernicious type, both in hospital and private practice, for the last four years and have found it most satisfactory ... If the treatment by suggestion is to be successful ... two essentials must be observed: the patient must come into hospital; a promise must be obtained from the husband and all other relatives not to visit the patient until the vomiting has ceased for 48 hours. These safeguards are based on sound psychological grounds. At home the patient's bedroom tends to become an axis about which the entire world revolves. In hospital the patient is one of many passengers on a ship whose quarter-deck I strut undenied. I keep the relatives away because I found in earlier cases that their advent to the sick-room was often the signal for a fresh outburst of vomiting. This is especially true in regard to the husband ... From the moment the patient enters the hospital she is denied the solace of the vomit-bowl. She is told that, in the event of not being able to control herself, she is to vomit into the bed; and the nurse is instructed to be in no hurry about changing her.

He tells women that they are to eat normally in the hospital, that nothing is wrong with their digestion, and in 'no circumstances' will he end their pregnancy. He did not deny that toxaemia caused some of the vomiting of pregnancy, but he considered it rare. In Atlee's view, the majority of cases were neurotic in origin and a way of getting attention. To prove his point, he described his treatment of a patient, newly wed, whom he found lying on the sofa when he visited. Beside the sofa was a 'particularly fine rug' that had been a wedding gift. Atlee told his patient that when she felt sick she was not to be sick in a bowl but on the carpet. That evening, after eating a good meal, which was the first she had been able to eat in some time, she felt sick and looked at the rug and was sick all over it. That, however, was the last time.[179] Atlee, through his 'suggestive method,' was assuming control in order to convince women that he could make them better. He was denying the physical origin of their vomiting. That his patient had been sick on her prized rug only once proved his point. Self-control was all that was needed.

Atlee's suggestions may have been extreme, but they were not without supporters. Dr Victor Harding described the favoured treatment at Toronto General Hospital: isolation, sedatives given 'to cover the neurotic factor,' and fluids to correct the dehydration.[180] William J. Stevens, an Ottawa physician, worried that too many women accepted the physiological nature of nausea during pregnancy and did little when it became more severe. At that point he agreed with Atlee that the patient needed rest, isolation, and 'complete confidence in the doctor and nurses ... and the exercise of the patient's will-power assured by the strongest encouragement.' He even suggested injecting some of the father's blood into the mother, on the theory that the blood of the foetus might differ from that of the mother but be the same as the father's. By injecting the mother with the father's blood, the woman could be desensitized to the 'foreign protein.'[181] In this respect, Stevens recognized the physical origins of the vomiting, but he gave no details in support of such a treatment.

Not all physicians agreed with Atlee. In 1929 an article in the *Canadian Medical Association Journal* noted that women were the only vertebrates that experienced vomiting of pregnancy and suggested that the knee-chest position helped alleviate the symptoms. What worked for animals might work for women; for this reason the article also advised continence in sexuality.[182] The use of animal imagery belittled women. It compared them to inferior species and found the women wanting, not quite up to the task of bearing children. But it did not suggest that the vomiting was a result of neurosis.

Even if the neurotic aspect was there, by the time it reached the stage of pernicious vomiting, the toxic factor had taken over. Indeed, most physicians, were coming to see the vomiting of pregnancy and the pernicious vomiting of pregnancy on a continuum largely caused by toxicity. As a woman wrote in the *University of Western Ontario Quarterly*: 'To assume that the majority of pregnant women are neurotic and that the vomiting is psychic is a diagnostic habit that is akin to classifying as "neurasthenia" all physical conditions that cannot be easily diagnosed.'[183] Atlee, however, remained unconvinced. He acknowledged that the post-mortems of women who had died of pernicious vomiting revealed that physiological changes had occurred. But he argued that the vomiting itself had caused them, not that they had caused the vomiting. He still insisted that the cause was neurotic in origin.[184] The division between physicians over this issue was more than theoretical. It affected treatment. Those adopting the toxicity model often turned to drug therapy as an antidote and in so doing privileged the science of medicine.[185] Atlee's position privileged the art or the physician's skill.

Eclampsia was one of the top life-threatening conditions of pregnancy. In the early decades of the century, physicians responded to it in a variety of ways: bloodletting, the use of morphia, subcutaneous injection of saline, use of hot packs, induction of labour, ice pack to the head, emptying of the stomach, and quiet.[186] In the interwar period, the emphasis shifted to preventing a full eclamptic state from developing, through regular blood pressure tests and urinalysis, the latter to test for the level of albumin. If the patient could be stabilized, physicians deemed that the pregnancy could go to term; if the blood pressure kept rising, they would induce labour.[187]

Toxaemia of pregnancy could lead to eclampsia and was a condition necessitating careful watching. In Toronto in the 1920s, the Burnside Lying-In Hospital had a special ward for patients with pernicious vomiting and late toxaemias of pregnancy, where a nurse-dietician supervised them.[188] Not all women could receive such treatment or get their pre-eclamptic state caught quickly. Mrs Alice Kellaher was a case in point. For two weeks before her admission to Halifax's Victoria General Hospital on 29 May 1921, she had noticed some blurring in her sight, 'especially on rising.' On the day before her admission she 'went almost completely blind and began to have convulsive seizures.' The next day her physician sent her to the hospital. According to the case history, 'examination of the urine showed a larger amount of albumen. The patient was prepared for operation' and a caesarian section was performed.[189]

At times physicians blamed their patients for the development of eclampsia. A doctor in Wolfville, Nova Scotia, who supported a low-protein and high-carbohydrate diet to ward off eclampsia, suggested that part of the problem was that too many pregnant women ate too much and did not exercise enough. A 1945 article in the *Canadian Medical Association Journal*, written by two American physicians, raised the racial issue when they pointed out that black women developed eclampsia more than white, even though both experienced the same rate of pre-eclampsia. The reason for the difference, they concluded, was that white women cooperated with their physicians in keeping appointments and keeping to their diets, whereas black women did not.[190] In neither case did the physicians probe the reasons for women acting the way they did.

Most physicians, however, were not interested in laying blame. They were more concerned with how to treat the condition so that it did not become life threatening. Helen MacMurchy acknowledged the value of a low-salt diet for women in a pre-eclamptic condition. Because it worked for them, she believed that all women in the last half of their pregnancy should refrain from adding salt to their food. By the late 1940s, the medical literature reported some experimentation with stilbestrol. Others, however, advocated a much quicker and more dramatic response to the situation of the mother. By all means try to offset the toxaemia, but if unsuccessful, therapeutic abortion was in order. The mother's life and health had priority.[191]

It was clear to many that because the symptoms of eclampsia can come on suddenly, 'pre-natal supervision cannot be too rigid or thorough during the last trimester.'[192] Close supervision did not necessarily mean keeping the patient informed. One woman recalled that in 1949 she had entered St Michael's Hospital, Toronto, with toxaemia, but no one had explained to her what this meant. The hospital staff simply informed her that she was going to have her kidneys flushed. Eventually a nurse came into her room and told her that they were going to induce labour, but she still did not understand what this involved. Contractions began, then stopped, but the next day she went into 'real' labour and gave birth to her first baby.[193] Nor did close supervision guarantee a happy outcome. Mrs Loewen, age twenty, had been under a physician's care since the second month of her pregnancy and had had monthly urine tests since her sixth. In her eighth month, she experienced 'terrific headaches during the last few days and edema during the last week. She had albumin in her urine from the sixth month.' She entered the Kitchener-Waterloo Hospital on 17 April 1945; labour was induced, and she gave birth to twins, both of whom died. Two days later she died.[194] All the prenatal care in the world could not prevent tragedies such as this from occurring. But physicians comforted themselves that care would limit their occurrence.

The goal of all prenatal care, whether in traditional or Western culture, was a healthy mother able to give birth to a healthy child. The interest Aboriginal society took in the work that pregnant women did, the food customs they followed, and even their interest in sex determination, reflects this goal. Canadian women of European heritage had their own traditions, but these too were designed to ensure a healthy mother and child. In both societies, the cultural habits and beliefs provided women with a sense of control over a force that was both dangerous and miraculous. Nowhere can this be seen more than in some women's continuing belief in maternal impressions. But the newer belief in medical science also provided many women with agency; it gave them different customs to follow to ensure their safe delivery.

The medical paradigm as part of Western culture was as all-embracing as the customs and taboos of traditional cultures. It was increasingly becoming part of the fabric of our society, and this intensification was particularly visible in the years following the First World War. Physicians had long been interested in the timing of conception, and after a more accurate understanding of the female monthly cycle was gained in the 1920s, the discussions of the role of sperm and ovum took on a less speculative form. Diagnosis of pregnancy, which many patients believed should be straightforward, challenged physicians to live up to expectations they could not meet, at least until the introduction of pregnancy tests in the 1930s. Even then, with the cost of such tests prohibitive, most physicians continued to put their faith in the signs of pregnancy – bodily changes which they could measure – as opposed to the symptoms of pregnancy as experienced by the pregnant women. Unlike the mothers-to-be, doctors were not particularly interested in predicting the sex of the child; rather, they attempted to understand how sex was determined. At times their search for causation seemed very similar to that of older beliefs, but framed in a scientific guise. Their reinterpretation of maternal impressions is an example of this. They became increasingly hostile to the continuation of such beliefs and by the interwar years had medicalized the pathways of impressions. They, rather than the families and local communities, became the interpreters of causation.

The most significant shift in prenatal care, however, was its very emergence. Going beyond the comparison of the problematic female body against the unproblematic male body, physicians caring for pregnant women compared them to the non-pregnant body and in doing so reinforced perceptions of pregnancy as being potentially dangerous. It was the doctor's responsibility to lessen this danger. Especially after the horrendous losses of the First World War and the influenza epidemic, the medical profession stressed the importance of regular prenatal visits. The problem was that the ideal put forward was difficult for the majority of women and their practitioners to meet, whether it was the number of visits expected or what needed to be checked and measured during the visits. The sense of frustration which physicians felt because of the gap between what the medical literature told them was the ideal prenatal regimen and what they were actually able to offer patients was accentuated by the fact that patients were not always willing or able to follow the physician's advice. That advice was extensive, covering many aspects of a woman's day-to-day life. Given in good faith, it was often based on an individual doctor's experience with his other patients. But its all-encompassing nature could mean that women who were unable to accommodate their lives to it were left with a feeling that they were not providing the best care possible.

The increasing emphasis on medical care and the advice given by physicians were rituals surrounding pregnancy and as much a part of Western culture as the food and activity taboos were for other cultures. But giving advice and providing care placed control of pregnancy more in physicians' hands than in the pregnant woman's. Educating women about their bodies had the added virtue (from the medical perspective) of enabling the patient to be blamed if she did not go to see the physician in time to be helped. As one physician admitted, 'When people continued to sicken and die with the best scientific medical care, we needed an alibi. So we sold them the idea that they did not come to us early enough or often enough. This had the additional advantage of being profitable; and there was just enough kernel of truth to lend credibility to a dangerously preposterous proposition.'[195] Prenatal care emphasized the abnormality of the pregnant state; healthy people did not go to see physicians. The encouragement of women to do so was partially the result of physicians' desire to keep track of the pregnancy. By constant monitoring of 'signs, symptoms, and test results,' they could reduce the chance of being surprised by complications in childbirth.'[196] But medicine could do only so much. It could not ensure that all women had enough to eat, worked and lived in safe environments, and rested enough. All that physicians could do was delineate the ideal care which they believed women needed and which doctors could partly provide. Childbirth itself became the testing ground. Had the care provided been enough?

CHAPTER FIVE

Childbirth

Presumably, when non-exposure of the vulva is adopted, it is done with the object of sparing the feelings of the patient, but, during the expulsion of the foetus, the patient is far too much occupied by her suffering to notice what is done, and, moreover, no sensible patient will object to a precaution taken for her own good, if the necessity for it is made clear to her. The patient's sentiments have in the past been too frequently considered to the detriment of her physical condition.

Henry Jellett, 1910[1]

Much of childbirth is socially constructed, surrounded by customs, taboos, and superstitions similar to those in the prenatal period. The physiological basics remain somewhat constant, but the context in which birth occurs directs aspects of the experience. A major aspect in the first half of the twentieth century was a tension over how physicians perceived childbirth. As noted in chapter 2, some acknowledged birth as a natural, physiological event and urged caution and patience, while others argued that natural and physiological did not necessarily mean unproblematic. Of course, trying to distinguish between the problematic and unproblematic birth was the challenge. For many in the profession, it led to distinguishing between women based on race, class, age, and cultural background. It also led to acceptance of the possibility of complications in any birth, even while acknowledging the safety of most births. This awareness of danger influenced doctors' perceptions of where the best place was for a women to deliver her child and who was the best person to be with her. It is clear that over time women increasingly gave birth in hospital rather than at home, and that by 1950 those in the birthing room with her were mostly strangers. Critics of hospitalization have created a romanticized view of home birth. But home birth varied significantly, depending on who was present – husband, friends, midwife, nurse, doctor – and hospital birth was not always to the woman's detriment.[2] Indeed, for many women it provided advantages. Nor was there a great distinction between what occurred in home births and hospital births – at least, those directed by physicians. In both, physicians paid attention to cleanliness, the position taken during labour, and finding standardized lengths for the stages of labour, though in doing so the degree to which they took control of birth and monitored it intensified over time. As the above quotation reveals, the sentiments of the patients were to give way to the primacy of the 'physical condition' as determined by the attending medical practitioners.

In the early years of the century, some physicians were adamant that birthing was in general a worry-free physiological process. In 1903 John McDonald from St Peter's, Cape Breton, argued that in most cases a physician did not need to intervene in the process of labour. Others agreed, estimating that 90 to 95 per cent of childbirth cases were normal (normal being defined as not necessitating intervention).[3] Nevertheless, physicians were to be present at all cases, because of the minority of women who might require their assistance. They were an insurance policy. As I. Clifton Edgar told the students and practitioners reading his 1907 text, the role of the physician was to be a watchful observer: 'In normal cases the object of the accoucheur is to find out, not how much, but how little interference is justifiable.'[4]

Not all physicians saw childbirth as normal. One of North America's best-known obstetricians, Joseph B. DeLee, asked: 'Can a function so perilous, that in spite of the best care, it kills thousands of women every year, that leaves at least a quarter of the women more or less invalided, and a majority with permanent anatomic changes of structure, that is always attended by severe pain and tearing of tissues, and that kills 3 to 5 per cent. of children – can such a function be called normal?'[5] Normal for him meant safe, painless, without repercussions of almost any kind. Such an ideal was next to impossible to achieve, and striving for it could lead some physicians to intervene even in unproblematic births.

Certain women were at risk. One of the strongest themes in the early medical literature was the belief that birthing was easier for Native women, women in peasant societies, and women in the past compared with middle-class urban women in the present. Little proof was offered to substantiate this belief; it had simply become conventional wisdom and seemed obvious. A typical reference was that contained in *A Text-Book of Gynecology* (1901), edited by Charles A.L. Reed: 'There is no doubt that between the women of aboriginal peoples and those who belong to the civilized races there are certain physical differences ... The reproductive function can be taken as an index. Savage women, as a rule, have but little difficulty in childbed, because they have large pelves and bear children with small heads.'[6] Several themes emerge from this assertion, which others picked up. The first was the creation of a binary: the savage, Aboriginal woman and the civilized and, left unsaid, white woman. The former had little difficulty birthing because there was little disproportion between her pelvis and the size of her child's head. Childbirth for such women was a natural process. The civilized woman, on the other hand, was clearly in a different situation: a smaller pelvis and a larger child's head. The size of head was a way of implying that the brains of civilized children were larger than those of Aboriginal children. Being more than a reproductive machine, civilized woman had lost her ability to give birth with ease. Childbirth, for her, had become a medical condition necessitating professionalized medicine.[7]

Only occasionally did a physician call this model of development into question. In 1905 L.W. Jones noted in the *Queen's Medical Quarterly* that he had attended two cases of childbirth among the Ojibwa and felt that both women had suffered 'as much as ... ordinary robust white women, nor was labor one whit quicker.'[8] But many did not let their lack of experience with other groups of women dissuade them from what they 'knew' was true. J. Clarence Webster in his 1903 text did not. Webster's view differed from Reed's only in detail in that he felt that the pelves of 'primitive and barbarian' races were smaller, but since the heads of their children were 'smaller and more conical,' birthing posed few problems. To explain, he used an animal analogy. 'It is interesting to note,' he wrote, 'that domestication is accompanied by increased difficulties in the labor of animals. Town-kept and stall-fed horses and cattle more frequently need help than those living on the plains.' The conclusion was there for anyone to draw, but just in case they could not, he added, 'The more artificial and luxurious women become, the greater is the percentage of abnormal parturition.'[9] A year later, A. Lapthorn Smith of Montreal added his own twist to the explanation. Modern women, he noted, were having difficulty because higher education increased the ability of their nerves to perceive pain; in addition, the pain of labour was greater for such women. Sitting at a desk all day caused the pelvis to become smaller and the abdominal muscles to atrophy, retarding the growth of the bones.[10] All resulted in more pain in childbirth. Higher education separated the civilized, woman from the uncivilized, based on both race and class.

With respect to the latter, in 1907 J. McArthur from London, Ontario, argued that 'the higher the social circle, or ... the greater the culture and refinement,' the more problems there were in birth.[11] Some held that differences also existed between rural and urban women. In 1909 Thomas R. Ponton of MacGregor, Manitoba, told of a patient who had just given birth to her third child. The first two had been born in England and attended by both nurse and physician, and during each birth the woman had nearly lost her life. Since then she and her family had immigrated to Canada and were living in a log house that was not properly plastered for winter. Nonetheless, the third baby was born without difficulty, and indeed Ponton had had little to do during the birth. His conclusion: a healthy and vigorous life on the Canadian prairie had strengthened the woman and consequently had made childbirth easier.[12]

Although the majority of births were unproblematic, no one ever knew with certainty which ones would not be. Because of this, the education of physicians prepared them to be on the lookout for complications. As well, careful record keeping helped them understand the parameters of a normal birth. Physicians noted the age of their patients, how many children they had had, and whether the births had been difficult or not. They drew co-relations between different variables. For example, older women often had more difficulty giving birth to their first child than younger women did. But what was an older mother? For Thomas Watts Eden the optimum age for a first birth was eighteen to twenty-three. Over the age of twenty-six, he said, a woman 'encounters greater risks, which steadily increase in gravity as age advances.'[13]

Hospitals, too, kept detailed records, and on these they developed a model of how a non-problem birth should proceed; births falling outside the norm were problematic. The hospitals carefully recorded the length of labour in its various stages and then designed guidelines for their physicians. Instructions for the nurses and house physician at the Burnside Lying-In Hospital, Toronto, in the first decade of the century were very clear about when to expect the various events to occur in a birth. The reasons for the instructions were equally clear: 'Our chief aim in making rules as to certain time records is to secure uniformity in methods of procedure.'[14] However, a physician who adhered to the rules too rigidly could become an automaton, someone who followed procedure without thinking about what he was doing and was not sensitive to the variations among women. Frederick Fenton of St Michael's Hospital, Toronto, was concerned about the problems of standardization with respect to the use of the pelvimeter, an instrument designed to determine whether a disproportion between the pelvis and the child's head existed. He noted, 'As soon as one commences to lay down definite rules for procedure based upon the true conjugate or any other diameter of the pelvic brim or outlet, then, I think, its usefulness is in a fair way to be lost and it may be the means of leading one into trouble.' In his view, the pelvimeter helped him be aware that there *might* be difficulty, but that was all.[15] Many physicians were torn between two models of medicine. One acknowledged the art of obstetrics, the need for the physician to be open to the endless variations within the process of childbirth; the other focused on the science of obstetrics, where the woman's body acted in a machinelike way and the seamless process of birthing was divided into stages. The former represented the reality faced by physicians, while the latter represented a way of dealing with that reality and was reflected in the urge to standardize treatment and to have guidelines and rules. Both models were necessary, and although they were not mutually exclusive, they were at times at odds with one another.

Throughout the interwar period and beyond, physicians continued to discuss the limits of safety in childbirth. Looking back on their careers, they tallied up the cases that had complications and noted the woman who had given birth to the most children, and the oldest and youngest age at childbirth, as if to see how much stress a physical body could withstand. Unlike physicians in earlier years, some were quite accepting of older women giving birth for the first time and did not feel that women in their thirties faced any serious problem. Percy Ryberg in his popular 1942 manual, *Health, Sex and Birth Control*, made it clear that the twenties were the optimum age but that probably no harm would result if a woman had a child in her thirties, though he advised checking with a physician first. Others were even more forgiving. In one issue of *Health*, D.E. Cannell posited that the difficulties of childbirth associated with women over the age of thirty-five had been exaggerated.[16] Both Ryberg and Cannell, however, saw medicine as the enabling factor in such births. Some physicians were not willing to go that far. J.W. Duncan and W.E. Gibson, both from the Montreal Maternity Hospital, argued that the best age for childbearing was under thirty. Their way of choosing this age was to look at the age of a male athlete when 'both powers of effort and endurance,' were highest. Since women in labour depended on effort and endurance, the transference of age from the male athlete to the childbearing woman seemed sensible, and they concluded that 'women over thirty are not good obstetrical risks; over thirty-five, poor ones; over forty, bad ones.'[17]

The 'effort and endurance' necessary and the 'risk' women underwent suggest an event that was potentially problematic. More than in the early decades of the century, physicians emphasized the need for vigilance and intervention in childbirth. Even when acknowledging the naturalness of birth and the need to have patience and let nature have its way, they often acted to the contrary.[18] The predisposition to intervene was strong. As seen in chapter 2, obstetrics and gynaecology had become coupled, and the latter stressed the pathological nature and weaknesses of the reproductive/sexual system of women. In addition, physicians understandably remembered their difficult cases, especially their failures, and the desire to avoid failure in future was a powerful spur to assume the worst-case scenario. As Winnipeg physician Ross Mitchell observed, 'Even the normal pregnant woman presents certain abnormalities.'[19] Physicians were trained to prepare themselves for these abnormalities. Birthing was both natural and pathological. W.W. Chipman of McGill University and the Montreal Maternity Hospital tried to convince his colleagues that the goal of every birth should be minimal interference, that 'the ideal delivery is, and must always be, the one that is spontaneous.' But for this to happen, women needed training. 'Pregnancy and labour are the supreme tests of a woman's fitness, physically, mentally, and morally ... The labour is not only a trial of her physical fitness, but also of her *morale*.'[20] For these athletics, the trainer of choice was the physician. Physicians had to perform a delicate balancing act. If they viewed birthing as physiological, they feared that not enough care would be taken; if they viewed it as pathological, too much interference might occur.[21] The question, of course, was where to draw the line. While the vast majority of births were unproblematic, there was no guarantee that any specific birth would be so; physicians had to be prepared, especially as the refrain that modern woman could not cope with birthing was still being sung.

In 1924 an editorial in the *Canada Lancet and National Hygiene* reported that 'two or three of Toronto's well-known specialists at the last meeting of the section of the Academy of Medicine on Gynecology and Preventive Medicine' made it clear that 'modern civilized women' were 'avoiding conception to escape the horrors and pains of labor and that pagan women [were] undergoing parturition with ease and little pain.' Two explanations for this were put forward. First, modern women were marrying at too late an age, some even in their thirties; as a result, the joints of their pelves were no longer flexible, causing hardship and pain during childbirth. Second, the diet of modern women was too rich, resulting in larger babies, which caused disproportion and resultant pain.[22] Two years later, the Toronto Board of Health was more general about the cause of the problem and blamed the modern, unnatural way of living for the development of 'sensitive nerves.' The modern body needed a modern approach.[23] Like DeLee in the earlier period, doctors seemed to believe that natural birth should be painless; because birth was not painless, it was no longer natural. The maternal mortality rates also were high in the 1920s and 1930s, and physicians were seeking explanations that did not reflect badly on themselves. They concluded that women had changed over time and were no longer able to experience birthing as a normal physiological process. But fortunately the very civilization that had ill equipped modern women for birth had also offered them 'the power to make motherhood the safest profession in the world' – the power represented by the scientific expertise of modern medicine.[24]

As in the previous decades, physicians in the interwar years and afterwards were specific about which women were having difficulty – women who led sedentary lives. First Nations women, rural women, and those who were active had less difficulty. Curiously, so did slim, blonde women, compared with 'short and stocky' brunettes. Some argued that Anglo-Saxon women had more problems than the 'foreign-born.'[25] Women who engaged in interracial relations also were at risk. Especially problematic, according to Dr Frank Walker, were Native women who became pregnant by white men. Harking back to earlier arguments about head size, he claimed 'that a half-caste child has a larger head than a pure blood Indian child, and parturition under these conditions is fraught with great danger to the mother.' Walker also linked length of labour to the eye colour of the parents, contending that labour was shorter when parents had similar eye colour. He also argued that labour was shorter when the child was female, because the female foetus inherited her mother's head shape, which conformed to the shape of the mother's pelvic canal.[26] Once physicians noted correlations, it became a short step to assume a cause-and-effect relationship. The irony of such views is that early feminist support of natural childbirth appealed to a very similar essentialist view of 'primitive' women, to which it was possible for all women to conform – they created an image of woman's body which all women were to meet.[27]

Such views primed physicians to intervene. Birthing may have been natural, but it required 'skilful and scientific management.' Part of the skill was knowing when to intervene. The list of potential complications seemed endless. Over the first fifty years of the twentieth century, medical journals seldom published articles on normal births. Rather, they published the offerings of physicians who had come face to face with birth difficulties in their practice and either had failed to meet the challenge but had learned from it or had overcome the challenge and wanted to share their victory with their colleagues. The unusual story captured the interest of the reader. Doctors gave tallies of their practice, both private and hospital, relating any complications or unusual occurrences, such as the birth of hermaphrodites, twins, or babies with 'deformities.'[28] They worried about precipitate labour, non-vertex presentations, women who suffered from primary inertia or who were RH negative or had health problems such as tuberculosis, heart disease, and syphilis. They feared the loss of the child and therefore focused attention on abortions, miscarriages, premature births, still births, and infant deaths. Even more fearsome was the death of the mother. Maternal mortality haunted physicians, and most Protestant physicians insisted that the mother's life had priority over that of her child.[29] Almost as fearsome was the danger posed by puerperal insanity. It was rare, but the literature devoted to it was not, especially in the early decades of the century.[30]

The physicians' fears about the possible complications attending birth affected their view of childbirth and in turn influenced their opinions on where a woman should give birth, who should be with her during birth, and what their own actions should be during birth. Much of the feminist literature on birthing has romanticized home birth compared with hospital birth. The former is seen as warm, caring, and personalized, whereas the latter is presented as technologically driven with little compassion for the wonder of the event itself. This polarization often compares the best of home births with the worst of hospital births. In fact, home births did not always ensure support, and the people present varied significantly. In contemporary society, we often have a nostalgic view of traditional cultures in which a birthing woman remained in her own home, cared for by other women who had gone through the same ordeal. For many this was the case, but for others isolation or separation was the rule. A woman of Tagish and Tlingit descent recalled that when she gave birth in 1917, she left her dwelling and made 'a little camp back of the main house, back of the main camp.' There she remained alone, though with the support of other women. But some remember isolation to the point where other women were not allowed to visit or be physically close to them.[31] Separation gave these women a chance to feel that what they were doing was important and significant. As well, it protected the family and the community from the blood associated with birth and its power to harm others. But the isolation also emphasized the impurity or messiness of the process. Florence Edenshaw Davidson, a Haida woman, recalled that 'they used to say they have the baby outside, not in the house because they have respect for their house keeping clean.'[32]

For some women it was circumstances, not culture, that conspired to leave them alone during birth. A tragic case occurred in 1918. On a blustery day in March, a woman living in northern Saskatchewan went into labour, and her young husband set out to get the doctor ten miles distant. When he arrived, the doctor was busy elsewhere, and by the time he was ready to leave, the weather had worsened. Not until the following morning did they arrive at the homestead only to find the wife dead.[33] Stories such as this convinced many Canadians that more medical services were needed. A less tragic case was that of an Inuk woman who recalled going into labour when she and her husband were travelling on the ice. He made her a small igloo, in which she gave birth; they had some tea and then started to move again so that they could reach land and build a larger igloo.[34] Both these cases remind us of the roles that husbands *could* play.

Despite these stories, most women delivering at home were supported by the presence of other women. Often when a woman went into labour, in both Native and non-Native society, women friends and relatives would arrive and take turns being with her and giving whatever support was needed, though this decreased significantly over time.[35] And, of course, in both cultures midwives could be present. Many commentators have pitted midwife-directed births, against doctor-directed births, arguing that the former gave women control over the process of birth. It did, but as seen in chapter 3, one result was lack of involvement on the part of husbands. As well, the question has to be asked, Which women had control?[36] In the case of a midwife-directed birth, the midwife was generally in control. The midwife was often older than the woman giving birth and thus was deserving of respect. She was also experienced and had the aura of expertise, for her place in the community had accustomed her to give advice on a wide variety of health issues. But because she was a woman known to the birthing woman – and, most likely, shared her class, education, and ethnicity – there was a connection between them that perhaps would not have existed with a physician. Also, the midwife could fit into the domestic regimen of the household more readily than the physician, who tended to arrive well after labour had started and left soon after the child was born.

Trained nurses, private or public, who attended home births were, of course, in a different position than helpful women or midwives. For one, they were usually younger. When Lucy Maud Montgomery had a nurse during her confinement in 1912, she was at first surprised by the youth of the woman, who was twenty-eight. She had, she wrote, expected someone 'old or middle-aged.'[37] What Montgomery had expected was someone whose age was more aligned with the popular conception of a midwife. Whereas the age of midwives gave them status, the youth of nurses may have worked against them and have offset, to some extent, the prestige of their training. Nurses' interest in professionalizing and separating themselves from the domestic work that midwives did also made the relationship between nurses and their patients more distant. As noted in chapter 3, although midwives were paid, most did not earn their living from what they did – rather, it was a vocation. While this may have been a motivation for many nurses, the reality was that they made their living from nursing and some charged fees beyond what many families could afford.[38] In addition, they had medical training, which had inculcated in them a sense of the 'right' way a birth should proceed. As a result, some nurses had a rather dismissive attitude about the conditions in which they found many of their patients, and they were determined that these women should be instructed in the proper way to live.[39]

Unlike midwives and nurses, physicians directing a home birth had authority because of their training and expertise. Like nurses, they were often outsiders, not part of the woman's personal network in the same way that friends or even a midwife could be. While some may have been very much a part of the local community and may even have delivered the woman herself, their training still created distance. And most physicians would have had little in common with patients who were working class or immigrant. Most significant was gender. Toronto's Adam H. Wright in his 1908 obstetric textbook warned student readers that they had to take care how they appeared to women and to take into account the gendered divisions: 'Very few modern surgeons think of operating either in hospital or private practise without wearing a fresh gown or apron of some sort. Obstetricians do not so commonly prepare themselves in this way; many of them simply take off their coats and roll up their sleeves within sight of the patient, and look sometimes as if preparing for a fight. The sight of a big, muscular doctor thus preparing to treat a poor, delicate, little woman, generally causes fear and trembling.' His solution was for the doctor to prepare himself out of sight of his female patient.[40]

Physicians also had the authority of law behind them. As early as 1892, the Criminal Code had made 'failing to obtain reasonable assistance during childbirth' a crime. Constance Backhouse has argued that the legislation 'reflected the increasing social and medical control that was being exercised over birthing.'[41] Similar provincial legislation in Ontario reflected a concern about the high infant mortality rates of maternity homes, which sometimes were known as 'baby farms.' Legislation had required private maternity homes in Toronto to improve their standards, with the result that few could compete with the hospitals that still provided considerable charitable care. Indeed, public maternity homes, which received government grants, could offer more resources or were seen to do so.[42] There was little opposition to medically assisted birth, and by the turn of the century it was becoming the norm.[43] And support for it expanded. The British Columbia Commission on Health Insurance, 1919–21, recommended that the state give a woman thirty-five dollars on proof that she had had a qualified physician (or if this was not possible, a nurse) attend her at birth. In the 1920s organizations such as the National Council of Women advocated medical assistance during childbirth and argued that maternity benefits could ensure this for all women.[44] Such support for the medical profession sent out the message that women needed professional help in giving birth. Few women seemed opposed. Rather, their concerns about the presence of physicians revolved around what the physician did or did not do, and the cost. Women often resented when a physician arrived just in time to 'catch' the baby. Even when the physician arrived after the birth, he still charged for his time. Most upsetting were those who refused to help a woman unless they were paid. In addition, physicians did little to help the mother after the birth, unlike neighbour women and midwives. For many working-class women, this was a significant issue.[45]

Whether alone or attended by husbands, friends, midwives, nurses, or physicians, the majority of women early in the century gave birth in their homes. Hospital officials knew and accepted this. Some institutions, such as the Montreal Maternity Hospital, set up clinics so that women would have the choice of delivering in the hospital or in their own homes with all the medical care that hospital personnel could provide. These births were those that physicians predicted would be free of problems. Women who were expected to have complications were to deliver in the hospital. While home births, through the hospitals, were only a small percentage of the hospital-controlled cases – at the Montreal Maternity they represented only 16 per cent of the cases in 1901, 30 per cent in 1916, and 14 per cent in 1920 – nevertheless, they represented a significant outreach attempt on the part of institutions introducing them.[46] Directed through a hospital program, home births were among the most medically cared for in the country. In order to obtain the services of the hospital, a woman had to agree to go to prenatal clinics (once these clinics were set up) and was thus medically supervised throughout her pregnancy. She had both the security of modern medical expertise and the comfort of home birth. Hospitals benefited as well. As the 1905 *Annual Report of the Montreal Maternity Hospital* pointed out, the work of its outdoor department was 'an invaluable means of training nurses and students to adapt themselves to conditions different from those to which they have been accustomed in hospital, and thus to make them more efficient and resourceful in private practice.'[47] This was especially significant in a period when the majority of births did occur at home.

There were significant benefits for the woman in a home birth directed by a physician. She was in a familiar setting, she could be surrounded by people she knew, and because she was in her own home, she and her family potentially had more say in how she was treated. As well, she had access to pain relief through a physician-directed birth. A physician's presence could, in the early years of the century, represent status and modernity with its appeal to science. However, some of the family's privacy was given up with the presence of a physician. Because he delivered the woman in her home, he was able to know more about her and her living situation than physicians delivering in a hospital were able to know.[48] For the physician, the disadvantages of a home birth were obvious. The birth was taking place in an environment that he could not totally dominate; nor was it set up for his convenience. And if the patient and her family had more say, he had less. He was under surveillance of the patient and her family. Physicians argued that in a home birth too often family and friends urged intervention to limit the woman's pain and too often physicians succumbed to the pressure.[49] Most physicians resented not being able to control who was in the birthing room. J. Clarence Webster in his 1903 text told his readers that 'unnecessary persons should be excluded,' and J.S. Fairbairn in his 1924 book railed against 'officious friends and other sources of disturbance.'[50]

In the early years of the century, practitioners were either ambivalent about or hostile to the presence of husbands. But with home births, doctors did not have the power to ban the husband from the birthing room. After all, the physician was the interloper. Adam H. Wright in 1908 told medical students how he coped with this problem:

> It occasionally happens that a husband desires to be present during labor, although why he should do so I could never understand. My custom is generally to allow him to be present if he wishes during the first stage, although I much prefer his absence. He can do no good and is apt to be intensely alarmed on account of his wife's suffering. Under such circumstances he becomes sometimes almost an intolerable nuisance, and it will keep one pretty busy assuring him that this is not the first time in the history of the world that a woman has suffered so severely. During the progress of the second stage I generally say, quietly, 'You had better leave the room now, we are getting near the end,' without giving any reasons why. He almost invariably leaves when so instructed without making any trouble. If by any chance he should insist upon remaining, I have nothing more to say.[51]

Nonetheless, the presence of the husband close by could be important for physicians. Some pointed out that if there were difficulties with the labour or abnormalities, the physician could advise the husband rather than the patient.[52] This protected the patient from becoming upset and ensured that the head of the family knew what was happening in case anything untoward occurred. If it did, he was prepared; if it did not, then the physician appeared to have successfully saved the situation.

For the physician, there were other drawbacks to home birth. He spent a great deal of time travelling to his various patients, especially in rural areas, and once in a patient's home was under pressure to remain, even if his attentions were not needed immediately. The conditions in patients' homes were not always comfortable. Home births meant that he could not carry the equipment that physicians increasingly believed was necessary for good obstetric care, nor was he surrounded by a support network that he could draw on as he could in a hospital. He had to adapt to a wide variety of situations. While trained to perform certain procedures, he found that the reality of the situation made some problematic. Each physician adapted his technique to his own individual practice and followed the customs that worked for him. But, over time, physicians tried to approach the hospital standard placed before them as the epitome of good care.[53]

At the beginning of the twentieth century, home births dominated; by mid-century hospital births did (see table 1). While only 17.8 per cent of births in Canada took place in hospitals in 1926, by 1940, 45.3 per cent did. The shift to hospitals was occurring elsewhere as well. In New Zealand half of the births took place in hospitals as early as 1926, and by 1940 the same was true in the United States. Britain, however, did not reach that percentage until shortly before 1950.[54] Within Canada rates varied significantly from province to province. In 1926, when just under 18 per cent of all births in Canada took place in institutions, only 2.7 per cent did in Prince Edward Island, but 48.2 per cent did in British Columbia. Ontario did not reach the 50 per cent mark until the late 1930s, and Quebec not until the 1950s.[55] The switchover to hospital births in urban centres could be swift but it was occurring in rural areas as well.[56] Despite these statistics, home births continued in most parts of the country and in some still dominated. In addition, home and hospital were not the only locales for birthing. In some areas, maternity homes existed.[57] This was particularly the case in the prairie provinces and represented a midway point in the transition from home to hospital birth. As Laurel Halladay has argued in her study of maternity homes in Saskatchewan, they existed in rural areas where the population was large enough to need maternity care but was not initially large enough to attract physicians – or, in later years, to provide a tax base necessary to build a hospital. Even the rates charged were transitional, somewhere between that of a midwife but not as expensive as a physician or hospital, considering the care received. These homes provided extended stays for women before birth, particularly in winter, when women would enter well before their due date to ensure that they would not be caught at home by a blizzard. The women who ran these homes often had practical experience and had served their communities as midwives before deciding to come into town to set up a home. Whereas midwives who went into patients' homes could remain independent, maternity homes, being in the public eye, often depended on the goodwill of physicians. Indeed, often physicians were the instigators of these homes, for they cut down on the travelling necessary to reach many women in their own homes. But these maternity homes were not to last. The passing of the Mutual Medical and Hospital Benefit Association Act in 1938, which provided private health insurance, led to a decline in clientele; the Second World War reduced the availability of the nurses who had often worked in the homes; there was increased regulation with more bureaucracy, which wore down many of the owners; and the introduction of the hospital services plan in the 1940s meant that women could travel to wherever they wanted in the province for care. Indeed, the elimination of these homes was one of the goals of socialized health care.[58]

As more women went to hospital to give birth, pressure on the facilities increased. In 1906 only twenty-five women had their babies in the Vancouver General. The next year 121 did so, and by 1916 there were 661. In the early years of the Depression the hospital could not meet demands for its services, so it refused to

TABLE 1
Percentage of hospital births for Canada, 1926–1950[59]

1926	17.8	1940	45.3
1930	26.6	1945	63.2
1935	32.2	1950	76.0

accept normal cases on the public wards and arranged for the City Relief Office to help charity patients remain at home by providing doctors' fees of twenty dollars and VON fees of ten dollars.[60] In large centres, hospital maternity cases were at times overwhelming. In 1930 in Montreal, 2,642 women entered the Royal Victoria Hospital to give birth.[61] Hospitals across the country felt similar pressure and the postwar baby boom only exacerbated it. The 1949 *Report on the Survey of Hospitals in Nova Scotia* noted: 'The present over-crowded, and often noisy labor-rooms will require modernization with provision of more room for patients while in labor.'[62] Not only were more women entering hospital to give birth, but obstetrics increasingly became an important function of hospitals. In Ontario 16.6 per cent of patients entered general hospitals for reasons related to childbirth in 1938; by 1947 the number had risen to 27.2 per cent. Women dominated the patient roster of hospitals. A sampling of patient records from the discharge books of the Royal Jubilee Hospital, Victoria, for 1927, 1935, and 1945 reveals that the percentage of adult patients who were women increased from 42.6 per cent to 58.52 and 61.49 per cent, respectively. Of adult women, 19.87 per cent entered for reasons linked to pregnancy or childbirth in 1927, whereas in 1935 the number was 22 per cent, and in 1947 it was 37.37 per cent.[63] Some hospitals, however, were slow to accept pregnant women and support the medicalization of childbirth. Hôtel-Dieu in Quebec City did not do so until 1939.[64]

Who these women were changed over time. Traditionally, nineteenth-century hospitals, as part of their charitable orientation, had catered to unwed and poor women. By the end of the century, the numbers of married women were increasing. At the Montreal Maternity Hospital in 1902, the number of married and unmarried childbirth patients was 144 and 92, respectively. In

1919 there were only 96 single patients, along with 1,317 married and 17 widowed. At the Ottawa Maternity Hospital, 20 per cent of all births at the turn of the century were to unwed mothers; by 1915, only 3 per cent were. Linked to the increase in married women was the rise in paying patients. At the turn of the century, approximately 45 per cent of women at the Ottawa Maternity Hospital were non-paying patients, whereas by 1915 only 30 per cent were.[65] A decrease in time spent in hospital before delivery also signalled the shift in obstetric clientele. A significant stay in hospital before delivery indicated one of three situations. The first was complications that necessitated medical supervision, a relatively rare occurrence. The second and third situations addressed the clientele: poorer women whose home situation did not lend itself to good care, and unmarried women who had nowhere else to go. In 1902 the average length of time spent in the Montreal Maternity Hospital before delivery was 15.2 days. By 1919 the stay before confinement for all patients was only 1.1 and for patients who entered early (for whatever reason), only 3.8 days.[66]

For the physician, a hospital birth was more convenient than a home birth, as Joseph B. DeLee explained in his 1913 text: it 'relieves him of a great deal of actual labor, it saves him many hours of tedious waiting, it lightens the burden of responsibility, and the knowledge he is prepared for all emergencies gives him a feeling of security which reflects itself in his work. The drudgery inherent in obstetric practice is thus largely eliminated, and the field becomes more inviting to the best men in the profession.'[67] Hospitals were an environment set up for doctors' convenience and control. No longer would they have to 'cope' with the homes of the poor. Poor women would be saved from themselves and their environment.[68] A case described in the 1904 *Union médicale du Canada* illustrates the kind of control doctors lacked in home births. Dr L.J. Trudeau had delivered a farmer's wife of her third child. Two days later she was suffering from headache and abdominal pain, and Trudeau recommended vaginal douches of boric acid and gave the woman's husband the equipment needed for the douching. The woman worsened and died, and it was only subsequently that Trudeau discovered that the husband had been using the equipment on two of his cows, which also had puerperal fever.[69] But hospital birth had its drawbacks: although the removal of the woman from her household might make medical sense, for the family left behind it could create problems. Nonetheless, as hospitals became more available and hospital birth more popular, physicians felt freer about insisting that their patients go to hospital. Since many physicians tried to emulate hospital conditions in their private practice, it made sense that they would want to have the 'real' thing if possible.

Not that physicians were unaware of some of the problems hospital birth posed. Harold Atlee believed that as hospitals increased in number and as more women gave birth in them, interventionist obstetrics increased. He argued that hospital facilities gave physicians security to intervene more than they might have done in a home birth.[70] In 1937 the Committee on Maternal Welfare of the Canadian Medical Association agreed, stating in its report that:

> The inefficient hospital ambushes its patients with two sinister dangers: The first is cross-infection and is the inevitable hazard where the hospital organization does not ensure the complete isolation of each patient ... The other danger appears when the convenience of hospital equipment encourages injudicious interference and needlessly radical procedures. The hospital must undertake to protect the patient from both of these disadvantages and can do so with efficient organization.[71]

In 1939 the Dalhousie University Public Health Centre reported in a study of its home and hospital births that the latter had a much higher rate of low forceps births, which it attributed to the teaching responsibilities of the university.[72]

Besides the medical care, the human care received could be problematic in hospitals. When births switched from home to hospital, physicians had more control over who could be with the woman in labour. No longer did they have to put up with the presence of friends or even husbands. Marion Hilliard of Women's College Hospital would not allow husbands in the delivery room. She had done so once, and that unfortunate man had fainted almost immediately, necessitating one nurse to help him and forcing others to step over and around him in order to care for his wife.[73] Some institutions specifically prohibited husbands being present. Even when they did not, several women interviewed recalled that their husbands had no choice but to be absent – they had to stay home and take care of their other children.[74] By the end of the twentieth century, the situation had changed remarkably. Of hospitals surveyed in 1993, 99 per cent of those responding stated that they encouraged the involvement of the women's partner during vaginal births.[75]

While in hospital, many women worried about the well-being of their families and about the cost of their stay.[76] Given the limited number of hospitals in the early decades of the century, women had often travelled long distances, which was not only tiring for them but also limited contact with their families. On the public wards of some hospitals, patients were not allowed access to private physicians but were assigned to staff members. Thus, if they had had contact with a sympathetic physician during their pregnancy, they were not allowed to have him with them during birthing. As well interns, who did not have much practical hands-on experience, often delivered public patients.[77] Moreover, staff insisted that the woman wear hospital attire. The regulations of the Burnside Lying-In Hospital in 1906 instructed nurses and the house physician to undress the woman 'at once' and place 'her cast-off clothing ... in a receptacle, from which it is to be taken for fumigation.'[78] This regulation reflected class assumptions about unwed or non-paying patients. It also reflected the reality of the poor, who might not be able to maintain the same level of cleanliness as the more wealthy. Another problem was that while in hospital, women were isolated from people they knew. The staff could not spend time with them, and because there was no previous history between them there was more chance for emotional distancing. For unwed mothers, the social disapproval of their situation could result in a less than supportive environment.[79]

Irma Avery recalled that when she was in St Michael's Hospital, Toronto, her labour was very long and the hospital staff would not let her husband in the room, though they did allow a priest, whom she did not know and did not want. When Jennie Graham entered hospital for her first labour at the end of the period under review, she remembered telling the nurse at some point that something was wrong, to which the nurse replied, 'What do you know?' Graham had the wit to come back with, 'But it's happening inside me. I do know.'[80] Some physicians were sensitive to what it meant for a woman to lose control of the birth situation,[81] but other than acknowledging the problem they could do little to alter the procedures. Maternity homes on the prairies and elsewhere perhaps provided a happy compromise. They were able to give the physician a more controlled environment than a home without the institutional trappings of a hospital. Many women found the homes a woman-centred environment. They made friends during their stay and even years after could recall the women who were giving birth there at the same time. They laughed and cried together, supporting one another in good times and bad.[82]

Nonetheless, there were advantages for women in a hospital birth. Much in a hospital setting gave the patient the feeling that everything that modern medical science could offer was available to her. She had access to educated and trained personnel whose status was high in society. If giving up some control over birth to the medical profession was the price one had to pay for 'modernity,' many thought it was worth it. Canadians had developed faith in science, faith in a knowledge they did not have but which they believed physicians did. The locus of medical knowledge and especially the technology that facilitated use of that knowledge was the hospital. For many women, hospital birth meant painless birth.[83] With hospitals' sliding scale of charges, a hospital birth could even be cheaper than hiring a nurse and physician to oversee a home birth. In 1921 an Alberta farm woman decided on a hospital birth because her home was simply too crowded. After the Second World War, living conditions in many homes were even more crowded.[84] Such an environment was not conducive to the kind of care that physicians argued women deserved in childbirth. A hospital stay also provided rest from a woman's domestic responsibilities. W.W. Bauer in a 1945 article in *Maclean's* argued that a home birth 'takes more preparation in advance, and much of this falls upon the mother herself. It involves the necessity of getting help while the mother recovers. It requires arrangements for caring for the baby, who would otherwise be in the hospital nursery.'[85] While true, the habit of hospitals separating mother and child became a concern, and by the early 1950s some hospitals instituted 'rooming-in' policies to let the two stay together. Newell Philpott from the Royal Victoria Hospital, Montreal, held that rooming-in made a woman 'vitally aware that she possesses a baby.' It also allowed both parents to become accustomed to caring for the child. However, rooming-in was for a privileged few who could afford a room of their own. As Philpott noted, 'While the cries of their own baby did not disturb women, the cries of others did.'[86]

Despite the increase in hospitalization for obstetric cases in Canada and the support of physicians for it, long after the trend began physician support for home births could still be found. In 1931, for example, John W.S. McCullough from the Ontario Department of Public Health gave his blessing to home births in 'simple cases.' In 1934 Dr J.R. Dean declared in the *McGill Medical Undergraduate Journal*: 'There are no obstetrical cases that, with proper equipment, cannot be handled in the home of the patient with safety and with as good results as are obtained in the hospital.' In 1942 Percy E. Ryberg in his advice manual to women declared: 'Confinement should not be regarded as being a hospital affair, unless conditions are abnormal.'[87] What did occur however, was a narrowing of cases which physicians deemed suitable for home birth and an emphasis on home birth being surrounded by medical control through nurse and/or physician and medical technique. Some believed that first-time mothers who were older should be hospitalized, whereas others argued that all first-time mothers should be. A 1935 American text estimated that 25 to 30 per cent of childbirths required hospital care in order to ensure proper treatment.[88]

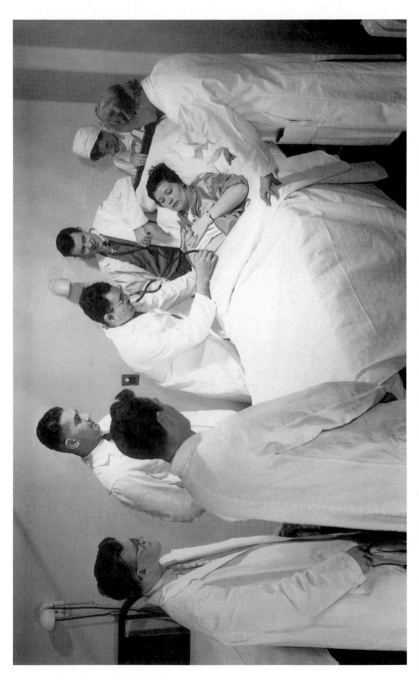

Medical education: medical students examining obstetrical patient; Dr Banting supervising, 1950.

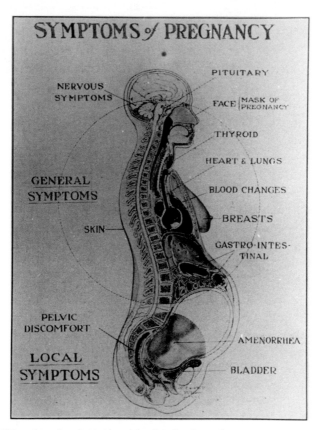

Fig. 70.—Diagram showing the wide distribution of symptoms which must be considered in the diagnosis of pregnancy.

Diagnosis of pregnancy was problematic in the early years of the century, and even thereafter.

Chatelaine's Baby Clinic

Conducted by
John W.S. McCullough, M.D., D.P.H.

No. 2. PRE-NATAL CARE

CLOTHING

The clothing of the expectant mother should be light and warm enough for the season. Underclothing should be changed frequently - once a week at least. The clothing should hang from the shoulders and not from the waist or abdomen. Corsets should not be worn after the third month. A maternity belt fitting firmly around the hips and under the abdomen may be used to suspend the stockings. Garters which impede circulation in the legs, and the elastic of knickers, should not be worn. Comfortable shoes with low, broad heels should replace the high-heeled ones in common use.

Physicians did not often discuss maternity clothing. Dr McCullough's advice was as extensive as any other medical suggestions concerning clothing.

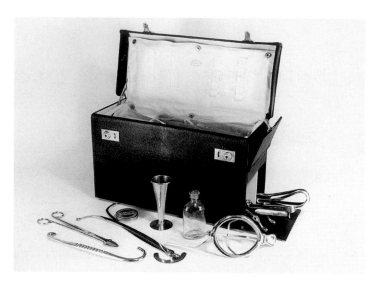

Obstetrical instrument case, 1940s. Contains rubber apron, surgical needles package, petroleum jelly canister, graduated bottle, midwifery strap, stethoscope, blunt hook and crochet, perforator, and pelvimeter.

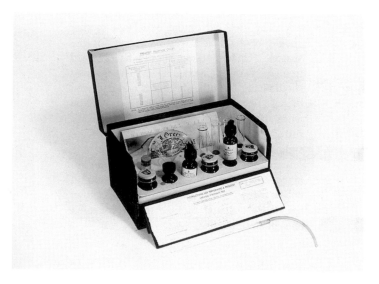

Pregnancy test by Bell-Craig Ltd., 1950. The accurate diagnosis of pregnancy was important for both the woman tested and the physician.

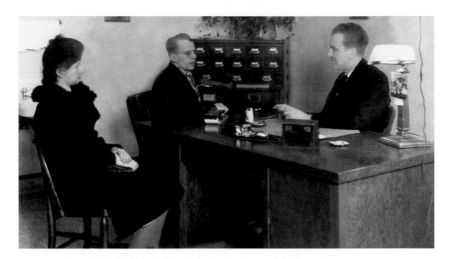

'The husband should accompany his wife on her visit to the doctor, at the beginning of her pregnancy, and obtain first-hand information' (Ernest Couture, *The Canadian Mother and Child* [Ottawa: Child and Maternal Hygiene, Department of Pensions and National Health 1939], 35). Couture's book was one of many advice manuals directed at pregnant women.

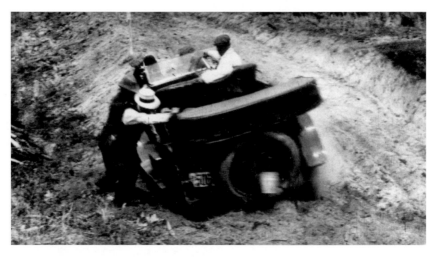

Car bogged down on the Cariboo Road, July 1914. The hazards of automobile travel in the early years of the twentieth century suggest why many doctors discouraged pregnant women from taking long trips.

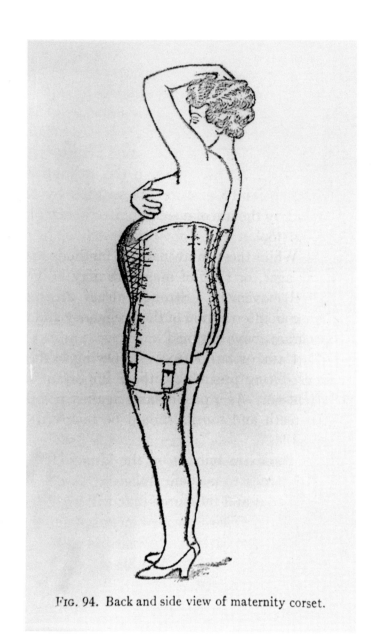

FIG. 94. Back and side view of maternity corset.

Some women liked the support a maternity corset gave them.

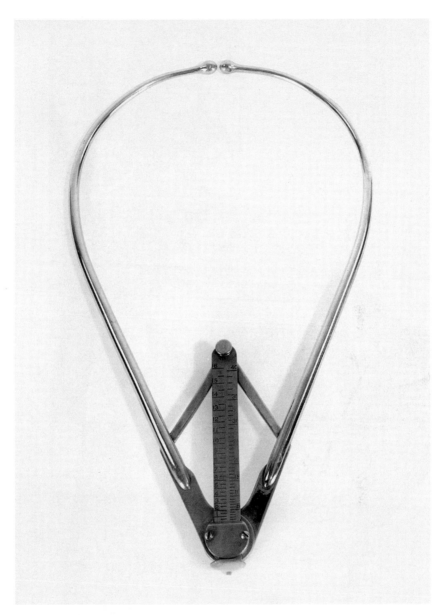

Carsten's pelvimeter, c. 1915. A pelvimeter helped the physician determine the pelvic dimensions in order to judge whether there was a disproportion between the size of the baby and the woman's pelvis.

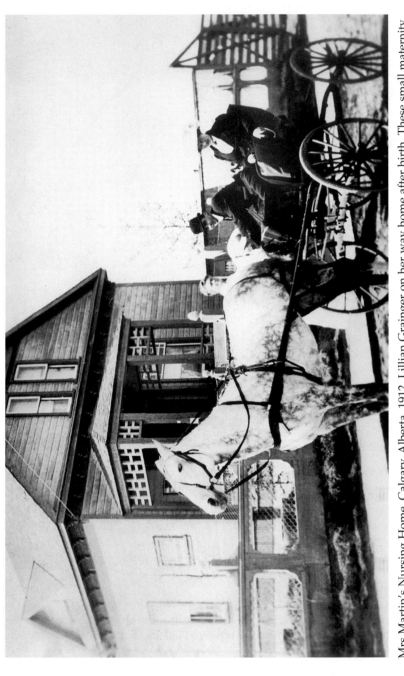

Mrs Martin's Nursing Home, Calgary, Alberta, 1912. Lillian Grainger on her way home after birth. These small maternity homes often combined the intimacy of home birth with the security of knowing that medical practitioners were available.

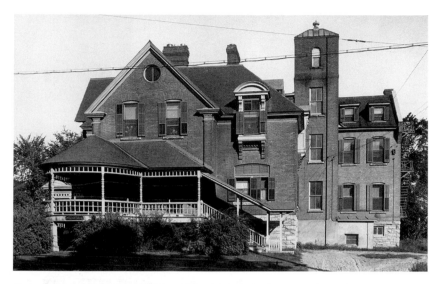

Ottawa Maternity Hospital, c. 1920. Although the size of medical institutions was increasing, particularly in urban centres, this hospital still has pretentions to a home-like atmosphere.

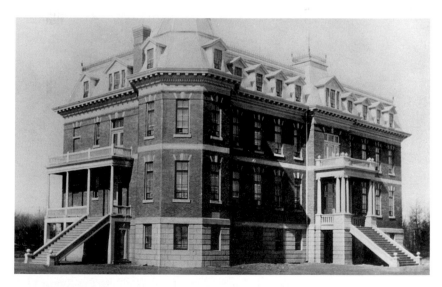

Maternity Hospital, Edmonton, Alberta, c. 1900–25. This hospital has a more institutional feel than Mrs Martin's Nursing Home.

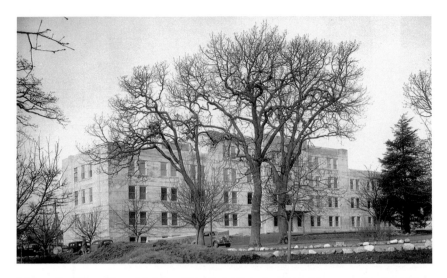

Maternity Wing, Royal Jubilee Hospital, Victoria, 1946. Compared to Mrs Martin's Nursing Home, the 'modern' maternity hospital could be overwhelming to the woman giving birth.

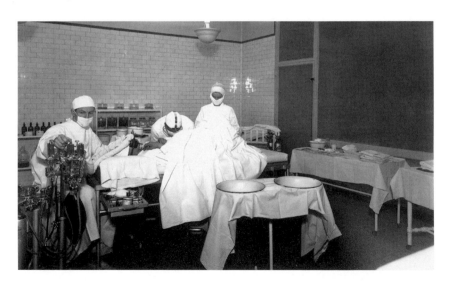

Hospital Delivery Room, Ottawa General Hospital, 1939. Note the concern for cleanliness. The atmosphere is obviously quite different from that of a home birth.

Controlling pain was an important part of medical midwifery. There was
extensive debate over what form of pain control was best.

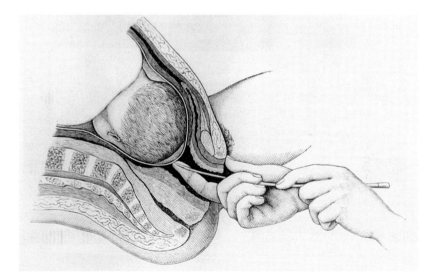

Instrumental puncture of the membranes. At times, the membranes did not
break on their own. In such cases, some physicians helped nature along, sometimes using their fingernail or, in this case, an instrument.

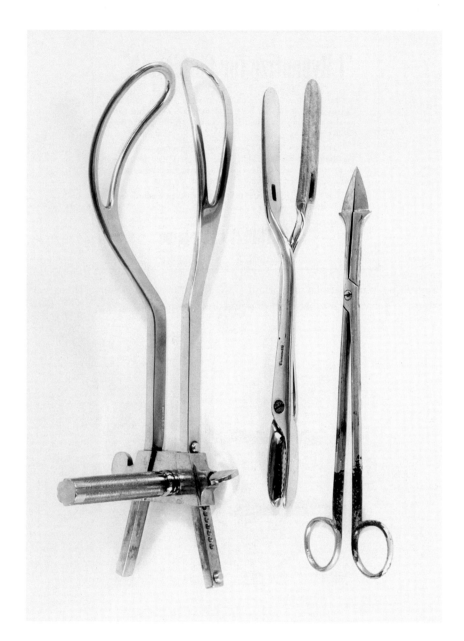

Various obstetrical instruments: (left to right) Mann obstetrical forceps, 1940s; Craniotomy forceps, c. 1915; Smellie's perforator, c. 1906.

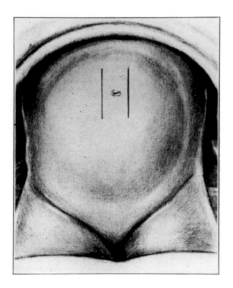

Classical caesarian section. The sites of incision in the abdominal wall.

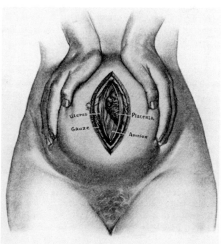

FIG. 1237.—CONTROL OF THE HEMORRHAGE IN CÆSA-
REAN SECTION BY THE HANDS OF AN ASSISTANT
GRASPING EACH BROAD LIGAMENT.

Caesarian section in the early years of the century was a dangerous operation.
As this drawing indicates, haemorrhage was a possibility.

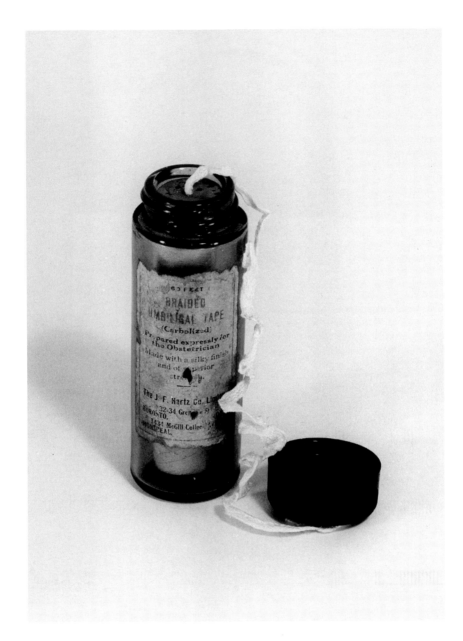

Braided umbilical tape bottle, c. 1930. Doctors used the tape to tie the umbilical cord before cutting it.

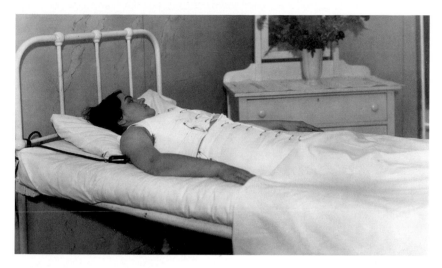

'Immediately after the birth the mother can be made more comfortable by means of carefully applied binders' (Couture, *The Canadian Mother and Child*, 63). Many physicians found the maternity binders of little use.

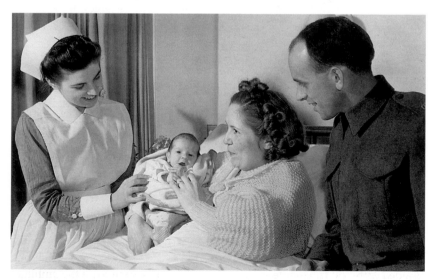

Obstetrical department, 1940. The happy result of childbirth.

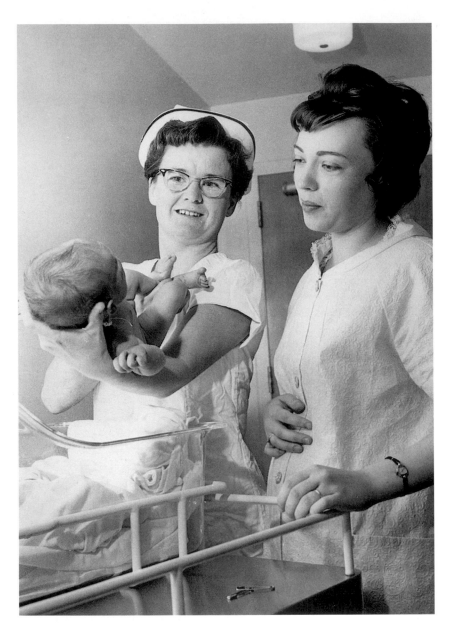

Nursery, 1950. A nursing instructor shows a new mother how to bathe her infant.

But what was proper treatment? Even for unproblematic births, the preparation was considerable. Birth has always been surrounded by extensive rituals and customs, no matter what the society or context. If there was any watchword surrounding hospital birth in the early decades of the century, it was cleanliness. Everything had to be clean – the woman, her dress, her bedding, the person who attended her, and any instrument used.[89] Doctors hoped such precautions would reduce the chances of infection. On entering a hospital, staff prepared the woman as if she was undergoing major surgery. First they bathed her and sometimes clipped or shaved her genital hair. In 1906 the superintendent of the Montreal Maternity Hospital recalled that some doubters had questioned the willingness of women to undergo the latter procedure but that when he explained the reasons to the women, they did not put up any opposition.[90] In a hospital setting, it would have been difficult for women, especially if they were charity patients, to oppose those in authority.

After the shaving, hospital staff sterilized the woman's genital area, often by scrubbing it with green soap and sterile water, using alcohol afterwards and then applying a towel soaked in a bichloride solution.[91] But it wasn't only surface cleanliness that was important. Physicians insisted that the women take some sort of enema so that they would not have a bowel movement during labour. This, they hoped, would lessen the chances of infection, as well as making the process less dismaying for both patient and physician. At the turn of the century, one physician recommended taking castor oil, which would not only clean out the large bowel but would help bring on labour. Some preferred a soapsuds enema, while still others were not specific, insisting only that some form of enema was needed.[92] There was also debate about douching. The superintendent of the Montreal Maternity Hospital argued that there was little evidence of its efficacy and maintained that streptococci were 'never normally present in the vagina'; but other hospitals, such as the Burnside, believed that a douche was helpful. After internal cleansing the woman was not allowed to use the toilet.[93]

Like the patient, the attending physician had to be clean and sterile. Surgeons had shown the way, and the medical literature encouraged obstetricians and others delivering children to ensure that their clothing was clean, and to disinfect their hands and wear gloves.[94] All this preparation was not limited to hospital births. In 1910 A. Edmond Burrows of Harriston, Ontario, gave an excellent summary of what physicians considered the optimum preparation in private practice:

> The Patient should be instructed to take a hot soap suds bath on the approach of labor. The bowels should be moved by a soap suds enema ... After the physician has given his hands the first scrub the pubes and vulva are shaved or clipped. The patient is then placed on a sterilized Kelly pad, and washed thoroughly with spirits of green soap ... The area is then flushed off with bichloride solution 1–4000 and covered by a sterile pad, wrung out of bichloride solution. The bladder is emptied, if necessary, by a catheter, using aseptic precautions. All superfluous clothing should be removed from the bed as these are usually filled with dust, and are a prolific source of infection. All drapery, curtains and table-covers should be removed for the same reason. A freshly laundered sheet is pinned over the mattress which should be hard. Frequently in the country a feather mattress has to be removed. The patient is covered with a freshly laundered sheet, the room should be warm enough so that this will be sufficient covering.[95]

It is unlikely that all these preparations were made, but Burrows presented them as what a good physician should do.

The increasing number of women experiencing hospital births in the interwar period and beyond received the standardized care that physicians in the medical literature had been urging. Compared with the earlier period, hospital instructions were less general and left little room for variation.[96] Shaving the genital area had become the norm, and enemas remained customary.[97] Obstetricians, disadvantaged in status compared with surgeons, focused on this issue as one that differentiated the two. W.J. Stevens, the attending obstetrician of Ottawa Civic Hospital, pointed out that the surgeon had 'a sterile operative field' on which to work whereas the obstetrician had 'an unsterile field,' having at times to deal with faeces and urine.[98] Private practitioners continued to emulate hospital techniques as the standard of good care. Recalling his rural northern Alberta practice, Alvine Cyr Graham made a point of mentioning the accommodations he had to make because of the conditions he found, but also his determination to proceed as much as possible as if the home birth were occurring in a hospital, especially with respect to cleanliness. Shaving or clipping genital hair were procedures that were also advocated in rural practice. Whether in hospital or at home, an aseptic birth was the goal. It had become one of the hallmarks of modern obstetrics and one of the advantages that physicians proudly pointed to when comparing the present with the past.[99] Winnipeg's Ross Mitchell detailed the ideal:

> To prevent infection from the patient, the vulva and lower abdomen are shaved, and these parts, together with the inner side of the thighs to the knee and the perinaeum, are washed with soap and water, then sponged with lysol, 1/200, or painted with alcohol and acetone solution of mercurochrome. Particular attention is paid to cleansing the folds of the prepuce of the clitoris. Finally the patient is draped with sterile sheets, leggings, and towels.

Mitchell then described the care which physicians at the Winnipeg General Hospital took over their own cleanliness: 'The hands and forearms are scrubbed with running water, soap, and a sterile brush, the nails cleaned with nail file or orangewood stick, and the scrubbing repeated, using a second brush. The total scrubbing lasts seven minutes. The hands and forearms are then washed in alcohol.' Both physicians and nursing staff wore gowns and masks to protect the patient from infection.[100] However, the clothing emphasized their separation from the patient even more. Nevertheless, the overwhelming emphasis on cleanliness may have had an appeal for women who were more than familiar with keeping their own households clean. They could translate the care they took in their homes to the care they would receive in hospital.

Physical and psychological support for the birthing woman was something that traditional birthing attendants understood. Among some First Nations, women physically supported the woman in labour.[101] This would have been impossible for Western physicians, who had to maintain a certain decorum because of their gender and training. They had to make the woman feel safe by other means. One turn-of-the-century textbook warned the attending physician not to add 'fear or despair to the suffering' of the woman. Whatever he might have to tell her relatives, 'he should, after his examination, give his patient the impression that all is satisfactory.' Throughout the birth, the physician should to remain 'quiet and confident,' and 'his manner, while firm, should be sympathetic and gentle.'[102] In hospitals this type of demeanor was more difficult to maintain. Adam H. Wright worried that modern hospital obstetrics was losing the art of caring and was focusing too much on the science.'[103]

In the years following the First World War, physicians continued to put forward a variety of ideas about what would keep a woman calm and encouraged. Most still deplored the idea of letting the patient have friends around, who might interfere and upset her. For some, the sense of security was not connected with what happened in the labour room so much as with the education that took place before labour, which assured women that childbirth was a joyous experience, not something to be feared.[104] Harold Atlee believed that letting women participate more would give them a sense of control and consequently reduce their tension. He advocated a more natural childbirth that emphasized a close relationship between patient and physician so that the woman would feel she was being cared for by someone sensitive to her needs. According to Martha Crosbie, one of Atlee's patients, he was successful. It was not just his support for natural childbirth that she admired but also his ability to explain what was happening and 'his enormous compassion for his patients ... plus his ultimate aim of giving childbirth the importance it deserved.'[105]

One complaint of modern critics of obstetrics is that physicians do not allow women to choose their position during labour and delivery. The accepted preference is for the woman to be on her back, a position more convenient for the physician than for the woman; indeed, it actually works against gravity and inhibits delivery.[106] Interestingly, a survey of Canadian hospitals in 1993 discovered that 63 per cent of those responding allowed women to choose their own position and that when they did, 62 per cent (mean) chose a semi-recumbent position.[107] As noted in chapter 3, variation in positioning existed in traditional society. Some women chose to sit, others to stand, kneel, or squat, or lie on their sides. Rarely were women on their backs. By the turn of the twentieth century, the position favoured in North America was for the woman to be on her back, although in Britain lying on the left side dominated. In Canada some adopted this custom. R.E. McKechnie of Nanaimo, British Columbia, for example, explained that the lateral position was of benefit for both the woman and the physician: 'To begin with, the patient is less exposed, and even the most unrefined woman appreciates attention to this detail. In using forceps everything is in favor of this position.'[108] However, most of the medical literature that Canadian physicians were reading and writing did not agree with him. J. Clarence Webster in his 1903 text acknowledged that there were some problems with the woman lying on her back – at times the placenta remained in the vagina as a result – but his solution was not to place the woman in a sitting or squatting position. Rather, his aim was to assist nature so that the woman could 'be delivered, in the highest states of civilization, in the recumbent position.'[109] Adam H. Wright admitted that with the woman on her back she was exposed more than she might wish, but he considered this a 'small matter when compared with the benefits to be derived.'[110] It is unclear how exposed the woman actually was. Photographs from early in the century show that women were heavily draped and not much exposure occurred. Wright might be suggesting that the woman felt more vulnerable on her back than on her side, particularly when her legs were strapped so that she could not close them.[111] Although aware that women in other cultures took differing positions, J. Clifton Edgar in 1907 stated that there was little to learn from them: 'Custom rather

than instinct appears to dictate the choice of these obstetric attitudes.'[112] He did not seem to appreciate the irony that the supine
position was culturally constructed as well.

In the interwar period and afterwards, the choice of position
narrowed further, at least, as reflected in the medical literature.
Fewer references were made to positions other than recumbent.
In the 1920s Dr Helen MacMurchy, when giving advice to neighbour women who were forced to stand in for a physician, advocated that the woman in labour be on her left side. Few of her
colleagues agreed – the woman on her back was the favoured
position in both North America and continental Europe.[113] Where
discussion about position did occur, it strongly rejected the squat
position. Paul T. Harper in his 1930 text stated:

> Gravity plays an insignificant part in dilatation. For this reason
> there is no advantage in keeping the patient about during the first
> stage. The upright position and walking about may *incite* contrac-
> tions; but they add in no way to their efficiency ... Rather, much
> walking about, premature straining and, especially, the pulling on
> straps divert blood from the uterus to the muscles of the legs,
> thighs and the back. By so much they *retard* labor. On the other
> hand, the dorsal position throughout labor conserves physical
> strength, makes it possible to keep the field clean, and it affords
> ample opportunity to palpate contractions and, therefore, to judge
> of actual progress being made.[114]

Nor was Ross Mitchell impressed by the squat position. He held
that in long labours it was exhausting and resulted in lacerations
and prolapse (ignoring the fact that many women lying on their
backs also suffered from lacerations and prolapse).[115] Alfred C.
Beck in his 1947 text made an interesting analysis of the traditional position that women took and why physicians rejected it.
He admitted that if left on their own, women would choose to
squat and that there were real advantages to this. For one, the
position provided support for the abdominal wall and allowed
the outlet to increase in size. He claimed, however, that the dorsal
position was introduced to maintain an aseptic routine. The in-

triguing point here is that he did not suggest making the squat position aseptic. Clearly, there were other reasons why physicians liked to place the woman on her back. It kept her passive and, as R.W. Johnstone made clear in his textbook on midwifery, it eased intervention and also monitoring.[116]

One aspect of birth carefully monitored was length of labour in its various stages.[117] The length of each stage could vary from woman to woman and from one pregnancy to another. Records of the Ottawa Maternity Hospital for 1896–1915 (4,674 cases) show that the mean number of hours in labour for the first stage was 11.98, with 0.25 the minimum and 96.0 the maximum. For the second stage 1.64 hours was the mean, with 0.017 the minimum and 36.0 the maximum. For the third stage 13.1 minutes was the mean, with 1.0 the minimum and 36.0 the maximum.[118] Clearly, the range for each stage was broad, but physicians were looking to establish a norm. Adam H. Wright in his 1908 text laid down his parameters: 'A labor has been unduly prolonged when it has lasted twenty-four hours or longer. The most serious protracted labors are those in which the second stage lasts longer than four hours. The dangers to both mother and child increase in almost geometrical progression (doubled each hour) as the hours roll on beyond this limit.'[119] Noteworthy about Wright's statement is the assurance with which he makes it and the trappings of precision that exist in it. Anyone reading it would assume that these were rules from which little deviation could occur without great harm to either the mother or the child.

For Helen MacMurchy in the early 1920s, the first stage of labour (from the discharge of blood-stained mucus to full dilation) could last from six to sixteen hours for a first child, although up to twenty-four hours was known; it was usually from two to twelve hours for any subsequent births. James Robert Goodall, obstetrician to the Homeopathic Hospital in Montreal, said in his 1932 text that no rule could pertain to all cases but that physicians were beginning to think that the second stage of labour should be shortened to a maximum of two hours.[120] On the other hand, G.C. Melhado, also from Montreal, recognized that while the average labour for a first-time childbirth was eighteen hours and for a subsequent birth twelve hours, 'it is equally true that many labours lasting a considerable longer time terminate spontaneously without any obvious deleterious effect on the child or mother.'[121] G.A. Hendry from Nova Scotia agreed up to a point: slow labour could indicate problems; as well, physicians had to respond to the fact that women and their families did not appreciate a labour lasting twenty-four hours, let alone forty-eight.[122] At times, however, a woman had to wait, not on nature but for the doctor. Two women interviewed who had their babies in hospital said that they were ready to deliver, but the nurses encouraged them to hold back – or literally kept their legs together – so that the doctor could arrive in time to deliver the baby.[123]

As this chapter has suggested, a variety of customs surrounded childbirth. Depending on who was involved in the birthing, we deem some natural, others superstitious, and still others scientific. Over the years being studied, physicians explored the tension between seeing birth as unproblematic or seeing it as potentially rife with difficulties. Most physicians acknowledged that the majority of births fell into the first category, but unfortunately they could not always predict which ones would fall into the second. But it is clear that many saw the percentage of unproblematic births decreasing over time. One reason they gave to account for this was the difficulties modern woman was experiencing in giving birth. Although she was able to exert her rights in many fields, her ability to give birth without trouble had apparently declined. This decline was also linked to factors such as race, class, and age. In making distinctions between women, physicians went beyond creating a binary and acknowledged the diversity among them, though they created a hierarchy of birthing ability which more often than not was inverse to a woman's status in society. Another reason was the higher standard being used to judge what an unproblematic birth was. The definition of the latter had emerged over years of record keeping, which helped form a normative model of childbirth. When there was an easing of that model, such as a willingness in the interwar period to entertain the ideal of older women having problem-free birth experiences, it reflected a belief in the advance of medicine that had enabled it and also in the security that the increased monitoring of birth had provided.

Once a normative model of birthing exists, the pressure is on physicians to develop a normative or accepted response to it. As long as childbirth remained in the home, they were less able to do so; however, hospital births increased significantly over time and by 1950 represented the vast majority of births. In the hospital, a doctor's wishes held sway more than in the patient's home. But we should not exaggerate the disadvantages of hospitalization or the advantages of home birth. Depending on who was there and the particular situation, home birth could be terrifying, just as hospital birth could. I have argued in this chapter that there is a danger in overromanticizing home births – they varied too much for generalization; and they could be as medicalized as any hospital birth. Nor should we assume that there was consensus among physicians about the preferability of hospital births. Well into the 1940s, some continued to argue that under a practitioner's care, home birth was safe.

Whether in home or hospital, physicians cared for their patients as best they could. Over time, the care became more uniform, less variable. Emphasis on cleanliness became more rigid and instructions more detailed. The position of the woman during labour was less open to choice. And the time of the various stages of labour became more precise. The result was that increasing numbers of women were having a similar birth experience.[124] The medical gaze focused on the body and how it acted, and it reacted, and it did so in a manner somewhat divorced from the specific person involved. Standardization led to a series of conventions and interventions – bathing, shaving, enemas – even for unproblematic births. For problematic births intervention became even more intense and for many physicians worrisome.

CHAPTER SIX

Obstetrical Intervention

The friends should be told that it is necessary to give a little help, a euphemistic way of stating that one advises the use of forceps. The patient need not be informed, and the friends should not be allowed to be alarmed about it. If they refuse to allow forceps to be employed the practitioner must unwillingly acquiesce, but if he has tact he will soon be able to persuade them to allow him to do what is advisable.

David Berry Hart, 1912[1]

One of the major criticisms of modern obstetrics is that too much intervention accompanies childbirth. But what would non-interventionist childbirth be like? The usual response is that it would be more natural. Yet as we have seen, a host of customs and activities surround childbirth no matter what the culture. The same is true of interventions, though they are of a different nature and degree. In Canada, medical practitioners have directed a range of interventions that are familiar to most of us. Pressured by time constraints, financial rewards, and patient demands, physicians have had to balance the dangers accompanying intervention against the consequences of not intervening in cases of problematic births. That there has never been unanimity about what to do and when is clear. Disagreement among physicians arose about examining women after labour had commenced, inducing labour, managing the pain of labour, using forceps, performing episiotomies, and encouraging the expulsion of the placenta. In examining each of these, several overarching themes emerge. First, doctors were not uniform in their perception of intervention and debated the pros and cons of various types. If, as some critics have suggested, doctors wanted to control birth through intervention, there was no unanimity about how best to exert that control. Nevertheless, the rational or scientific view of the body meant that physicians believed control was possible.[2] Second, no matter what intervention an individual physician advocated, it often led to others. There was a symbiotic relationship between specific interventions. Third, as the above quotation from Hart makes clear, intervention was not a matter of hospital as opposed to home birth; what distinguished interventions was not where they took place but who directed them. Compared with the interventions of First Nations people and midwives, those of medical practitioners were broader and more intense.

As we have seen, there were various beliefs about what was best for the pregnant woman in order to protect her well-being, that of her child, and her community. Because childbirth is generally without danger for most women, but not all, any culture will take steps to offset the dangers, to intervene in the natural process that the woman is undergoing. For example, First Nations people were concerned when the birthing process was too long, because it could exhaust the woman and place stress on the child. To help nature, the Dene placed a towel boiled in spruce-bough liquid around the middle of the woman and had her drink a herbal brew. These measures, they believed, encouraged a quick birth, helped with the afterpains, and loosened a retained placenta. Among the southern Kwakwa Ka'wakw (Kwakiutl), labour could be induced by drinking the juice of stinging-nettle roots. The Mi'kmaq believed that a special bone found in the heart of the moose, ground into powder and cooked in a broth, was good for the spasms of childbirth.[3]

In Western society, midwives also intervened. If the baby needed to be turned to a better presentation, some midwives would do so. Others were known for expanding the vagina in order to ease the child's emergence, while still others were willing to induce labour by giving the woman a dose of castor oil. One midwife related how in order to help the birth along she would push down on the woman's abdomen. For the afterbirth, midwives' interventions were very similar to those of Native people. For example, some made a brew from juniper bushes to help with the afterpains and rid the body of 'corruption.'[4]

Physicians knew that at some point in their careers they would have to intervene in childbirth, and much of their education focused on when and how to do so. The challenge was in distinguishing between preventative or curative intervention and 'meddlesome midwifery.' Physicians were well aware they were walking a tightrope. Yet as already noted, many believed that modern women needed their assistance; others pointed to the increasing number of older women giving birth as an explanation for intervening – older women simply experienced more childbirth complications.[5] These beliefs became part of 'the collective medical consciousness' and did not always 'warrant formal analysis of benefits, harms, costs, and outcomes.'[6] Consequently, meddlesome midwifery could be the result. Other factors also encouraged intervention, as the Toronto physician M.H.V. Cameron explained in 1919:

It is axiomatic that no one not possessed of patience and unlimited time for the case in hand, can practice obstetrics with the highest success. The busy man, with many calls to make, who takes a confinement as an interruption to his busy afternoon is less apt to practice 'a masterly inactivity' than he should be. The weak man who cannot resist the importunities of the patient or her friends is less apt to refrain from meddlesome measures designed to hasten a delivery that might otherwise complete itself if given time. The unfortunate man who, for want of training or experience, fails to recognize the normal, is more apt to become panic-stricken and seek to terminate labor by manual dilation of the cervix or by premature rupture of the membranes or other means not called for in the circumstances, were he but certain of his diagnosis.[7]

The time issue was important; linked to it was other business the physician missed because of the time spent with labouring women. Nor did the comparatively low pay that many physicians received for attending childbirth encourage patience. Intervention earned the physician more money. The more a physician did during birth, the more he could charge. At the turn of the century, private obstetrical practices revealed a stronger correlation between intervention (instrumental, hand, medicinal) and paying patients than for non-paying. The records of the Vancouver General Hospital for the years 1931 to 1941 did so too: more intervention occurred on private wards than on public.[8] Many physicians throughout the twentieth century argued that women and their families demanded a quick end to labour pains. In some cases, physicians simply became exasperated by the patient and wanted to end everyone's ordeal as quickly as possible. Such seems to have been the case with Lorna Moschini, who in 1901 at the age of twenty-two was giving birth to her first child at the Montreal Maternity Hospital. Her record states: 'Patient complained severely of pains would not assist in bearing down cried out loud with each pain showing plainly her neurotic character.' Her cries placed the physicians on edge. The result was a resort to chloroform and forceps.[9]

Medical literature warned physicians to expect the unexpected. This was particularly the case after the First World War, perhaps a reminder that despite the advances being made, childbirth could still be deadly. In 1931 L.C. Conn, professor of obstetrics and gynaecology at the University of Alberta, told his colleagues that disproportion was always a possibility. The lesson to be drawn was: 'We must consider every obstetrical case as a possible case of disproportion. Consequently, we should be on our guard at all times.'[10] Physicians reading this could take away the impression that it might be best to assume disproportion before waiting for it to be proved, and therefore to intervene. Similarly, the hyperbole surrounding any new advance in obstetrics not only informed physicians of what was happening in the field but also encouraged them to take advantage of it in the name of curative intervention. X-ray pelvimetry was an example. In 1948 A.H. Maclennan, in the *Alberta Medical Bulletin*, waxed eloquently about its use, which he called 'one of the greatest contributions to obstetrics in the past 10 to 15 years.' He assured his readers that the technical aspects of its application were now standardized and that physicians should use x-rays as an aid in deciding whether surgical intervention was necessary.[11] At the same time, the physicians who were concerned about intervention reminded their colleagues that any intervention increased the risks to mother and child. Some feared that although the graduate in medicine was warned about the dangers of interference, he had also 'been told of surgical obstetrical procedures which the tyro is eager to apply and which applied without the restraining influence that training and experience alone can give, are directly dangerous to the patient.' Patience was necessary in order to give nature a chance.[12] Summarizing the situation in 1951, F.B. Exner concluded: 'We have sold the public the idea the *most* medical care is the *best* medical care, a highly dubious proposition that even the doctors (who have the most to gain by believing it) are beginning to doubt.'[13]

While it is difficult to judge in hindsight whether or not intervention was necessary, we can determine what was occurring from the perspective of practitioners. In general, physicians estimated that most births did not need intervention. The *Annual Report of the Montreal Maternity Hospital* for 1914 recorded that in the external department (which handled women who birthed in their own homes), spontaneous births numbered 385 and 'artificial' births 27. Thus, 93.5 per cent of births required no intervention.[14] But these births were the ones predicted to be uncomplicated beforehand. In 1924 W.W. Chipman, professor of obstetrics at McGill University, reported:

The total number of confinements during the past year in the Montreal Maternity were: In the In-door Service 1,354. In the Out-door Service 379. Total 1,733 cases. Of this total, 1,536 patients delivered themselves spontaneously; and only 197 required assistance. This assistance took the form of forceps extraction in 172 cases, and a version and extraction in twenty-five cases. This mechanical assistance in the 197 cases represents a percentage of 11.5.

This is not so far from the general statement that 90 per cent of all deliveries are spontaneous, provided they are wisely left to themselves. It is true that within these figures are not included fifteen cases of Caesarean section, but as an offset to this, it is to be remembered that in hospital we deal with the abnormal and complicated cases.[15]

Even with the fifteen caesarean cases included, 87.9 per cent of cases were spontaneous. Although this was not as high as that recorded ten years earlier, it is still impressive. The lower number included both hospital births and hospital-directed home births; the former would have included women brought to the hospital from home because of complications. In 1939 the Dalhousie University Public Health Centre's prenatal clinic reported that over eleven years its home deliveries had been 98.5 per cent spontaneous and its hospital deliveries 86.9 per cent.[16] Hospitals took great pride in providing figures that emphasized the lack of intervention, though their definition of intervention was selective. For example, they might note forceps births but not always births in which anaesthesia was used.

Many hospitals and private practitioners did not have such high rates of non-intervention. Early in the century, Dr Almon intervened in almost 30 per cent of his private practice cases. In the 1930s the Vancouver General Hospital indicated that 28 per cent of its births were outside normal parameters.[17] It is often difficult to compare Canadian statistics with those elsewhere because the definition of normal/abnormal birth and what constituted intervention varied. But based on its own figures, between 1910 and 1921 a Boston maternity hospital saw intervention (forceps, version, caesarian section, mechanical induction) increase from 29 to 45 per cent of its deliveries.[18] In 1928 the intervention rate in a hospital in London, England, seemed comparatively low – 8.86 per cent – but it included only forceps use, caesarian section, and instrumental induction of labour.[19]

One type of intervention that raised concern in the early medical literature was physicians examining their patients too often during the first stages of labour in order to keep track of what was happening. Unless physicians followed aseptic precautions, hand intervention could be the origin of infection. It could result in damage to the mother and a slower recovery. Nor was it conducive to protecting a woman's sense of decorum or privacy. J.F.W. Ross, an associate professor of gynaecology at the University of Toronto, disagreed, especially with respect to the third stage. In the March 1900 issue of the *Canadian Practitioner and Review* he wrote:

> We are told that there must be as little examination with the finger as possible. We are told that the interior of the uterus must not be meddled with except on certain special occasions when it is indicated (whenever that may be). We are told that it is a dangerous doctrine to promulgate among students that, while the patient is anesthetized ... the finger should be passed up into a depressed uterus for the purpose of inspecting its interior. I believe that this teaching is all wrong and that there is no danger to the patient from the introduction of the aseptic finger into the puerperal uterus.[20]

His colleague at the University of Toronto, Adam Wright, vehemently disagreed with him and in the same issue of the journal penned a rejoinder: 'The chief aim of my life as a practitioner and teacher of obstetrics has been to fight against such methods. Fearing that the views of a man of Dr Ross' ability and position would carry sufficient weight to influence some young practitioners, I am entering this protest against the procedures which he advises.'[21] Such a strong personal response was unusual in Canadian medical circles, in which physicians tended to couch criticism in general terms and almost never directed it at a particular colleague. It reflected the seriousness of Wright's concern and his worry that Ross's position as a teacher would make his words more acceptable. But students needed to be taught, and at times teaching hospitals admitted that they examined women frequently so that students could learn.[22] While such procedures were educative, they also sent out a message that many doctors did not like. For instance, an editorial in the *Hospital, Medical and*

Nursing World in 1928 worried about hand examinations and the improper use of gloves.[23] But there were still those who seemed to follow Ross's earlier teachings. A 1940 text made the point with respect to the first stage of labour: 'Aseptic vaginal examinations performed by competent men in a good environment have not decidedly increased the morbidity, and the advantages obtained are a more detailed study of the fetal head.'[24] What physician was going to assume that he was not competent? However, by the 1940s, vaginal examinations had become rare; rectal examinations had taken their place.[25] Nonetheless, medical literature continued to debate the issue well into the late twentieth century.[26]

Version was another form of hand intervention. In consisted of shifting the position of the child to a more favourable presentation. Version helped in cases of disproportion or contracted pelvis, and some even argued that it could offset the use of forceps and shorten a woman's labour – and, as a corollary, benefit the busy general practitioner by saving him time.[27] In Dr Almon's turn-of-the-century practice, almost 70 per cent of his hand interventions consisted in turning the child.[28] Although the safety of the procedure improved, care still had to be taken because of possible rupture of the uterus when podalic version (turning by the feet) occurred after prolonged uterine contractions. Karl M. Wilson from Rochester, New York, worried that the wrong message was being sent. In a 1936 issue of the *Canadian Medical Association Journal* he explained that when leaders of the profession adopted intervention such as versions as a prophylactic measure, the average physician was liable to do so as well so as not to appear 'behind the times.'[29] Staff at Montreal's Royal Victoria Hospital agreed and in 1948 made a point of mentioning that the six versions and extractions done at the hospital were emergency procedures.[30] Nevertheless, some physicians favoured versions. A single doctor alone was the source of most of those done at the Vancouver General Hospital before 1933. When he no longer practised, the rate decreased significantly.[31] Dr Geggie's rural Quebec practice averaged a 2 to 10 per cent version rate a year.[32]

The purpose of intervention was to offset complications and maintain control over birthing. Nowhere was this more obvious than in the induction of labour when the physician made the decision that nature was not proceeding as it should. Some inductions were clearly life saving, for instance, when a woman was suffering from eclampsia and only a quick birth would end it. At times, however, the decision to intervene did not appear to be so medically necessary. For example, in the early decades of the century, physicians worried about a woman going beyond the expected term of her pregnancy. But how much beyond the expected term was too long? For most of the period under review, little accuracy existed in knowing the date of conception. Consequently, estimates of term were just that – estimates – and they could be woefully inaccurate. Dr Henry Langis's turn-of-the-century Vancouver practice revealed that the difference between expected date of labour and actual date (excluding premature births) varied from less than a day to as many as forty, the average being ten days.[33] Yet some physicians spoke out with authority, denying much leeway. In 1909 Adam H. Wright insisted that labour should be induced within three days 'after the patient has reached term as a matter of routine in all cases.'[34] He clearly believed that pregnancy had a definite term, that he knew how to calculate it, and that each woman had to conform to it. It did not seem to matter that there was no immediate danger for either mother or child, or that there was little obvious reason for a three-day period of grace rather than one, two, four, or more. His attitude revealed a potential repercussion of standardizing the experience of pregnancy – intervention. As well, it reflected some physicians' belief in the science of medicine – that the term of pregnancy could be calculated precisely (even if that was not the case). And it indicated the, at times, arbitrary nature of where a physician might draw the line between pregnancies that necessitated intervention and those that did not. Two years later, Wright addressed the issue in response to criticism received:

One of the objections raised is that we cannot always tell when the patient has reached 'term.' For instance, there may be evidence to show that conception has occurred, not shortly after the last menstrual period, but a little before the next period should have commenced. In such a case, or in any case of doubt, the accoucheur may obtain evidence by both external and internal examination which may assist him in arriving at a correct conclusion. If the matter still remains doubtful, it may be well to wait for one week before inducing labour. It is safer, however, to induce labour one or two weeks before 'term,' than two weeks after.

While Wright was now willing to wait a week rather than three days, his description still paved the way for intervention. Instead of responding only to a woman whose pregnancy had gone beyond term, he makes it clear that intervention before term is preferable. But since you cannot predict which pregnancies will go beyond term, all pregnancies became candidates for early induction. While Wright's confidence in his ability to calculate term correctly may have been comforting to students and patients alike, it was based on a faulty understanding of the female cycle and thus was likely to be incorrect – though Wright could not have been aware of this. Ironically, while Wright opposed Ross's hand intervention in labour, he is here advocating it in pregnancy in order to determine the date of conception. Thus, in order to know when to intervene (induce labour), other intervention became necessary. Wright certainly convinced himself. By the end of the article his earlier conciliatory stance has disappeared and he returns to his 1909 position 'that it would be well for both mother and child to make it an ordinary matter of routine to induce labour in all cases within a few days after term.'[35]

Physicians had specific time limits in mind with respect to each stage of labour, and they often found it useful to intervene to speed up labour. The urge to do so was partially a consequence of making comparisons between surgery and childbirth. Physicians were impressed that surgeons could keep their field of work sterile while the obstetrician had more difficulty. The fact that labour lasted from hours to days (if all the stages were taken into account) meant that obstetricians simply did not have the same kind of control over the birthing process that surgeons had over their cases. As well, speeding up labour limited the time women were in pain. The methods used for this and the induction of labour were often the same.[36]

Dilation of the cervix was a form of induction usually but not always resorted to after labour had begun. N. Preston Robinson of the County of Carleton General Hospital recounted in 1902 that at times the cervical dilation was a painful and tedious process, so he helped things along by dilating with his fingers, which he felt saved the woman hours of suffering. Helping along labour also led some practitioners to break the bag of waters, the amniotic sac (which one student physician at the Montreal Maternity Hospital did with his fingernail).[37] While Barton Cooke Hirst in his 1912 textbook described breaking the bag of waters, he made it clear that this should not be a common occurrence. In turn, Toronto physician M.H.V. Cameron condemned both cervical dilation and the breaking of waters as the response of a physician who was in too much of a hurry.[38] Yet some physicians continued to use one or the other procedure. For example, Dr Geggie favoured manually dilating the cervix to save time even in normal births, arguing that improvement on nature was part of medical practice. Speeding up labour would preserve the strength of the patient.[39]

At the turn of the century, R.E. McKechnie from Nanaimo, British Columbia, advocated the use of ergot to encourage labour if pains were weak. His attitude about its dangers seemed somewhat cavalier: 'If ergot can cause stronger pains, then use it, and pay little heed to the possibility of rupture uterus from tetanic contraction. In most cases it won't happen and if the pains do become too strong they could be controlled by chloroform and the birth brought to an end through forceps.'[40] As with Wright's combining hand intervention and the induction of labour, one form of intervention could lead to others. More popular than ergot was pituitary extract (pituitrin). The extract increased the intensity of contractions and prolonged them, thus shortening the intervals between pain. B.P. Watson, obstetrician and gynaecologist at Toronto General Hospital in 1913, noted that the extract's adoption had been swift and widespread and that such being the case doctors often used it indiscriminately. The best indication for its use was weak uterine contraction, but he considered that it was also helpful for 'size or malposition of the head, face and breech presentation, twin pregnancy, and minor degrees of contraction of the pelvis.' While Watson was willing to expand the indications for its use, he argued that it could offset other operative intervention.[41] S.P. Ford agreed, noting that since he had started using pituitary extract, his use of forceps had decreased significantly.[42] John Hunter of Toronto, on the other hand, preferred to use forceps rather than resort to ergot or pituitary extract.[43] Both ergot and pituitary extract were given intramuscularly, and once injected, their effect was difficult to control.[44] Nonetheless, only a few in Canada spoke out against it, and in many parts of the world the use of pituitrin was almost routine, especially in Cuba, Puerto Rico, South America, and Germany.[45]

Pituitrin continued to be popular in the 1920s. But it could be dangerous. Helen MacMurchy's report on maternal mortality in 1925–6 implicated the use of pituitrin in 21 per cent of maternal deaths, five of them for induction but most of the others for augmentation of labour.[46] Some physicians worried that too many manufacturers were making unsubstantiated claims for pituitrin and that their colleagues were overlooking the dangers of uterine rupture, being in a hurry and too busy to give nature a chance. Even *Chatelaine* got into the debate and told its readers that most Canadian physicians condemned its use.[47] Perhaps so, but some physicians continued to use it. Dr Geggie did so on a regular basis (see Figure 1) in combination with chloroform. Reacting against the criticism of the use of pituitary extract, M.T. Sullivan of New Aberdeen, Nova Scotia, made the bold statement in 1925 that he had used it in every case for the past fourteen years unless it was contraindicated by pelvic obstruction, and he claimed that he had yet to see a case harmed. As some others had in the past, he argued that it cut back on the use of forceps. Meanwhile, some physicians used other interventions to lessen their use of pituitrin.[48] So the cycle of intervention continued.

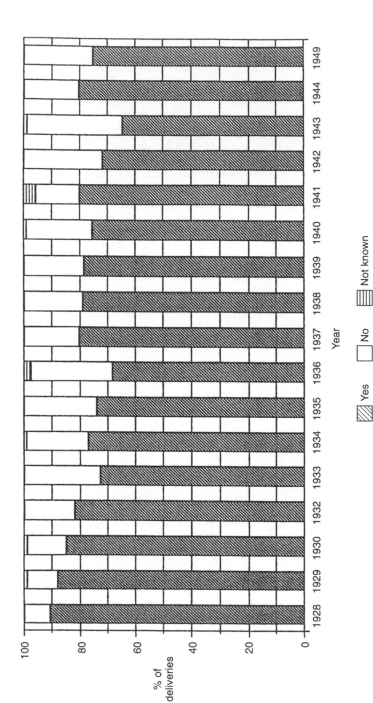

Figure 1 Pituitrin usage in Dr H.J.G. Geggie's obstetrical practice, 1928–1949

Source: Jayne Elliott, '"Endormez-moi!" An Early Twentieth-Century Obstetrical Practice in the Gatineau Valley, Quebec' (MA thesis, Carleton University, 1997), 173

Support for pituitrin to induce labour also continued. Trying to negotiate his way through the vast literature on it, Harry Beckman of Milwaukee in 1931 examined its use with reference to the teachings of Dr Watson of Toronto:

Despite the belief that pituitrin is dangerous when used to induce labor, a large number of physicians do so use it and apparently with safety. Since I fancy they have for the most part been emboldened to do so by the work of Watson, of Toronto, his latest report will be summarized here ... The indications for the induction in Watson's cases were pregnancy prolonged beyond the term, pregnancy toxemia and eclampsia, distress or discomfort before or at term, and antepartum hemorrhage, the greatest number coming under the first head. The question of true post-maturity of course is open to discussion, for, as R.W. Holmes well said once before the American Gynecological Society, 'We know not when pregnancy begins therefore we cannot definitely fix the day of confinement ...' A recent questionnaire sent out by Scott (1926), one of the Toronto group, has revealed the fact that Watson's method is being very widely used, but that there is almost unanimous opinion among those employing it that the originally proposed dosage is too large, and they either use smaller doses throughout or start with smaller doses and increase slowly. It was also shown that the procedure is occasionally followed by death of the infant, owing, for the most part, to the tetanic contraction of the uterus that sometimes follows the use of pituitrin.

Beckman believed that the dangers of pituitrin demanded more care: not only was there the danger of tetanic uterine contraction, but it could also result in premature separation of the placenta, fatal compression of the foetus, foetal asphyxia, deep laceration of the cervix, and rupture of the uterus.[49] G. Leslie Watts of the University of Toronto asserted that the Burnside Lying-In Hospital still used Watson's method of induction. But unlike Watson, Watts considered that induction for postmaturity was a rather hit-and-miss-affair, since it was almost impossible to know when the end of the pregnant term was – a fact he blamed not on the impreciseness of medical science but on the carelessness of women in keeping track of their last menstrual period. Even when postmaturity was established, induction was not the answer, claimed Watts, since it usually led to labour that was 'slow and unsatisfactory.'[50] For other physicians, however, postmaturity was still one of the more popular reasons for induction. A study of the Vancouver General Hospital in the mid-1930s revealed that private practitioners favoured induction for postmaturity more than staff physicians did.[51] W. Pelton Tew of London, Ontario, estimated in a 1940 paper that postmaturity occurred in one out of two hundred pregnancies and that it was more likely to occur among older women, women who had begun puberty late, women carrying a male child, and women leading sedentary lives. As well, 'women in winter [would] be more likely to go beyond term and women with low blood oestrin or high progesterone.'[52] The list of indications was expanding. Since there was little way of anticipating which specific woman would need induction, all were potentially at risk. And that was the problem. A study of five hospitals by Mr A.J. Wrigley of Guy's Hospital, London, England, revealed that 50 per cent of all cases of induction had occurred because of a mistaken diagnosis of disproportion.[53]

By the interwar period, physicians had begun to use thermal agents, or electrical and mechanical methods, to induce labour.[54] The mechanical means included packing the vagina and cervix with gauze, the introduction of a hydrostatic bag into the uterus, and the introduction of a catheter or bougie into the uterus.[55] In looking at the cases of induction by bag or bougie at the Montreal Maternity Hospital between 1923 and 1927, Walter Fletcher of Montreal determined that there had been 240 cases, 86 per cent by bag and 14 per cent by bougie. The indications for bag induction were toxaemia (including eclampsia, albuminuria, hypertension, and pernicious vomiting; 47 per cent), disproportion (20 per cent), and haemorrhage (including placenta praevia, premature separation of the placenta, and low implantations; 14.1 per cent). The bag inductions had a maternal mortality rate of almost 2 per cent and an infant mortality rate of nearly 23 per cent; in addition, maternal morbidity was 29 per cent. For cases induced by the bougie, no maternal deaths occurred, but infant mortality was 15 per cent and maternal morbidity 18 per cent.[56] The correlations that physicians made between various methods and outcomes were not to suggest cause and effect. Given the seriousness of the conditions of the women, this would not have been accurate. But they were warnings to one another that induction was a serious step to take.[57]

Physicians were appreciative of the value of induction in some cases. William Johnston recalled that when he first began his practice in Lucknow, Ontario, in the interwar period, a colleague called on him to help in a case of eclampsia. The young woman was convulsing, so the physician gave her chloroform and began dilating the cervix, first with one hand and then the other. Finally a six-pound baby was born, the convulsions ended, and the mother seemed to recuperate in the normal way. As Johnston recalled, it was 'a masterful performance.'[58] However, some worried that their colleagues were becoming too willing to induce labour for non-medical reasons. As Henri Guyot of the Winnipeg Medical Society observed, 'Today, it seems, induction of labor has almost become routine treatment in certain hospitals, mostly for the convenience of the patient or the doctor.'[59] Guyot's concern was understandable. Because of its dangers, critics feared the induction of labour in unproblematic cases. They accused physicians of being lured by the attraction of the procedure. As one critic noted, such births 'are at first sight spectacular and dramatic, and therein is their danger ... In a sense, they provide for the woman a vicarious labour, inasmuch as the obstetrician takes upon himself the main delivery ... No, this may be brilliant, but it is not safe obstetrics, and disastrous indeed, would be the result if these procedures were generally employed.'[60]

Nevertheless, induction remained popular. One physician interviewed recalled that in her early years of practice in the 1950s it was not uncommon for physicians to induce their patients two weeks before the beginning of the hunting or fishing season if their patients were near term. If the induction did not work, a caesarian was performed. But she added that at other times it was the patient herself who wanted the induction. Dr Marion Hilliard also induced to meet the desires of her patients – for instance, when a woman wanted to have her child on a special day. One of her patients recalled going to the hospital for an injured toe and, since she was near term, Hilliard gave her the choice of staying in hospital and having the birth induced rather than having to return in ten days' time, when the likelihood was that she would go into spontaneous labour.[61] That patients may have acquiesced in or even demanded intervention is not surprising. They did not remain passive throughout labour or in the decision making about it. This was especially true with respect to the use of anaesthesia.

Pain management was one intervention that appealed to physician and patient alike early in the century. The amount of pain a woman could endure depended on its severity and her own pain threshold. One Newfoundland woman recalled being in labour for four or five hours, at which point she had to send for the doctor, who used forceps to end the labour. Mrs Roy, age thirty-six, entered the Montreal Maternity Hospital on 15 March 1902, having previously had ten pregnancies – three full term and seven premature; all her labour had been difficult. In this case she had slipped and fallen on her back and had been in labour pain for approximately ten days. When the pain finally became too much to bear, she entered hospital and delivered twins. Ruth Howard recalled having been in labour for twenty-seven hours, during which time she was 'terrified,' since she had no idea what was happening, and no one had told her anything. Certainly, the pain, the length of labour, and not knowing increased her fear. Jane Rutherford remembered that she had entered hospital after her waters broke but had trouble bearing the pain and, in consequence, was given anaesthesia.[62]

Controlling the pain of childbirth had been a major breakthrough in the mid-nineteenth century, but the introduction of anaesthesia was not the end of the story. Early in the twentieth century, physicians kept searching for the perfect anaesthetic, one that would both eliminate pain and leave mother and child safe. From the physician's perspective, a pain-free patient was a calm patient, one more willing to take medical direction.[63] Some physicians even argued that anaesthesia might end racial suicide, the reasoning being that too many women limited the size of their families because of the pain they had to endure in childbirth. Less pain meant more babies. Using the same reasoning, others felt that it would cut down on criminal abortion.[64]

Physicians were sensitive to the issue of pain and the pressure placed on them by their patients to do something about it. Adam H. Wright described how he had explained to a woman who asked for pain relief that although he was quite prepared to give it, the child would be better off if he did not. He found that this advice was often enough to encourage a woman to persevere and endure the pain.[65] Some physicians agreed with Wright that anaesthesia was unnecessary in normal labours; others, not having been trained in its use, avoided it. The Burnside Lying-In Hospital, concerned about anaesthesia being used too frequently, directed the house physician not to use it without the permission of the attending physician.[66]

But these views were unusual. Most physicians were more than willing to give relief from the pain of labour. This approach was reinforced by the belief that modern woman could not bear pain as well as women had done in the past. Physician entrepreneurs publicized pain relief. Dr J.H. Dye, for example, advertised in the *Weekly Manitoba Liberal*: 'To WOMEN WHO DREAD MOTHERHOOD Information How They May Give Birth to Happy, Healthy Children Absolutely Without Fear of Pain – SENT FREE.'[67] Frederick Fenton of the University of Toronto was dismissive of those such as Wright who wanted women to endure pain stoically. Fenton contended that it would not help them physically and could be harmful: 'Long continued or oft repeated great pain invariably results in more or less shock and exhaustion.'[68] Joseph B. DeLee, in his popular 1913 textbook, went even further. While he no longer used anaesthesia in the first stage of labour, he did to the surgical degree (that is, giving the woman the amounts of anaesthesia a surgeon would use in order to operate) in the second stage. DeLee assured his readers that the patient usually woke up just after the child made its first cry.[69] DeLee never stopped to consider that perhaps the mother might want to hear the first cry of her child. While most physicians did not advocate DeLee's procedure, medical literature by the second decade of the century assumed the use of some kind of pain alleviation, usually consisting of whiffs of anaesthetic to get the woman through the most extreme pains (or, as physicians phrased it, giving the patient anaesthesia to the obstetrical degree). In 1914–15 hospital staff gave approximately three-quarters of the patients in the Ottawa Maternity Hospital some form of anaesthesia, either chloroform or ether. The records of the Kingston General Hospital are similar: more than 80 per cent of patients had anaesthesia between 1916 and 1920.[70] The issue for physicians was not whether but when to intervene and provide pain relief.

Discussions of what kind of anaesthesia to give became a major issue in obstetrics. Since none seemed to satisfy all needs, tradeoffs occurred. For example, one textbook at the turn of the century compared chloroform and ether:

> For mere obstetric analgesia chloroform is generally preferred. It has the advantage over ether that it is pleasanter; the necessary quantity, too, is less bulky, and is, consequently, more conveniently carried in the obstetric bag. On the other hand, it is not so safe as ether, and possibly it impairs the strength of the uterine contractions more than does the latter agent. It is a powerful vasomotor depressant and its too free use may paralyze the arteries and incapacitate the heart. Theoretically it is especially dangerous in the third stage of labor.
>
> For obstetric operations in which full narcosis is required, chloroform, as a rule, gives place to ether. By some obstetricians the latter anaesthetic is preferred for general obstetric use. It is not less manageable than chloroform for all obstetric purposes, and, as its advocates believe, it does not weaken, but rather stimulates, the uterine contractions.[71]

How was a physician to make a decision? If he chose chloroform, the contractions would decrease in intensity and prolong the labour, which might encourage him to intervene in other ways.

Yet chloroform was easier to carry and 'pleasanter' for the patient. As Everett S. Hicks from Port Dover, Ontario, pointed out, chloroform was the anaesthestic of choice for a country doctor. Nonetheless, by the second decade of the century, ether was becoming increasingly popular in unproblematic births, as well as in cases where forceps were used or caesarean sections made.[72]

Physicians kept trying different types of pain relievers, looking for the elusive perfect one. Among those mentioned in the medical literature were chloral hydrate, opium, heroin, and morphia alone or in combination with hyoscine. A combination of nitrous oxide and oxygen attracted many advocates. Claims for it were impressive: some deemed it safe to use throughout the entire labour, easy enough for a nurse with little training to control; or the patient herself could administer it with the proper machine. It had no harmful effects and even obstetric operations could be performed under it. The only contraindication was threatened rupture of the uterus.[73] It appeared to be the elusive perfect anaesthetic. Unfortunately it was expensive.

Anaesthesia had an intimate and symbiotic relationship with other forms of intervention. Some procedures necessitated its use. For example, physicians felt that the use of forceps required it, even to the surgical degree. In turn, its use often necessitated intervention. Chloroform could reduce contractions, and this in turn led to the use of forceps to put a stop to what had become a tedious and oftentimes dangerously prolonged birth. One Toronto physician worried that with the increased use of anaesthesia, inexperienced doctors were more prone to curettage in the third stage of labour, since they knew they were not going to cause the woman pain.[74] Anaesthesia could also control the dangers of other procedures and encourage their use even more. R.E. McKechnie from Nanaimo, British Columbia, told his colleagues in 1901 that ergot could speed labour that was taking too long. Acknowledging that ergot could result in excessive contraction and the rupture of the uterus, he comforted them by pointing out that the use of chloroform would control 'excessive action.'[75] But it could also prevent dangers such as the convulsions of eclampsia.[76] Anaesthesia, then, could relieve the woman of the pain of birth, it could allow for life-saving intervention, and it could also encourage and even cause intervention.

Many of the issues of concern to physicians in the early decades of the century continued, to preoccupy physicians in subsequent years. Older forms of pain management continued, and newer ones were added. Chloroform and ether remained popular, although the effect of both (especially the former on the liver and kidneys) tended to limit their use to the operative degree.[77] Chloroform seemed more popular in England, whereas ether reigned in the United States.[78] The list of what was available kept getting longer: chloroform, ether, chloral, opium, morphine, nitrous oxide, cocaine (applied locally), morphine-scopolamine; pantapon, heroin, and vinyl ether, etc. But none was perfect. Betty Lawrence reported having undergone hypnosis.[79] Physicians could be found to make claims for each. H.J. Shields of Toronto insisted that pride of place went to nitrous oxide.[80] W.J. Stevens of the Ottawa Civic Hospital argued: 'Undoubtedly the greatest advantage made in obstetrics in recent years is the perfection of rectal synergistic analgesia ... intramuscular injections of morphine and magnesium sulphate and colonic instillations of an ether mixture, given at the commencement of real labour.'[81] As Stevens's statement reveals, the challenge was deciding not only what to use but which combination. In the first stage of labour, doctors at the Burnside Lying-In Hospital often used heroin alone, or in combination with sodium amytal or nembutal if they deemed a more powerful sedative advisable. In the second stage of labour, they gave a choloroform and ether combination.[82] In the United States such a 'cocktail mix' of anaesthetics essentially put the patient to sleep until after the birth.[83] Canadian physicians did not seem to go that far, at least not as a matter of course. But whatever the focus, the medical literature is replete with articles by physicians relating their use of new, old, or combination pain relievers which they felt they had discovered or rediscovered.

The search for the perfect pain reliever continued. Caudal analgesia became quite popular in the 1940s. It did not cause the woman to lose consciousness or control over her muscles, and reports claimed that labour was shortened and that the children born were more active.[84] Stories of its success appeared in popular literature informing women about its benefits so that they could ask their physicians for it. In the 5 June 1945 issue of *Saturday Night*, Anne Fromer introduced it to her readers in an article entitled 'Childbirth without Pain.' She told of a husband coming to see his wife after she gave birth: '"Hello darling," he whispered in a sickroom undertone "how are you feeling?" His wife laughed and took a large bite of toast and marmalade. "Much better than you look," she said. "A day's shopping tires me a lot more than this."' Yet caudal anaesthesia was not without difficulties. Fromer noted that a physician had traditionally been able to check on the progress of labour by the degree of pain being experienced and, in consequence, go about his other duties until needed. With caudal anaesthesia, because the woman was not experiencing pain, the physician had to stay waiting for the birth to occur; in wartime few physicians in civilian life had the time to do this.[85] Unlike the popular press, the medical press was more cautious in its endorsement. One Montreal physician insisted that keeping the mother awake was a disadvantage – if she gave birth to a deformed child she could not be prepared for the shock of seeing it.[86] In addition, caudal did not work on all women; it was time consuming to administer; and eventually it was acknowledged to have resulted in some maternal deaths.[87]

While the use of so many anaesthetics and analgesics (drugs that relieve pain) seemed to have a frenetic quality, one medical commentator remarked that the multiplicity of agents represented 'praiseworthy zeal,' although he admitted that this also revealed that the perfect pain reliever had yet to be discovered.[88] And as Maxwell Yates pointed out in the *Alberta Medical Bulletin* in 1950, many of them had only localized popularity. 'Nothing has been developed to displace the generally used ether and chloroform as it was in use in the days of Queen Victoria,' added Yates, though he reported that at the University Hospital, Edmonton, they had used something called trilene in 600 cases with satisfactory results.[89] Making one's way through the array of pain relievers was not easy. Physicians warned one another to fit the specific drug to the specific patient.[90]

Some attempts to find the perfect anaesthetic had unfortunate repercussions on the woman and child. Two Edmonton physicians related their experience in giving a combination of nembutal and paraldehyde, with the possible addition of more nembutal. They comforted their readers by saying, 'The adverse result of any restlessness that may occur [after delivery] is obviated by two measures. Side boards, 12 inches high, are placed on the bed, to be left for 12 hours, and a restraining sheet, 12 inches wide, is placed both under and over the patient's chest and tied to the sides of the bed, in such a manner that while she may lie comfortably on her back and turn to either side she cannot rise up sufficiently to fall out over the sideboards.' Just in case anyone was concerned about the child, these two assured them: 'It is our conclusion that these sedatives do not increase the incidence of fetal mortality. The babies are rather sleepy for 24 to 36 hours after birth, and may at first not nurse well.'[91]

Despite the problems connected with choosing the right agent for pain relief, physicians deemed the advent of anaesthesia a major advance. It certainly reinforced the view of the physician as hero – he took pain away. One psychology book, designed specifically for medical students, stated that the refusal to give anaesthesia was 'a sadistic impulse to inflict pain and witness suffering.'[92] As in the earlier period, a few physicians hoped that alleviating the pain of childbirth would encourage women to have more children, and some even suggested that puerperal insanity would decrease, since fear of pain often brought on the mental suffering that caused it.[93] Few women would have disagreed about the benefits of pain relief. Alma Miller from Carlyle, Saskatchewan, recalled that during the difficult birth of her child in 1946 she was given anaesthesia: 'Don't ask me what happened after that. All I know is that I came to and there was a little white faced baby there! And I was glad for it.'[94] One physician remembered his French Canadian patients pleading, 'Endormez-moi!' Yet some studies have suggested that some women had mixed feelings about its use.[95] It could take away from their birthing experience. Childbirth was not something Esther Thomas remembered fondly. She was in labour for three days and no one bothered to tell her what was happening. Finally, doctors gave her anaesthesia and when she woke 'presented' her with a child. In addition, her face was burned as a result of the anaesthesia.[96]

Anaesthesia remained part of normative childbirth in Canada, although one nurse made it clear that elsewhere this was not the case.[97] The records of the Nickle Pavilion of Kingston General Hospital reveal that anaesthesia was used in more than 90 per cent of cases by 1929 and 97 per cent by 1940.[98] The maternity homes of Saskatchewan gave most of their patients anaesthesia. The only exceptions were those where non-nurses were in charge of the birthing.[99] Women who had home births did not receive anaesthesia quite as often. Dr Walmsley's practice in Prince Edward County, Ontario, in the 1920s had only a 20 per cent rate of chloroform use.[100] But many physicians who still delivered women at home tried to keep up with the latest advances. A.B. Campbell from Bear River, Nova Scotia, reported in the *Nova Scotia Medical Bulletin* that until September 1930 he had used only chloroform or ether in labour. However, in 1931–2 he gave fifty-five of his patients hyoscine, and between 1932 and 1934 he gave sixty-one nembutal and hyoscine. He noted: 'Following the Refresher Course, when Dr. E.K. Maclellan gave us the full technique for using rectal ether, I attempted to use that method. I found it impossible to get even fair results unless I had a trained nurse on the case, or else went early and stayed with the patient until the labor was terminated ... In June, 1931 I read an article by Dr. Ashbury Somerville, on the use of hyoscine-hydrobromide alone to produce amnesia in labor ... A few days after I read Dr. Somerville's paper, I used his method.' Another general practitioner told his colleagues of the success he had had with lumbar anaesthesia.[101] Dr Geggie of Wakefield used pain relievers on a regular basis during the first stages of labour. In addition, he used an anaesthetic to counter the uterine stimulant he gave many of his patients in the hope that the balance would encourage rapid delivery with minimal trauma. Altogether, he used an anaesthetic in over 80 per cent of his cases[102] (see Figure 2). These

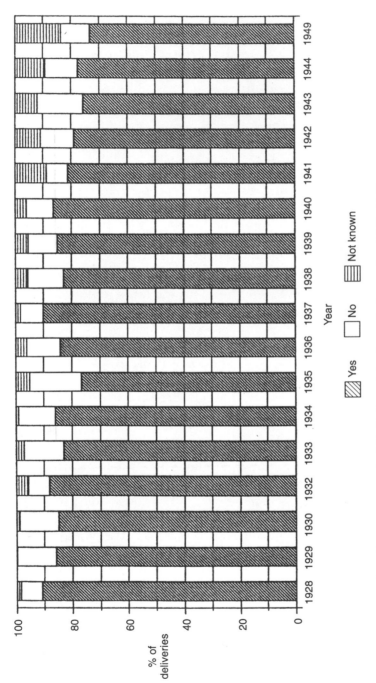

Figure 2 Chloroform usage in Dr H.J.G. Geggie's obstetrical practice, 1928–1949

Source: Jayne Elliott, '"Endormez-moi!" An Early Twentieth-Century Obstetrical Practice in the Gatineau Valley, Quebec' (MA thesis, Carleton University, 1997), 172

and other examples reveal that pain alleviation occurred in all types of practice and that physicians could very quickly take up most of the new forms of anaesthesia.

The idea of painless childbirth kept being reconfigured. In the years after the Second World War, some physicians took an interest in natural childbirth, by which they meant pain management without anaesthesia. While natural childbirth emphasized the woman managing the birth, it was essentially physician directed and controlled. Nonetheless, it represented a different orientation toward birth; and those, such as Harold Atlee, who were among the first to introduce it were rightly proud of doing so. For Atlee, it was a way of giving birth back to the woman.[103] Most of the references to natural childbirth in the interwar and immediate postwar years refer to the system developed by Grantly Dick Read in his book *Childbirth without Fear*.[104] Underlying Read's theory was the belief that fear caused tension and that tension caused spasm in the cervix, resulting in pain. The goal was to encourage women not to fear childbirth and its pain. A very close relationship between the physician and the patient over the period of the pregnancy was necessary so that the patient would understand what was happening during birth. She had to be trained. It necessitated the patient's trust in her physician and the willingness of both physician and patient to spend time with one another – something not always possible. The physician was often too busy with his practice, and many women could not afford to pay for the time. Nor did the results of Read's method impress everyone. Even Atlee believed that natural childbirth could not live up to the claims of pain relief made for it. Mary Percy Jackson, when discussing her work among Métis women, pointed out: 'Whatever Grantly Dick Read may say, most women, even half-breed Indians, welcomed analgesia through the second stage, and the old women, watching their granddaughters have their babies without pain, are enthusiastic for the method.' Some who were enthusiastic about Read's method thought that at the moment of birth a local anaesthetic helped.[105] Others, however, were less than enthralled with having their patients awake during childbirth. One doctor who encountered a woman using the

Read method recalled: 'I walked in and this woman was lying on the delivery table perfectly relaxed and calm. I figured either she was full of sedatives or had no business being out of the labor room, but when I examined her I discovered she was in the last stage of labor. She argued about it, but we gave her gas and put her down right away.'[106] He clearly was unable to cope with an alert patient.

One of the most fascinating episodes in the history of anaesthesia was that of twilight sleep, the use of a scopolamine-morphine combination. The morphine lessened the sensation of pain and induced a light sleep, while the scopolamine produced amnesia. Introduced to the medical world in Germany between 1902 and 1906, it reached its peak of popularity in the second decade of the twentieth century and then faded. American women especially were attracted to it as a result of it being described in the popular press. There was even a Twilight Sleep Association in the United States.[107] In Britain doctors did not engage in it much, except in nursing homes or for middle-class women.[108] Some historians have seen twilight sleep as an example of the success of patient demand – but if it was, the success did not give the patient much power. As a modern analyst has commented, 'It strengthened the position of the male doctor in the delivery room, it fortified the idea that advances in the management of childbirth were dependent on science, and it underlined the notion that in modern times childbirth should take place in hospital and not at home.'[109] While there is little evidence that doctors followed it very much in Canada, literature on it certainly existed.

Adam H. Wright made one of the earliest references to it in 1909. In an article that reviewed obstetrics over the preceeding decade, he noted: 'Many of us have used the combination of morphine and hyoscine (or scopolamine) with varying results.' He did not think it was applicable to private practice but felt that in future it would have a significant place in obstetrics. Four years later he had basically rejected the combination.[110] In the early months of 1915 the *Canadian Practitioner and Review* printed a series of articles by Drs Gordon Gallie and W.A. Scott analysing the use of twilight sleep in the maternity wards of Toronto General Hospital. While twilight sleep actually eliminated the memory of labour pain for 60 to 70 per cent of women, Gallie and Scott warned of specific problems: on the general ward service of a large hospital, many women entered too advanced in their labour for the morphine and scopolamine combination to be used; in addition, the staff was often too busy to give the 'prolonged personal attention' necessary. Their conclusion was that 'the method is proper in general practice ... where the finances of the patient permit the transfer of a complete working force to her room for the entire duration of labor.' Since the physician had to individualize treatment for each patient and remain with her throughout, most physicians found its use impractical. In the October issue of *Canada Lancet*, Gallie and Scott were more positive. The advantage of twilight sleep from their point of view was that it provided women in the first stage of labour with pain relief that was traditionally given to women only in the later stages. They also maintained that women recuperated faster after twilight sleep than otherwise. Since twilight sleep necessitated patient cooperation, they argued, 'better results [were] obtained in private practice among the more intelligent type of women.' The second stage of labour was often lengthened, they noted, but physicians could offset this with a 'small injection of pituitary or a little pressure on the fundus.' Thus, intervention led to intervention, though Gallie and Scott said that with some patients twilight sleep obviated resort to forceps. They also warned that as a result of its use, some babies showed oligopnoea (hyperventilation) and asphyxia, but a hot bath could overcome both. The caveats regarding twilight sleep were significant. Their conclusion: 'We do not think that the method should be commercialized by promising it to any particular patient who asks for it. We simply tell our patients that if suitable cases they will be given it.'[111] Gallie and Scott were not the only ones trying twilight sleep during these years. J.A. Kinnear of Toronto did so and argued that a competent nurse could supervise it so as long as the physician was close by in case labour advanced faster than anticipated. Similarly, Gordon G. Copeland of Toronto Western Hospital stated in May 1917 that he found it valuable 'where indicated' but that he really preferred nitrous-oxide-oxygen.[112]

Doctors did not seem to be as enamoured by twilight sleep as the popular press and many women were. An article reprinted in the 1915 *Canada Lancet* pointed out that the non-medical literature on it was one-sided and could not be trusted; scientific articles were more balanced, and their conclusion was that twilight sleep hindered labour and adversely affected the respiratory ability of the newborn.[113] Many physicians dismissed it as a fad demanded by women 'in the so-called higher circles of life.' It appealed to the commercialism that many did not like to acknowledge was part of medicine. The fear was that any inexperienced physician who promised this 'painless labor' could find himself taking the place of 'the most experienced physician who refuses to imperil his patient's safety.' Moreover, these inexperienced physicians could charge from five to ten times the normal fee.[114] In 1916 J.W. Duncan, assistant obstetrician at the Montreal Maternity Hospital, tried to minimize twilight sleep's innovative appeal by pointing out that trying to obtain amnesia was not new in obstetrics or in medicine in general. He did not reject it out of hand, however, but discussed which women were the most suitable candidates; he concluded that the primiparous were, because their labour tended to be longer, giving the drugs time to work. Like Gallie and Scott, he stressed the importance of having a skilled obstetrician at hand and the need for each patient to have individualized and constant attention. His final conclusion was that investigation into twilight sleep should at least continue.[115] Despite this call, its critics were gaining the ascendancy. The American literature reprinted in the Canadian medical press was largely negative, and the Canadian literature also was moving away from twilight sleep. While there would still be people dazzled by twilight sleep who would continue to use it, the consensus of much of the medical press was that it was a fad whose day had gone.[116]

In the interwar period, when twilight sleep was mentioned it was often as something physicians had tried and found wanting; or it was listed as one response among many that physicians could offer women in childbirth. Harry Oxorn thought that after the war women began demanding painless childbirth in larger numbers but noted that twilight sleep became a generic term to represent the giving of opiates, barbiturates, or rectal ether.[117] Commentators treated the morphine-scopolamine combination itself as a passing historical fad. In 1924 Wesley Bourne of the Montreal Maternity Hospital noted that staff had not used twilight sleep for a long time.[118] But even with the general dismissal, there were still references to it from time to time. Ross Mitchell of the Winnipeg General Hospital, while not endorsing it for general use, pointed out that it was more effective than morphine alone and that it was better suited for hospital than for home births.[119] Others focused on which women might benefit from it: women pregnant for the first time, those who had flat pelves, or those who were 'neurotic and frightened.'[120]

Whatever the form of pain relief, the relationship with intervention and the medicalization of birth was at times clear. As an American physician openly acknowledged in the *Canada Lancet*, anaesthesia had 'acted directly and positively toward the development of the art [of obstetrics] itself by making possible manipulations and procedures which were before impossible or unthought of.'[121] Some pointed to the increased use of forceps as a result of anaesthesia; still others, the increased use of episiotomies and even caesarean sections.[122] But impact was not always a one-way street. Ross Mitchell, for example, advocated an injection of morphine and with scopolamine when labour became bogged down. His hope was that by giving the woman a chance to rest and sleep, she would better bear the pains of labour and that this would lessen the pressure of family and friends for the physician to use forceps to end labour quickly.[123]

While anaesthesia may have obviated the use of forceps in some cases, forceps almost always necessitated (for humane reasons) the use of anaesthesia. The indications for forceps use were many. In 1901 at the Montreal Maternity Hospital, there were 7 forceps cases out of a total of 229 confinements, or 3 per cent, for the following reasons: neurasthenia, contracted pelvis, bony tumour, arrest in cavity, and arrest at outlet. Some physicians argued for forceps use only when the cervix had been dilated for two hours or in prolonged labour. Others insisted that in premature births, forceps could act as a way of protecting the 'soft fetal head.'[124] Advocates referred to it as the 'most valuable though most dangerous instrument.' The author of an article in the March 1918 issue of the *Canadian Practitioner and Review* preferred forceps over drugs: the reactions to the latter were too individualized to be predictable.[125]

Despite the long history of forceps use, at the turn of the century it was a procedure that some still viewed as unusual and needing explanation.[126] Lapthorn Smith of Bishop's University argued that forceps had saved hundreds but also had killed or maimed thousands. He accused physicians of being too anxious to put an end to labour – their fee was so low that they could not afford to spend the time waiting for nature to take its course.[127] While acknowledging the dangers in their use, Frederick Leavitt of the University of Minnesota said that Smith was exaggerating and that as long as the physician took aseptic care, forceps were safe.[128] However, Leavitt was taken to task for raising the question 'May we not safely use the forceps in every case?' K.C.M. responded to this in the *Canadian Practitioner and Review* of 1903: 'We do not like the nature of this question. Physicians should not aim at demonstrating what they *may* do or what they *can* do, but rather at what they *ought* to do in the interests of the patient.'[129] Joseph DeLee criticized physicians who used forceps in order to save a woman the pain of the second stage of labour. The attending physician should allow the woman to make a trial of labour and only when this proves impossible should he use forceps in otherwise normal births. Yet DeLee himself was a great believer in the use of outlet forceps. He used scopolamine in the first stage of labour, waited for the cervix to dilate, then gave the patient ether, did an episiotomy, and lifted the foetus out with forceps.[130] Some physicians connected the high rate of maternal mortality to forceps use, especially in high forceps births when the head was 'not engaged in the brim.' Others felt that too many of their colleagues ignored the dangers because they did not see the 'stretching and tearing' caused by the forceps and simply comforted themselves that their patients did not die.[131] Worried about the dangers inherent in their use, the Burnside Lying-In Hospital forbade its house physician to use forceps without the permission of the attending obstetrician.[132]

What was the rate of forceps use? At the turn of the century, looking at his last hundred cases, L. Bentley of Toronto felt comfortable in saying that he had used forceps in 35 per cent of them. Others' rates were not as high, some being as low as 6 per cent. Between 1912 and 1914, the Ottawa Maternity Hospital had a 27 per cent forceps rate, and this declined to 20 per cent in the following years.[133] In 1914 B.P. Watson of the Burnside Lying-In Hospital recognized that frequency of use differed from physician to physician and from hospital to hospital. However, he seemed pleased to note that at the Burnside the rate of forceps use in public cases was 22.2 per cent whereas for semi-private patients it was 57 per cent.[134] Clearly, forceps use varied widely.

Many of the themes of the early decades continued in the interwar years, suggesting the difficulty medicine had in controlling practice. Although the medical literature warned of the dangers of forceps, there were still complaints from physicians about colleagues who had used forceps too early, causing lacerations, which suggests that many engaged in procedures that did not have the approval of the profession as a whole.[135] Helen MacMurchy echoed Lapthorn Smith in pointing out that forceps had saved lives and also asking how many they had destroyed. Her 1925–6 study implicated forceps in 19 per cent of maternal deaths.[136] Forceps use could also lead to maternal morbidity. Mrs Mavis Booth, age thirty-seven, entered Victoria General Hospital in Halifax on 1 March 1921, suffering from a lacerated perineum and prolapse of the uterus. She had had a forceps birth nine years previously, at which time her record had noted that the perineum became torn but no repair had been done. She had since had two more children and had begun to notice the prolapse.[137] While the record does not specifically blame her problems on the forceps birth, the vast medical literature did make connections between forceps use and health problems such as sepsis and lacerations, and eventual gynaecological difficulties.[138] Harold Atlee feared that physicians resorted to forceps too often and for the wrong indications, although he comforted himself in the belief that by the 1930s high forceps use at least had declined and forceps technique had improved.[139] An editorial in the *Canada Lancet and Practitioner* in 1928 castigated readers: 'We believe doctors are too often anxious to bring labor on in order to relieve the woman of her agony and allow him to get on with his other work. We think men do not spend the time at confinements which they used to. Nature is not given a chance.'[140] But waiting on nature could have tragic consequences. One Newfoundland woman whose previous births had all necessitated the early use of forceps believed that she had lost her child because the physician covering for her usual doctor did not use forceps soon enough.[141] This case raises at least two questions. Why did the woman's doctor not tell his replacement about the woman's case history? And why did the woman not mention it herself? She apparently did not feel that she could make suggestions. Deference paid to physicians was such that she could not question what the replacement practitioner was doing; though, of course, no one actually knows why she lost her baby.

One of the reasons for physician concern about forceps in the interwar period was the perception that it took skill to know when and how to use them. Physicians worried about both the deficiencies of obstetric education and the high maternal mortality rates, for which they felt they were being blamed. Textbooks detailed the care and time needed to train a medical student to use forceps properly. Textbooks also went over the indications for forceps use in an effort to limit how often doctors used them, but at times the descriptions were so general that they allowed a fairly wide interpretation. A 1935 major obstetrics book listed seven indicators: too weak pains to bring about delivery; delay caused by disproportion (did not say how much disproportion); when the uterine force direction was abnormal; delivery 'hindered' by the soft parts of the mother; 'when it is necessary to deliver the mother quickly'; when the child needed to be born quickly; and when the child was having difficulty being born because of 'certain malpositions of the head.'[142] Yet many births could fall into one or more of these categories depending on the woman's ability to endure pain and on the doctor's skill (or lack) in assessment. Cases at the Royal Victoria Hospital, Montreal, indicate that forceps were used for 'maternal distress' or 'delay,' but it was unclear what these terms actually meant.[143] The issue was not whether the patients needed forceps – some clearly did – but the vagueness of the guidelines and the language that opened forceps use to abuse. On the other hand, too close adherence to rules could also lead to intervention occurring without thought to the specifics of a particular case.

Some doctors were not concerned about forceps use. H.M. Little of McGill University made the extraordinary statement: 'My own practice is to deliver a great many of my primiparae with forceps.' He recognized that his was a 'radical' position but felt it was necessary to offset what he viewed as the real radical-ism of the 1920s – the too frequent resort to caesarian section.[144] Little clearly believed that one intervention would lessen resort to another. But it could also lead to another. As already noted, forceps necessitated the use of anaesthesia; in turn, the increased use of anaesthesia generally was encouragement to resort to forceps.[145] Ross Mitchell believed that increased aseptic proce-dure gave physicians the confidence to intervene and to respond safely to their patients' demands to 'do something.'[146]

What were the rates of forceps use during the interwar years and beyond? In his rural practice A.F. McKenzie from Monkton, Ontario, used forceps in 18 per cent of cases. Dr Walmsley from Prince Edward County, Ontario, had a 13 per cent rate, whereas his friend Dr Geggie in his Gatineau Valley practice had only a 9 per cent rate. The Montreal Maternity Hospital's record in 1923 was 9.92 per cent.[147] The Winnipeg General Hospital had a 7.7 per cent rate in the mid-twenties and for the period 1923 to 1933 a slightly higher rate, 7.96 per cent. Considering this too high, Ross Mitchell assured colleagues that most forceps cases were low forceps and 'done in many instances for teaching purposes.'[148] The Vancouver General Hospital in the mid-1930s had a 10.26 per cent rate. The rates of some institutions could be quite high. In 1930 the Royal Victoria Hospital, Montreal, had a forceps rate of

20 per cent; in 1948, 38 per cent. The Kingston General Hospital records revealed a 49 per cent rate in 1929, 40 per cent in 1935, and 45 per cent in 1940. The rate of high forceps use had declined at the Kingston hospital but the percentage of cases undergoing c-section had increased.[149] These statistics can be compared to those elsewhere. In 1934 in the United States, forceps were used in almost 20 per cent of all deliveries, but the rates varied from 0.5 to 80 per cent. European clinics were averaging 3 to 4 per cent.[150] In the 1920s, even Queen Victoria's Jubilee midwives in England had a rate of 6 per cent; and before the Second World War, British rates soared to 50 per cent or more, based on the belief that the second stage of labour needed to be short. By the 1950s, however, it had declined to 5 per cent.[151] The reasons for the differences are not clear. But Canada was influenced by both British and American attitudes, as reflected in its use of medical textbooks from both countries. Its orientation to Europe through its British heritage offset, to a degree, the American orientation to intervention and perhaps even the short-lived high rate in Britain.

What is intriguing about the range of rates is their association with other factors. As noted, Ross Mitchell linked the high rate at Winnipeg General Hospital to its teaching function. A study of births in Manitoba, 1939–40, revealed a rate of 24 per cent for women who had had adequate prenatal care but an 18.6 per cent rate for those who had not.[152] A physician at the Royal Victoria Hospital in 1948 noted that on the private and semi-private wards most of the births were forceps and almost all the patients had episiotomies.[153] At the Vancouver General one staff physician linked the combined use of barbiturate drugs, low forceps delivery, and episiotomy for first-time mothers.[154] He felt that this lessened induction of labour. Thus interventions became clumped together.

Forceps and episiotomies often went hand in hand in the early decades of the century. In 1911 H.M. Little of McGill accused his colleagues of causing lacerations with their too anxious use of forceps.[155] One way to offset perineal lacerations was to perform an episiotomy. Even when physicians did not use forceps, however, lacerations or tears could occur. A physician from London, Ontario, raised the familiar argument that the perineum was vulnerable because modern women were not fit to bear children.[156] Those espousing episiotomy felt that a clean cut they could suture afterwards healed faster than an uneven sutured tear. Opponents, however, held that episiotomies should be done only when it was clear that a laceration was going to occur. But the problem was that the physician did not know when a laceration would occur.[157] Lapthorn Smith of Bishop's University had a compromise to offer the episiotomy/no episiotomy debate. He placed sutures in the perineum before birth; then, if a tear occurred, it was easy to bring the lacerated edges together. If no tear occurred, the physician could easily remove the sutures.[158] While not common in North America in the early decades of the century, episiotomy was more so in Europe, especially in Austria and Germany.[159]

Evidence suggests that in the 1920s, 1930s, and 1940s episiotomies became more common. Lacerations from birth were still an issue for many within the profession, especially as a cause of future problems if they did not heal properly. Robert Ferguson of London, Ontario, considered it good obstetrics especially in primiparae. A Newfoundland midwife recalled that in the interwar period the local physician would perform an episiotomy if the mother was a 'young person' or if labour pains were not strong and the labour was taking too long. Joseph DeLee used it routinely in these years. Herbert M. Little of McGill held that 'episiotomy has proved its value and is to be preferred over distention of the perineum.' For Little, fear of tear no longer motivated its use; simple distention of the perineum did. Jennie Graham remembered that her physicians preferred to cut an inch rather than have her tear half an inch.[160] Supporters were especially hostile to the growing popularity of natural childbirth in the late 1940s, for unless a woman was anaesthetized, they could not do an episiotomy.[161]

The records of the Montreal Maternity Hospital suggest that episiotomies were a matter of course. In 1930 the hospital claimed that the vast majority of its first-time mothers underwent episiotomy. Between 1936 and 1939 the rate was 77 per cent for primi-parae; the overall rate was 47.3 per cent.[162] Looking at the increase in episiotomies from 1933 to 1941 at the Vancouver General, F. Sidney Hobbs focused on three explanations: 'a more uniform method of teaching in the medical schools, whereby most students are now taught to do episiotomies instead of getting lacerations'; 'use of the barbiturate drugs combined with a low forceps delivery and episiotomy'; and 'more doctors confining their work to this speciality, particularly in the last ten years.'[163] Another factor was that physicians more often performed them on paying patients than non-paying.[164] Ian Graham, who has examined the rise of episiotomy in the United States and Great Britain, has argued that the shift occurred in the late 1920s and early 1930s, when the leading voices in obstetrics became advocates. Other reasons for its adoption included the increasing tendency to see childbirth as pathological; the shift to hospital birth, which encouraged intervention; the desire of physicians to control the uncertainty of birth; and the alignment of obstetrics with gynaecology and thus the transformation of obstetrics.[165] By the late twentieth century, rates in Canada had declined somewhat to 63 per cent for primiparous and 42 per cent for multiparous women.[166]

Yet not all physicians were converts. One woman in the interwar period recalled that the response of her physician to the tear in her perineum, a result of her first delivery, was rather cavalier. He apparently told her that repairing it did not make sense until after she had finished childbearing.[167] The Lamont Clinic in Alberta discouraged episiotomies as late as 1948.[168] At Montreal's Hôpital de la Miséricorde, episiotomies were rare – maybe 3 per cent – but lacerations or tears approached 48 per cent.[169] Mary Percy Jackson did not find that episiotomies were needed for Métis women; she found that they seldom tore:

> In eighteen years I have only had to stitch three torn perineums in Metis women (one stitch apiece). I don't know whether it is because they are so young when they start having babies (aged 15 to 18 usually) or if it is the absence of fear and nervous tension

during labor, or whether they are simply made of better stuff than white women. Whatever the cause, their perineums stretch like good pre-war elastic. It is really impressive to see a woman deliver herself of the enormous head and shoulders of a 13-pound infant without the smallest laceration of perineum or vagina.[170]

While such experiences could confirm the advantages of natural childbirth with its control of fear, they could also confirm the medical perception that Native women, unlike their white counterparts, were simply more capable of delivering children without interference.

While most of the interventions of childbirth focused on the first and second stages of labour, physicians did not ignore the third stage. The main concern was prompt and complete expulsion of the placenta. In 1901 an American textbook advocated the use of ergot to aid this. Acknowledging that such assistance was not necessary in true physiological cases, the authors, Egbert H. Grandin and George W. Jarman, argued that few women were able to undergo childbirth 'in a strictly physiological manner.'[171] Many hospitals in England, Scotland, and Ireland, however, had prohibited the use of ergot before expulsion of the placenta.[172] To ensure that the placenta was completely expelled, others advocated using a finger examination, douching after birth, or curetting the uterus after the placenta was expelled.[173] Others routinely did an internal examination at the end of the third stage of labour, checking for lacerations that needed mending. But as the authors of one text pointed out, after going through childbirth, most women present deviations from the non-pregnant norm; physicians should restrain themselves and only examine those women whose cases are 'exceptional and urgent.'[174] As noted with other areas of intervention, one form often replaced another. James R. Goodall of the Royal Victoria Hospital, Montreal, explained in 1914: 'The tendency is to pass from the more heroic forms of attack to the milder forms of treatment. There has been a gradual slow change from sharp curette to dull instruments, later a slow substitution of digital removal for the instrumental cleaning, and lastly the abandoning of the manual invasion for the douche cleansing method, and today that conservative tendency is making itself still further felt in a policy of total abstention from interference.'[175] But in the interwar period there were still some physicians who did not wait for the physiological expulsion of the placenta. Whereas past physicians had resorted to ergot, pituitrin was now used; but some warned that just as the dangers of ergot had finally been recognized, those of pituitrin would eventually be as well.[176] One Newfoundland physician had his own way of encouraging the expulsion of the placenta – tickling the lower part of the abdomen.[177]

Childbirth procedures in most societies are interventionist. Even a brief examination of childbirth among First Nations people and those directed by midwives underscores this fact. Only the nature of the intervention varies, and its degree. Within the medical and social culture in which Canadian physicians worked and lived, several factors encouraged intervention. Time was money, and in order to save money, doctors might try to reduce time spent at the bedside. Intervention was an expression of skill, and doctors charged more for cases in which they deemed intervention was necessary. They also succumbed to the pressure of their patients to 'do something.' The medical literature constantly alerted physicians to the dangers of intervention but also glorified it in appropriate cases. Intervention was part of medical culture: if intervention was not a possibility, why would a physician be needed?

It is not always possible to evaluate whether interventions in the past were necessary. But it is possible to discern commonalities stemming from the medical discussion of intervention. It is clear that many physicians were concerned about the degree of intervention that was occurring. In the early decades of the century, some were concerned about the examination of women after labour had begun. Over time, vaginal examinations did decline, but rectal examinations took their place. Versions, which had been popular with some, needed to be justified by mid-century. The induction of labour raised a number of issues. Few would criticize it for women suffering from eclampsia, but for an arbitrary definition of postmaturity the decision was not as straightforward. And once made, for whatever reason, induction led to other forms of intervention. Expediting labour was similar. The use of pituitrin became popular in the interwar years, and this popularity was enhanced by the broadening of indications for its use. While not all physicians agreed with the ease with which many of their colleagues adopted pituitrin, they could identify with the urge to shorten labour.

Pain management in a variety of guises underscores doctor-directed birth for the entire period under study. What changed was the form of pain relief that an individual practitioner could use. But despite the myriad choices and the faddish nature of some, as with many interventions, pain relief had a symbiotic relationship with others – some procedures demanded its use, and its use resulted in others. Pain management occurred in all types of practices – home and hospital – and was symbolic of a doctor-dominated birth. Even when women seemed more involved, as in the case of demanding twilight sleep or participating in natural childbirth, a close look reveals that their agency was severely limited. Other interventions, too, pick up on the above themes. Forceps use generally required the use of anaesthesia, but as some practitioners argued, it could alleviate the need for pituitrin to speed up labour. As with any form of intervention, physicians had to balance between the dangers of using forceps and the help they afforded. The former was of major concern, and despite perpetual warnings in the interwar period about the skill needed to operate them, the indications for their use could be vague, leaving incredible discretion to the practitioner. Forceps and episiotomies clearly went hand in hand, and the latter became a way of offsetting what might occur – tears or lacerations of the perineum. While most of the interventions listed focused on the first and second stages of labour, aiding the expulsion of the placenta in various ways was popular as well.

As argued in this chapter, physicians were certainly not agreed on the need for the various interventions discussed. But while each physician could make individual decisions, the statistics from hospitals and private practices suggest that there was an inexorable drift toward increased medicalization of childbirth. It may not have been as high as in the United States – figures on forceps use and discussions of twilight sleep suggest that – but neither was it as low as in some European clinics. But rates may be only one indication of reality. The perception of it was another. Certainly, the perception of physicians was that intervention was increasing, although they differed on which ones they supported and whether the increase was posing problems for both their patients and themselves. Nowhere was this highlighted more than in the medical discussion of caesarian section.

CHAPTER SEVEN

Caesarian Section

In recent years, due largely to improvements in technique the safety of Caesarian section has markedly increased. This has resulted in a widening of its indications, so that today there are few obstetrical complications which may not, on occasion, be best dealt with by abdominal section.

A.W. Andison, 1947[1]

The above quotation suggests that caesarian section had not always been as popular as it later became. It also suggests a popularity and acceptance that readers early in the twenty-first century might misinterpret. Compared with figures late in the twentieth century, the rates of c-section at mid-century were not high. Nevertheless, they had increased over time, and some physicians were expressing concern about the fact and urging their colleagues to curb their excitement about the dramatic procedure. But the excitement was understandable when the alternative to c-section is remembered – mutilating surgery on the foetus in the hope of saving the mother. C-sections gave the child a chance to be born live, and for Catholic physicians and patients especially, this was the only moral decision they could make. For other physicians, c-sections allowed them to reconfigure the definition of risk. Whereas early in the century c-section had posed too much of a risk for the mother, by the interwar period physicians were arguing that it had become the saviour of both mother and child. The meaning of skill, too, changed. The skilled practitioner went from being the surgeon who performed the surgery to one whose knowledge of obstetrics would allow him to judge when surgery was necessary. Determining this was never exact, for the indications for c-section broadened over time, forcing individual physicians to choose which indications they believed to be the most significant. C-sections also faced practitioners with the choice of sterilizing a woman in order to offset the dangers of a future c-section or of performing repeated surgeries.

Caesarean section has a long history. But because of its high maternal mortality rate in the early years, it remained a rarity even at the turn of the twentieth century. This was not to last. As early as 1904 an article on 'Major Obstetrical Operations' in the *Canadian Practitioner and Review* noted that the procedure was 'becoming very popular.' Two years later, H.L. Reddy of the Women's Hospital, Montreal, confidently maintained: 'While Caesarean section is a grave operation I do not consider it any more severe, or as much so, as many of the operations of daily occurrence by surgeons in every great hospital, although it may be a little more spectacular.'[2] Physicians began to stress its simplicity and lack of difficulty, touting it as one of the significant advances of modern obstetrics.[3]

While many doctors in the interwar years continued to embrace c-section, an increasing number deplored what they saw as a bandwagon effect. In 1930 C.B. Oliver of Chatham, Ontario, argued in the *Canadian Medical Association Journal* that the ease and simplicity of the procedure attracted adherents, which in turn attracted emulators. He suggested that if consultation before surgery was mandatory, fewer c-sections would occur and those that did would have better results. Yet in the same year and in another journal, Oliver praised c-section to the skies.[4] Other physicians worried that too many of their colleagues resorted to c-section when vaginal births were possible. Still others feared that too many doctors were depending on it to overcome the difficulties they faced in managing childbirth.[5] In 1932 H.B. Van Wyck of Toronto General Hospital and the University of Toronto comforted himself that at least the situation was not as 'extreme' in Canada as it was elsewhere. In the United States, for example, c-section rates reached as high as 14 per cent in some hospitals and were 3 per cent for the United States as a whole, with some American experts estimating that three-quarters of them were unnecessary.[6] In the mid-1930s, one hospital in Kansas City had a rate of 32 per cent. In the late 1940s, some hospitals in the United States and Great Britain were reporting rates as high as 8 or 10 per cent.[7]

How did physicians explain the trend? Some claimed that it reflected the shift in obstetrics from 'a medical to a surgical speciality.'[8] H.O. Howitt of Guelph, Ontario, noted that c-section had already passed through several phases with the pendulum going back and forth until the mid-twenties, when there was a 'conservatism' regarding it.[9] But conservatism seemed more rhetorical than real as concern about the 'caesarian section problem' escalated.[10] But what was the solution? Frederick G. McGuiness of Winnipeg General Hospital, picking up on Oliver's point, suggested that hospitals should institute a rule that any major obstetrical procedure must require consultation with a staff member. The Winnipeg General did so and had a c-section rate of only 0.79 per cent.[11]

The incidence of c-section in Canada in the past seems minimal compared with what later occurred. In the early 1980s the rate was 15 per cent (although higher in teaching hospitals) and by the early 1990s it had reached 20 per cent. In the early 1990s the rate was even higher in the United States: 25 per cent, with half of them deemed by some as unnecessary.[12] But physicians in the interwar period were reacting to the increase they had seen. At the Royal Victoria Hospital, Montreal, the rate was 1.8 per cent in 1927 but by the late 1930s, 3.3 per cent. At the Burnside Lying-In Hospital, Toronto, the rate reached 5.78 per cent in 1929, although it had decreased to 1.90 by 1937. The caesarean section rate at the Montreal Maternity Hospital was only 0.47 per cent in 1912 but was 1.04 in 1915 and 4.5 per cent by 1940. Vancouver General Hospital's rate in the 1930s was approximately 3 per cent. Even Winnipeg General Hospital, which prided itself on its low rate, experienced an increase in the 1930s.[13] The national rate was 2 per cent of hospital obstetrical cases (which of course meant a much lower rate for the entire obstetrical population) in the interwar years, but it was 5 per cent in the late 1940s. Henricus J. Stander thought that in any maternity clinic the rate should not be higher than 4 per cent and in private practice not more than 1 per cent. Others considered that any rate above 3 per cent warranted a reassessment. Yet, as seen, rates varied from hospital to hospital; they also varied from physician to physician. Paul T. Harper in his 1930 obstetrics text noted that 'training, aptitude and individual preference' accounted for certain doctors performing c-sections.[14]

Who received c-sections? Despite all the emphasis on prenatal care, it did not obviate the need for surgical intervention. In 1939–40 the c-section rate for those with adequate prenatal care in Manitoba was 1.1 per cent and for those without it only 0.6 per cent.[15] Of course, those who knew or suspected that they would have difficulties may have self-selected themselves and sought prenatal care. More c-sections were performed in urban areas than in rural.[16] Specialists – the physicians perhaps more willing to do surgery – were concentrated in cities where access to hospital facilities gave them the support c-sections necessitated. Also, physicians in urban centres would be more likely to meet colleagues and discuss what the latest advances were. Unlike the rates of forceps use, the c-section rates in teaching hospitals were low, at least on the public wards. The significant increase in c-sections was among private patients. For example, at Toronto General Hospital the rate on the public ward in the late 1930s was 2.7 per cent but on the private ward it was 7.4 per cent. The same discrepancy was true for Winnipeg General Hospital at the end of the period.[17] The Toronto General Hospital private ward figure was much higher than that at two comparative New York hospitals, the New York Nursery and Child's Hospital and the New York Lying-In Hospital, which had private ward rates of 3.8 and 4.9 per cent, respectively.[18]

What accounted for the higher rates on the private wards? Surgical births brought in more money to the physician than normal births, and private patients could afford the cost. One physician associated lower fertility rates with private patients and linked these lower rates with increased c-section rates as a way of ensuring a safe birth.[19] Also, as more middle-class women entered hospitals, there was simply a larger population on which to operate. None of the above speculations, however, provides a medical reason for the increase in c-sections. In fact, medical reasons would suggest that there should be a higher rate of c-section among poorer women whose health had been under-mined by malnutrition, resulting in birth complications.

In the past, alternatives to c-section could be gruesome. At times vaginal birth is problematic and indeed impossible with-out putting the life of the mother or her child at risk. Physicians (outside Catholic circles) generally gave priority to the life of the mother, which meant that they sometimes faced sacrificing the life of the child in order to save the mother. Embryotomy, or dismemberment of the child (usually but not always after the death of the foetus), was one certain way to increase the mother's safety when vaginal birth was life-threatening for her. In the early years of the century, the favoured form of embryotomy was craniotomy, puncturing the foetus's brain and removing its con-tents to facilitate delivery. Such a procedure was difficult for any physician to do.

Cases of craniotomy were rare. Montreal Maternity Hospital, for example, averaged only one craniotomy a year in the early decades of the century. But although not common, they were part of the physician's experience and training.[20] The 1907 edition of J. Clifton Edgar's obstetric textbook devoted eight pages to c-section but eighteen to embryotomy, which 'comprises eight dis-tinct operations, many of them complicated.'[21] In the period before birth control, some women who had severe pelvic dispro-portion could undergo several craniotomies. It is difficult to im-agine what their feelings must have been when they discovered that once again they were pregnant with a child to whom they would not be able to give birth. For these women, c-section was truly a life saver, for it gave them the possibility of having a live child. Physicians hoped that c-section would make embryotomy on a live child obsolete. H.L. Reddy told of a patient, Mrs R, aged thirty-three, who came to the Women's Hospital, Montreal, in

1905. Her previous and only pregnancy had resulted in a craniotomy, and her physician had told her that if she became pregnant again she would have to undergo a c-section. She did so and gave birth to a 8½ lb. baby girl.[22] It is unclear why Mrs R's physician insisted on a c-section. She did have a slightly contracted pelvis, but the safety of the surgery in 1905 was problematic. His insistence probably reflected his own unease about performing a craniotomy on a live child. Obstetric texts were taking this position. David Berry Hart in his 1912 *Guide to Midwifery* told his readers:

> Craniotomy should not be done on a living child ... Instead, some of the cutting operations, such as caesarean section, pubiotomy, etc., should be chosen. Craniotomy, therefore, is practically restricted to cases where the child is dead, or where the parents absolutely refuse to allow caesarean section to be done. In this case the medical man may have no other resource than to act against his own opinion. He should, however, refuse to repeat it in a subsequent case.[23]

For Catholic women, embryotomy resulting in the death of a live foetus was not an option. In 1907 H.L. Reddy told of one of his patients, Mrs M, aged twenty-six, who was pregnant with her first child. She had entered hospital after thirty hours in labour, and physicians attempted to extract the child with forceps but failed. As the case record reported, 'An uncle, a priest, who was present, forbade any operation to destroy the child.' A c-section was done and a living child born, although it did not survive. The mother recovered.[24] Frederick Fenton of the University of Toronto and St Michael's [Catholic] Hospital, Toronto, stated categorically: 'It must be recognized that craniotomy on the living child is no longer permissible.'[25]

Increasingly, embryotomy was becoming the procedure that had to be explained.[26] Nevertheless, annual reports of hospitals still listed them and medical literature occasionally referred to them as an option, especially in non-hospital births. A horrendous case was described in 1924. Mrs C lived fifty miles from

Fredericton and her physician arrived at her home early one morning to find her in labour. She had a difficult time and he could not extract the child and finally brought her to the Victoria Public Hospital the following evening. The case record described what the hospital staff saw: 'Physical examination found a complete laceration of the perineum with much bruised appearance. The uterus had within it the head only of a full term child. Her physician said that after much effort by version, he had gotten the child to daylight but could not deliver the head, so amputated it. The irony is that a caesarean saved the mother.'[27] Whether if done sooner it could have saved the child as well is unknown. O. Bjornson, professor emeritus at the University of Manitoba in 1935, told of a case where a physician had misjudged the size of the child compared to the pelvic opening of the mother. The result was a child unable to be born but labour too far along for a safe caesarian section; the physician's only choice was craniotomy on a live child.[28] The moral of the case for Bjornson was that physicians should take care in estimating pelvic measurements: good obstetrics could obviate embryotomies. Such narratives became the lore of medicine. No wonder physicians greeted (and continued to greet) c-section with relief!

In the early years of the century, the dangers to a woman undergoing c-section were so great that few such procedures were performed. Physician loyalty belonged to the woman, not the child, and physicians generally accepted only two exceptions to this 'rule.' The first was when the mother requested the section in order to save her child. Mrs A.F., for example, had already given birth to two children who did not live long because of birth injuries. In her third pregnancy she was 'intensely desirous that baby should be safeguarded.' Thus a c-section was performed at St Michael's Hospital, Toronto, and a healthy baby born.[29] That she gave birth in St Michael's suggests that she may have been Catholic and, if so, would have been influenced by the dictates of her religion. Also, given the pronatalist atmosphere of the times and her own desire to have children, she was willing to put her health, if not her life, in jeopardy in order to have a child. In this case, the result was successful. The second exception to placing the mother's life first was when the mother was dying and the child was still alive. Joseph Hayes of Parrsboro, Nova Scotia, told of one of his patients who had eclamptic convulsions. He bled her of a pint of blood, but even that did not stop the seizures. She became 'moribund' and, receiving the permission of her family, he cut open her abdomen to remove the child.[30]

While many physicians remained concerned about the maternal mortality rates of c-section, some convinced themselves that medical advances were doing away with the trauma of deciding whether or not to save the life of the mother by sacrificing the life of her child.[31] When physicians believed that c-section would no longer kill the mother (at least, in numbers that seemed to preclude the surgery), they rewrote the scenario to one of saving the child's life without losing that of the mother – or, in their version, saving both lives. But of course, the mother's life was not saved; it was simply not sacrificed absolutely. J. Clarence Webster, in his 1903 obstetrics text, told his readers that c-section was 'probably as safe for the mother as is embryotomy, and has the advantage of saving the fetus in the great majority of cases' – both of which claims are questionable.[32] Doctors held the power of life and death in their hands, but to kill deliberately, as in embryotomy, was a power they did not want. C-section changed the medical script from mother's life versus child's life (which for most non-Catholic physicians had a clear resolution – that the life of the mother must be saved) to a much more ambiguous one – the chance (no guarantee) of saving the life of the child and at the same time not losing the mother. Overlooked were other scripts: both could be lost, the mother lost and child saved, or the mother put through major surgery with no live child to show for it.[33]

What was the mortality rate for c-section? Unfortunately, there was little consistency in measurement or clarity about which measurement was used. Some physicians compared it to general mortality statistics, others to maternal mortality statistics, and still others to c-section deliveries. In 1904 an article in the *Canadian Practitioner and Review* estimated that it was 3 to 4 per cent (of women operated on) by 'skilled' hands when the woman had not been previously infected.[34] Such a figure bolstered the claim of the surgery's safety. In 1904, however, it was difficult either to ensure 'skilled' hands or to guarantee an uninfected patient. That physicians wanted the low rates to be true was understandable considering the alternatives to c-section. As a result, mortality estimates continued to stress the best-case scenario. Looking at the general maternal mortality rates at the Montreal Maternity Hospital from 1905 to 1909, H.M. Little noted that they included one c-section death. He did not think that fair. After all, 'there was evidently some fault in technique, such as is apt to occur with a major operation.'[35] A woman could die, then, from a 'fault in technique,' and if that were the case, her death should not be attributable to the c-section itself or to maternal causes. In 1906 H.L. Reddy of the Women's Hospital, Montreal, quoted the general maternal mortality rate of 10 per cent in cities and argued that 'in the hands of good operators [the c-section rate] varies from 5 to 7 per cent.' He concluded: 'This being the case the operation no longer deserves the discredit it rightly obtained in the days before asepsis when the death rate was 50 per cent.' He acknowledged that it was still a 'grave operation' but said it was no more dangerous than many operations taking place daily at 'every great hospital.'[36] Some deemed it safer than other procedures, such as a high forceps operation.[37] One procedure had superseded another.

In estimating the risks of maternal mortality from a best-case scenario – a skilled surgeon working in a great hospital, on an elective not an emergency c-section case – physician writers encouraged surgery. Indeed, the dangers of not being in a best-case scenario might prompt physicians to ensure that they were in one. For example, knowing that elective c-section was safer than non-elective might lead to an unwillingness to give women sufficient time to make a try at labour, or not to let them try at all, before deciding to operate. Increased elective c-section would lower the mortality statistics (from c-section), which in turn would encourage more physicians to resort to it. In this way, the section became part of normative practice. In the words of H.E. Kendall, writing in the *Canadian Medical Association Journal* in 1915,

Among the events marking the progress of the surgical art, the growth of the operation of caesarean section is a notable one. To the student of the eighties, its very name was awful and holy, and the procedure was to be thought of by the very bold only, after every other hope had fled. Now all one needs to guard against is infection, and the operation can be lightly selected, if suitable for the case in hand. In short, it is often good practice to cut the uterus and sew it up again instead of waiting unduly or dilating and tearing it when one desires to empty it quickly of its contents.

While acknowledging a maternal mortality rate of 10 per cent, Kendall noted that this was for both elective and emergency sections, and he argued that 'the two should not be mixed in statistics or in our minds.'[38] The language used is telling. Kendall stressed the art of the surgery, which in turn emphasized the skill necessary to perform it. But its dangers seemed to have vanished: it was an operation just like any other and could be 'lightly selected'; there was even a sense that a physician would prefer it, since the operator did not have to wait 'unduly' for nature to take its course.

In the interwar period the discussion of risk and what it meant continued. In 1924 Herbert M. Little warned his colleagues about the 'appalling maternity mortality' associated with the surgery and questioned whether improvement in foetal survival was significant. Others agreed and urged a more conservative management of birth.[39] Unlike other surgery, physicians did not perform it for illness; in most cases they did not operate because the patient's life was at risk; rather, they did it to save the child. But this was not the way in which many interpreted it. H.H. McNally of Fredericton, New Brunswick, told of one of his patients, Mrs S.L., in her thirties, a primipara at full term:

In labour when I was called; all day passed and the night without delivery. It was the next afternoon, after strenuous attempts at delivery she was removed through the town to the Victoria Public Hospital – a caesarean operation saved the mother, the child was lost. This woman called me again in labour with her second child, but would not submit to caesarean operation until an attempt was made to deliver. Again she was removed from her home to the hospital – a caesarean operation saved mother and child.[40]

The interesting aspect of these cases is the emphasis McNally placed on saving the mother in both and saving the child in one. In neither case did he give any indication that the woman would have died without a c-section; that is, an embryotomy could have been performed, but in that case the child *certainly* would have died. Of course, there was no guarantee about the outcome for the mother either, but there was no certainty that she would have died. It might be more truthful to say that the section in the second labour saved the child and in both cases the mother survived the surgery. Nonetheless, in the medical literature, physicians described the section as saving both mother and child even though the mother's life was very rarely at risk.

Although physicians emphasized the survival of mother and child, the general focus on high maternal mortality rates (from all causes) and the need to explain them in the interwar period directed attention to c-sections. A study of maternal mortality in Ontario in 1933 found that in 18 per cent of cases caesarian section had occurred, and that mortality in the operative group of births (which included more than just c-sections) compared with the spontaneous group was 8.2 per 1,000 and 2.3, respectively. Some estimated that c-section mortality was seven times that of natural delivery or, in absolute terms, '2.8% in clean cases, 6.2% for suspicious cases and 9% for unclean cases.' A study of Winnipeg General Hospital found that mortality rates from c-sections (elective and emergency) were as high as 30 per cent.[41] In New York City during the same period, c-sections were involved in almost 20 per cent of maternal deaths even though they represented only 2.2 per cent of deliveries.[42] What was an acceptable risk for the mother in order to save the child?

Much of the medical literature downplayed the possibility of maternal mortality and instead emphasized the almost certain death of the child without c-section. Paul T. Harper in his 1930 text told his readers that 'section is done primarily in the interests of the child.' He admitted that it was not as safe as vaginal birth for the mother and should not be done if the child was not alive. While true, a sleight of hand occurs, for one is left with the conclusion that there would be a living child at the end of a c-section. Indeed, Harper justified c-section when the mother was willing to assume risk to herself 'for the *certainty* of producing a live child.'[43] Yet there was no certainty, only statistical odds. In 1930 Winnipeg, with two hospitals, reported a maternal mortality rate of 10 per cent with c-section and an infant mortality rate of 25 per cent.[44] Physicians accepted that the *absolute* knowledge of the child dying without the surgery took precedence over the *possibility* of the mother and/or child dying. In 1922 A. Mackinnon of Guelph, Ontario, described a successful recovery from c-section of one of his patients: 'If we could feel sure of such a result in every case, in this day of excellent hospital advantages, how very many cases would we submit to caesarian section rather than deliver by the vagina with severe injuries to the mother and the probable death of the child.'[45] For him, the issue was no longer the certainty of the child's death without section but only its probability; nor was it saving the mother from death (even in rhetoric) but, rather, saving her from injury. In these various scenarios, physicians glossed over the high maternal morbidity rate caused by the surgery.[46] The certainty of the child's death was also stressed by the Catholic Church. In 1930 the papal encyclical *Casti connubi* prohibited sacrificing the life of a child in order to save the mother.[47]

The acknowledgment of risk to the mother seemed, at times, perfunctory. W.G. Cosbie of Toronto General Hospital admitted that mortality was ten times the rate of vaginal births but said that 'the indications for caesarian section included many of the gravest complications of pregnancy and childbirth and the deaths following the operation in many cases should be attributed to them rather than the operation.'[48] The surgery had become the subject whose rights needed to be protected. It had a life of its own separate from the reasons for its existence in the first place. By reifying the surgery, making it the subject, Cosbie and others took it out of human hands, making it less able to be changed or stopped. C-section could be safe if there were no birth complications, but the point of c-section was to mitigate those complications. If it could not, then it failed. But the rates had declined at Toronto General Hospital from about 5.78 per cent in 1930 to 1.7 per cent in 1938, close to the 1.6 per cent English rate for elective c-sections.[49] In 1949 the Royal Alexandra Hospital, Edmonton, was deservedly proud of the fact that its staff had performed 291 sections with not one fatality; indeed, the last mortality had been in 1935. Acknowledging that the section rate was increasing, A.H. Maclennan considered that it was 'not to be criticized,' given the non-existent mortality rate which the hospital had been experiencing.[50] The confidence this gave physicians such as Maclennan was clear. Physicians granted that the life of the mother came first, though they did so almost as a matter of form and with none of the urgency that had existed in the early years of the century.[51] Much of the medical literature suggested that c-section had become so accepted and so common that risk (meaning death) was only one of many factors that practitioners had to consider – a normal consequence of major surgery.[52] As seen, the consequences of risk changed significantly over time. In the early years of the century, the high maternal mortality rates as a result of c-section had meant that patients were the ones with power to insist on having the procedure. Few physicians had been willing to assume that responsibility. By the end of the 1940s, however, the scenario had altered. The doctor claimed that he would save both mother and child even though, in most cases, the mother was not at risk. Mother and child became one, and the one was the child; the child's risk became the mother's. It seemed irrational not to want to be saved and, from the doctor's perspective, not to want to save.

Linked to the concept of risk was the issue of skill, the survival of mother and child being its measurement. In the early part of the century, most critics of c-section had been surgeons, who emphasized the danger of the procedure and argued that it should be left to those with surgical skill, namely themselves. But a 'skilled practitioner' could have different meanings: being expert in techniques, being careful and alert, or being knowledgeable. Henry Jellett saw the 'nervous' physician as the problem – the man who went against his own judgment and allowed the woman 'every chance of delivering herself' even when he felt that this was not possible.' Jellett's words are telling. More often than not the medical literature described the physician delivering the child and not the woman. When vaginal birth was under criticism, Jellett described the woman as subject, as agent, causing dire consequences for herself.[53] The good or skilled surgeon would not let this happen. The skilled surgeon was in control. J.J.C., author of a tellingly entitled article, 'Midwifery Should Be a Branch of Surgery,' argued that a good obstetrician prepared each case as though surgery might occur. Childbirth was potentially a 'branch of surgery,' and for the safety of the patient practitioners needed to recognize that.[54] This view increased the prestige of those delivering babies, but the encouragement to prepare for the worst (which is what medical education prepared students for) was given with little thought about repercussions. A surgeon, was the ideal to emulate. The skilled surgeon in a hospital setting could ensure optimal conditions, but most private practitioners did not have the luxury of elective sections or control over the environment in which emergency c-sections occurred. A gulf clearly existed between the expert or specialist and the physicians who were on the front line of patient care.

The tension between general practitioners and surgeons increased over time as surgery dominated obstetrical training and hospital focus. A 1929 editorial in the *Canadian Medical Association Journal* argued: 'Obstetric teachers should redouble their efforts to impress on students that operative obstetrics is surgery, and very often major surgery, and demands, like major surgery, ideal aseptic conditions, skilled assistants, and more training than they receive in their undergraduate course.'[55] The message was clear: leave obstetric surgery to the experts. But who were the experts? In the early decades many had agreed that c-sections should be done by skilled surgeons, but by the mid-1920s some were suggesting that surgical skill was not enough. A 1924 article in the *Canadian Medical Association Journal* urged the surgeon to have some kind of obstetrical training before he operated on childbearing women.[56] A redefinition of skill was occurring. Physicians delivering babies had long felt themselves to be undervalued compared with surgeons. C-section was their chance to show that they, too, could perform spectacular feats without placing their patients at risk. C-section saved time and was even more dramatic than the surgery performed by most surgeons, since it involved two lives, not just one. Many encouraged one another to see obstetrics as a surgical speciality. But skill was necessary to know when to operate, and when not to operate, and in knowing what type of c-section was best.[57] So while skill in surgery was necessary, it was no longer enough. Opponents of c-section worried that it was taking the decision making out of obstetrics by normalizing how physicians reacted to problems. One text warned its readers: 'The operation must not be regarded as a blanket method of overcoming the difficulties encountered in obstetric practice.'[58] Another argued that c-section was the failure of the obstetric art, since 'section is *obstetrical* only in the narrow sense that a child is born as a result of it.'[59] Those who refused to operate were the ones to be admired. The skilled practitioner remained a constant ideal, but the meaning of skill had changed.

Nonetheless, the lure of the surgery remained. C-section saved lives in certain situations and was an aid to safer birth in others. Over time the indications for surgery increased. Physicians distinguished between absolute indications (those that did not give the physician any choice but to operate) and relative indicators (those about which a physician had to make a judgment call). The former, limited in extent, did not change all that much. The latter expanded considerably, thus raising the issue of medicalization of birthing and intervention in birthing. The results of both led to an emphasis on childbirth as a potential surgical occurrence.

Medical practitioners had a certain amount of choice in deciding whether relative indicators applied in a particular obstetric situation. Most, however, did not have much control over what the indicators were. The elite – the specialists, the teachers, the writers of textbooks – determined what these were. General practitioners did not have to apply the elite opinions to their own practices, but if anything went wrong they knew they would need to justify their actions by the literature available. Absolute indicators, on the other hand, were those about which almost all physicians could agree, for example, a situation in which the choice not to perform a section would result in the death of the woman. Extreme pelvic contraction so that even embryotomy could not occur was one, as was the existence of a pelvic tumour blocking the birth canal, or a cancerous degeneration of the cervix.[60] All were medical reasons for a section and did not change over time. Pelvic contraction, however, was seldom interpreted in the narrow terms set out above. As physicians became more confident about the surgery, pelvic contraction, where the birth was not possible without a craniotomy, became an accepted indicator. An easy way of determining this was to examine the woman's previous history. If she had already had a craniotomy, physicians believed that another one was likely. Such a decision, of course, really depended on the ability of the physician to measure accurately both the size of child and the pelvic aperture, a situation not possible in the early decades of the century. Nonetheless, pelvic contraction of a certain severity was an absolute indicator on which almost all could agree. In 1908 R.E. Webster of the County of Carleton General Hospital was very specific: 'the living child in a flat pelvis of a conjugate of 6.5 centimetres or less, or in a generally contracted pelvis of 7 centimetres or less – or in case the child is dead with a pelvis of 5 centimetres or less.'[61] When there was some element of contraction, but not absolute, the physician would allow the woman to try vaginal birth if she had not had a child before; but, as mentioned, if craniotomy had occurred previously, he would perform a c-section.

Physicians in the early decades of the century added other conditions to the list of indicators; but given the debate over these, they had to be considered relative. They depended on the individual physician and how he felt about the situation, the specifics of a particular condition in a particular patient, and whether alternative techniques existed which, for whatever reason, the physician or patient accepted or rejected. For example, in 1902 A. Lapthorn Smith referred to medical literature that supported c-section in cases of placenta praevia. Smith himself was dubious, since the surgery had to occur before haemorrhage began, and it was not always possible to know that the condition existed before haemorrhaging started. He also believed that if the child was alive, version offered it a chance of survival without endangering the mother. Five years later, he had changed his mind because of what he saw as the improvement in the 'technique' of c-section.[62] While some physicians followed a similar path, others were not convinced and preferred to sacrifice the child rather than have the mother undergo a c-section.[63] The division among Canadian physicians reflected that of physicians elsewhere. American practitioners were more sympathetic to c-section in cases of placenta praevia than the British were.[64]

Puerperal eclampsia also encouraged debate. Frederick Fenton of the University of Toronto, in a 1910 article on c-section in cases of eclampsia, argued for the procedure. Pregnancy had caused the eclampsia, so terminating it was the solution. A year later H.L. Reddy of the Women's Hospital, Montreal, described a series of eclamptic cases and listed various ways with which they could be dealt: 'We use hot packs, purgatives, drip salines, when possible and also oxygen. Delivery is performed by accouchement force [rapid forcible delivery], and lately, by caesarian section when the os and cervix are not dilated or easily dilatable.'[65] Joseph B. DeLee of Chicago agreed on c-section once the child reached viability, but he acknowledged that this made sense only if there was 'a well-equipped hospital' available.[66] At times, protracted or difficult labour became an indicator. H.L. Reddy described a patient who had entered the Women's Hospital on 15 March 1906. Each of her previous six pregnancies had gone to full term, but each subsequent labour had been longer and more difficult. When she entered the hospital she had been in labour ten hours, and after another nine hours concern arose about damage to the woman and child if physicians used forceps. A c-section was offered the woman, and she agreed.[67] Physicians were well aware that the indicators for c-section were broadening. As Thomas Watts Eden explained in his 1915 text, 'Owing to the present low mortality of caesarean section, the indications for its performance have been considerably extended in recent years. It is now performed under most of the conditions which were previously held to necessitate craniotomy upon the living child ... while owing to the uncertainty of the survival of the child after induction of premature labour, it is encroaching ... upon the field of this operation also.'[68] The language of Eden's statement is fascinating. The c-section appeared to have a life of its own. It was an aggressive subject, 'encroaching' on the territory of other subjects. In his description, the doctors performing the surgery seem to have disappeared.

A. Mackinnon from Guelph, Ontario, summarized the situation as he believed it existed in the early 1920s. While in the past contracted pelvis, eclampsia, and placenta praevia had been the major indicators, he said, now 'the indications for Caesarian Section ... embrace the following conditions, namely, tumours, impacted shoulder presentation, abnormal conditions of the child, undue rigidity of the cervix and vagina, grave diseases threatening the life of the mother and some cases of prolapse of the cord.'[69] A study of patients at the Burnside Lying-In Hospital between 1925 and 1939 revealed that disproportion was the most common reason for performing a c-section (34.4 per cent), followed by previous section, many of which would have been because of disproportion (24.2 per cent), and placenta praevia (11.9 per cent). Heart disease existed in 10.7 per cent of the cases, but most of these occurred in the early years. Other indicators were 'toxaemia, accidental haemorrhage, tumours of bony pelvis or soft parts, and ruptured uterus.'[70] While severe pelvic contraction continued to be an absolute indicator, 'slight contraction' could justify the surgery as well.[71] Indications continued to vary depending on the situation in which a physician found himself. In the 1930s, physicians at the Royal Victoria Hospital, Montreal, noted an increase in women with deformities of the pelvis, chiefly among refugees from Europe.[72] William Victor Johnston of Lucknow, Ontario, described his way of dealing with pre-eclampsia. He kept the woman in bed, put her on a salt-free diet, and checked her blood pressure every day. If the blood pressure rose he induced labour with quinine and pituitrin, and if that failed he ruptured the membranes. Only if that was unsuccessful did he resort to a c-section.[73] He had a small-town and country practice with little of the support network that many physicians living in large towns had. For him, indications for c-section had to be grave. For others, section became a way of relieving the patient. Mrs Jackson Hover entered the Kitchener-Waterloo Hospital on 2 January 1943, having previously had three pregnancies, the first two normal and the third leaving her with third-degree lacerations. During this fourth pregnancy she had been in bed for four months because of pernicious vomiting. She could not walk more than a few steps without being in pain in the perineal area. Her mother had died at the age of thirty-six from a c-section. An x-ray report confirmed that she was carrying twins and that the first twin was in a breech position. Her pelvis was small, but the case record noted, 'The heads should pass through the pelvis.' Nonetheless, she had a c-section.[74] This patient had already gone through so much in this pregnancy and was facing a difficult birth; for her and her physicians, c-section was an understandable choice.

Each physician worked out his own set of indicators, many of which overlapped, though some were individual. Harold Burrows did not broaden the indicators; rather, he stressed the main one – disproportion – and in doing so suggested that it should be given greater medical concern so that every pregnant woman would undergo pelvic measurement ' before submitting to the cruel test of natural labour.'[75] E.K. Maclellan of Dalhousie University disagreed, pointing out that an accurate measurement of the child was not possible.[76] M.E. Gorman from Lindsay, Ontario, wrote in 1930 that he would perform a section in the following situations: 'where there is a rigid cervix ... where there is disproportion between the head of the child and pelvis ... where there are twins ... where there is cardiac disease, or toxaemia.' M.G. Tompkins of Dominion, Nova Scotia, personally felt that c-section for eclampsia was no longer as popular as it had once been, but he did think it suitable for 'elderly' primaparae.[77] Others considered that the section was useful for women who could not bear the pain of birthing and consequently did not progress once they went into labour. 'Factors which are hard to assess correctly' also could be indicators, including 'poor physical and poor mental equipment, malnutrition, lack of rest, exhaustion from a previous labour or from repeated childbearing, anaemia.'[78] The assumption underlying such a list was that physicians would know when the conditions existed, and that they could measure them precisely. Many physicians saw no end to the broadening of indicators and indeed felt it an important advance in obstetric care.[79] Without a doubt, it normalized c-section as a procedure.

The decision to perform a c-section was not always made by the physician. Often patients or their friends had put pressure on him to operate. Even though the doctor performed the operation for indications that existed in the medical literature, he was usually not happy about it. Time and again, physicians mentioned to one another in the medical press, in a disapproving tone, demands by the patients and their families for a quick and easy end to the labour, as if this was not an important consideration. They accused women of being weaker in the twentieth century than women had been in the past and therefore unwilling to submit to the pain of childbirth.[80] Ross Mitchell felt that in some cases the fear of childbirth and pain actually became a medical indicator for the surgery: among women of a 'higher social class ... unless they are particularly well equipped physically for easy labour, and such is seldom the case, uterine inertia develops early in labour; the patient demands relief and the subsequent course of labour becomes a nightmare for all concerned. Such women, however, stand operation well and recover more quickly than after vaginal delivery.'[81] Given that Mitchell expressed concern about the increasing occurrence of c-section, his view of these women is intriguing. But how many women were demanding c-sections? The medical literature described few specific cases.[82] But the choice facing women, while a private one, was influenced by the society's persistence in defining the successful woman as a mother, and by the institutionalized medical profession's claim that it had a safe alternative to some of the more horrendous complications of childbirth. So it is not surprising that some women chose a c-section. But some did not. Mrs S.L. of Fredericton had already undergone one c-section and made it clear when she became pregnant again that she 'would not submit' to another. Unfortunately for her, the attempt at vaginal birth was unsuccessful and a section proved necessary.[83] What the case of Mrs S.L. and the references to patients demanding c-sections reveal is patient agency. Agency was clearly not expressed in the same way, but it was one more pressure on physicians.

The issue of patient preference raises interesting questions of how much power and influence patients had, and how much physicians and the patients themselves felt that they should have. Did the patient have the right to insist on surgery that might endanger her life? In the early decades of the century, physicians clearly felt that she did, especially if it was to save the life of her child. But did anyone else have the right to pressure her to have the surgery? Physicians would not see themselves as pressuring women, but when they could argue that the c-section maternal mortality rate was low enough to make it an acceptable risk to ensure the survival of the child, the women had less ability to refuse. At times, pressure came from less altruistic motives. As noted in the previous chapter, some physicians about to go on fishing or hunting holidays were known to induce labour in women near term. When that failed, c-section would occur. But it was not always the physician who exerted outside pressure. In 1922 H. Orton Howitt of Guelph, Ontario, told of a patient, age forty-three, who had a large fibroid blocking the outlet of the pelvis, preventing the vaginal birth of a live child: 'Her husband was a prosperous farmer, and dearly wished for an heir. It was thought that unless this child was saved, there would be little chance of another child in the future. By caesarian section, a splendid male child was delivered. The fibroid was removed, at a subsequent operation.'[84] The pressure to provide the husband with an heir was clearly a factor in the decision. We cannot assume that the woman disagreed, but the telling point in this account is the emphasis on the desires of the husband rather than the wife. Fortunately for the former, a 'splendid' *male* child was born. Howitt's case raises an additional indicator for c-section: an elderly primipara. In 1930 C.B. Oliver of Chatham, Ontario, explained his practice. If any woman was forty-five years of age and pregnant for the first time, he offered her the choice of a c-section, after explaining the dangers of vaginal delivery and the safety of the section.[85] In this case, there was no specific medical indicator for the c-section. The only issue was that the woman was older and her first pregnancy would most likely be her last. For Oliver and others, age was a medical indicator. The maternal role was so central for women that the idea of not having a child could appear more horrendous to both physician and patient than undergoing surgery. Determining risk was not only a medical issue but also a social one.

Two subsidiary issues linked to c-section were sterilization and repeat c-sections. When the danger of c-section was high, the former was in vogue; when safety became assumed, the latter was, for many, a matter of course. In the early years of the century , doctors were understandably worried about a woman having to undergo a subsequent c-section if she became pregnant again. The solution for non-Catholic physicians was to sterilize the woman at the same time as performing a c-section. As one turn-of-the-century text made clear, 'A very important point in favour of caesarean section is that the Fallopian tubes can be tied and divided, so as to prevent subsequent conception, whereas embryotomy may require to be performed ten or a dozen times.'[86] A present risk offset a future risk. And the future risk of pregnancy was strong because birth control was illegal.

At first glance, sterilization placed control in the physicians' hands. However, physician control was only apparent. In the early decades of the century, it became almost a mantra in the medical literature that a physician could sterilize a woman only at her request.[87] The gravity of ending a woman's childbearing potential in a pro-natalist society meant that physicians needed the patient's consent. It absolved the physician of responsibility; he was simply doing what the patient requested. But although physicians would sterilize the woman only with her consent, they did not always wish to do so. In reporting one of his cases in 1907, Lapthorn Smith mentioned being asked by the patient to sterilize her during a c-section; but 'during the exciting interest of the operation,' he forgot to do so. Not that he considered this a significant oversight. As he explained, 'Naturally the woman was disappointed, but the writer no longer considers the operation [c-section] a serious one' if done early.[88]

Most physicians were not happy about sterilizing women; it

went against social mores and deep-seated beliefs about the purpose of women and the family. But what choice did they have? When indicators for c-section were relative, D.J. Evans of McGill suggested that subsequent vaginal births were possible as long as the abdominal wound healed to withstand the pressures of subsequent pregnancy and labour.[89] As indicated by Lapthorn Smith's reaction, some physicians were willing to entertain the idea of repeat c-sections rather than sterilization. In 1911 an article (unsigned) in the *Canadian Practitioner and Review* argued that there was no reason for repeated c-sections not to occur and 'no logical reason why the patient should not become the mother of a normal family, with periods of quiescence and comfort between pregnancies, making the operation of sterilization unnecessary.'[90] Thomas Watts Eden in his 1915 text pointed out that some women might not be entranced by the prospect of a repeated section, in which case sterilization should be done. However, his own feelings were that sterilization, which he termed 'permanent mutilation,' was unnecessary, since he had known the surgery to have been done up to five times on the same woman with few ill effects.[91]

The debate on sterilization continued throughout the interwar period and beyond. In 1922 A. Mackinnon of Guelph, Ontario, reported on a discussion at the British Medical Association, where doctors had expressed concern about performing c-sections on young women who most likely would soon become pregnant again. The fear was that any subsequent pregnancy and labour might result in the rupture of the uterus, and consequently, many argued that, although 'regrettable,' sterilization was the best option for the safety of the woman. Mackinnon, however, was not convinced and maintained that with proper care the danger of rupture could be avoided: 'Until I see a stronger reason I will not sterilize any mother on whom I may operate.'[92] He clearly believed that the decision to sterilize was his and not the patient's to make. Others, while sympathetic to his view on sterilization, believed that the old dictum 'Once a Caesarean, always a Caesarean' had merit.[93] Dictums or rules such as this provided physicians with security, giving medicine an aura of objectivity and relieving a physician of personal responsibility. Responsibility lay with general consensus. Not all were willing to follow the rule, however – the art of obstetrics militated against this. The old adage had merit, but it was only a guide. Some argued that a previous section was not an absolute indicator of the need for another one; each pregnancy had to be judged on its own merits. Ross Mitchell in 1938 suggested allowing a trial of labour after a previous c-section. He claimed that this would appeal to those women who refused to get pregnant again if faced with a repeat section.[94]

In 1930 John J. MacPherson, at the annual meeting of the New Brunswick Association of Registered Nurses, discussed the optimum number of c-sections that could be performed on the same woman. He estimated two to three, although picking up on Watts Eden, he acknowledged cases where five had occurred. But what did he do with his patients when they had reached the optimum number? The answer was sterilization – done by others if not by him.[95] Even among Catholics, sterilization was more of an option than it had been. In 1947 Ross Mitchell reported: 'If the patient is a Roman Catholic and the surgeon believes that Caesarean hysterectomy is, for that particular patient, a safer procedure than any type of conservative section, he may in the opinion of some Catholic moral theologians, perform the operation. The uterus need not be diseased to justify its removal.'[96] While a number of caveats limited the opinion, it potentially gave significant power to the surgeon. But not all physicians recognized the limits of c-section. In one extraordinary passage of a 1935 edition of *Midwifery*, the authors noted:

Caesarean section can be repeated indefinitely – it has been done 6 times on the same woman – and the risk when performed under proper conditions is no greater than at the first operation. The practitioner may be urged by the wife or husband, or both, to do some mutilating operation to prevent conception, and may feel that his duty is to carry out the patient's wishes. The medical profession has never recognized that patients have a right to give its members such orders as to disconnect the Fallopian tubes from the uterus, as they might order their plumber to disconnect the supply pipe to their bath. The Fallopian tube cannot be replaced like a bit of lead piping. Should the child die and the parents desire another, or should the mother become a widow and re-marry, and her second husband wish for a child of his own loins, she may return to her surgeon with the pathetic and hopeless demand to be put right again. Such things have happened, but the chance of their occurring weighs but slightly in deciding the balance against mutilation. The question is to be decided on higher ethical grounds, and the practitioner has a duty to the State as well as to his patient. If the woman fears to undergo another operation, it is the parents' business to avoid future pregnancies, not the practitioner's to make them impossible. If their measures fail and pregnancy results, abortion is at any rate a less immoral procedure than mutilation, for it involves the destruction of one pregnancy only, and not the incapacity of child-bearing for the woman's lifetime.[97]

First there is a dismissal of the dangers of section, followed by the statement that the physician is under no obligation to do what the patient requests. This stance is a far cry from that in the early years of the century when the dangers of c-section made physicians more willing to accede to requests for sterilization. Now, the prestige and status of the profession had become such that patients were not to have control (although clearly some still did). As reflected in this quotation, a new power alignment had formed. The practitioner's responsibility was not only to his patient but also to the state.[98]

Fortunately for patients, not all physicians were so categorical. In 1940 Nathan Shaul of Toronto analysed his obstetric practice and reported that he had performed 26 sections out of 1,449 deliveries. Of these 26, one was because the woman had heart disease and 'sterilization was indicated,' and two had been because of the 'desire for sterilization.'[99] Shaul was willing to do a c-section for no other reason than to sterilize a woman at the same time. A vaginal birth had a lower risk factor than a c-section but would require a separate sterilization procedure. Thus, the patient's decision to be sterilized resulted in a physician making

a decision based on convenience – the patient gets two procedures at one time. How typical Shaul was is unclear. But certainly
the willingness to combine the two procedures (for whatever
reason) was not unusual in some institutions. Over 40 per cent of
the c-sections done at the Burnside Lying-In Hospital between
1925 and 1939 were combined with sterilization.[100]

Others, however, were concerned about the signification of
this trend. Henricus J. Stander, author of a 1936 text on obstetrics
published in New York, criticized a pattern he saw. Too often
women had c-sections and sterilization for what he considered
as non-medical reasons – the woman's insanity or feeble-
mindedness. He maintained that this was against all medical
practice. Physicians should not perform c-sections on 'normal'
women (by which Stander meant physiologically normal); sterilization of such women should be separate from the childbirth
process.[101] No evidence of or concern about such a trend occurring in Canada was found. However, L.J. Harris of Toronto made
a similar point when he criticized performing c-section on women
with heart disease so that they could be sterilized at the same
time they gave birth. He was not against the sterilization, but like
Stander he thought it should be done as a separate procedure.
Physicians should not perform a higher-risk procedure in order
to do a lesser-risk procedure at the same time, no matter how
convenient this may have been.[102]

The decision on whether or not to combine c-section with
sterilization occurred within the broader confines of medical culture and its demands. One of these demands, as seen in chapter
2, was financial. Samuel S. Peikoff in his autobiography recalled
one incident:

In the spring of 1924 and I was lying fully clothed on my bed in the
Interns' Quarters. My head throbbed as I suffered the agony of a
hangover after attending a drunken farewell party the previous
night. I burned with shame. Just then Joe Allen, the senior intern,
sauntered into the room. 'How do you feel, Sam. Oh boy, what a
party. After just three drinks you were sailing on the clouds. You
kept ranting and raving about that ignorant slob who butchered

that young mother. Her Caesarian section was mercenary and unnecessary. You were more euphoric by the minute.'[103]

We have already noted that physicians performed sections more often on paying than non-paying patients. A physician who agreed with Peikoff's reaction pointed out in 1936 that the increase in c-section rate was due to 'medical competition' and economics.[104] In the late 1930s, L.J. Harris of Toronto referred to the 'surgical outlook' that eschewed the pain of nature. Doctors succumbed to impressing the family with dramatic intervention. In Harris's words, 'One gets very little credit for a skilful, successful delivery from below, but even an unnecessary Caesarean section usually makes the family feel that the attendant has done something wonderful and has saved the mother's or the baby's life.'[105] Many factors contributed to the surgical outlook of medicine and of society in general: more and better hospital facilities; the increasing number of physicians doing surgery; a falling birth rate that raised the value on the birth of a living child; and 'modern impatience and meddlesomeness.'[106] The latter in particular was a theme expressed about so many medical procedures. The time of physicians had become limited; too many were no longer willing, according to their own colleagues, to be patient and let nature take its course. Their training had prepared them for problems, which led to defensive medicine. Peer pressure also was present. Prominent physicians constantly wrote about the value of c-section in a variety of situations, and their readers could not help but be swayed.[107] Harold Atlee recorded:

During the war we had a patient whose long and trying labour ended in section. Four years later she approaches us, again pregnant, and very anxious to avoid operation. In the meantime her pelvis had been x-rayed and found well within normal measurements. We gave her a trial of labour under close supervision and she delivered in 8 easy hours. The baby weighed 155 g more than the previous one. It then came out that her air force husband had been ordered overseas the week before she started her first labour, which had greatly upset her. With the present baby, the war was over, her husband safe home and her motivation towards normality complete. We have encountered similar cases. Hasn't the time come for us to search the pregnant woman's soul as well as her pelvis in these cases of difficulty?[108]

How a physician could be expected to keep track of his patients' lives, let alone their souls, was unclear, but Atlee considered it necessary to try in order to practise good medicine. While the hyperbole of Atlee's imagery may seem controlling, he was encouraging his colleagues to listen to their patients and understand the context of their lives. The family physician, more than any specialist, would be in the best position to do so.

C-section was a form of obstetrical surgery which by 1950 had become accepted. Its history in Canada shows the concern that many within the profession had about its popularity. The debate about it reveals the way in which religious morality could affect the medical choices made. Canadian c-section rates in general were lower than those in the United States but could vary in specifics – perhaps the most significant being between paying and non-paying patients. The acceptance of c-section by mid-century was a far cry from the fear it had engendered at the turn of the century when it had incurred high maternal mortality rates. As a result, physicians had emphasized the absolute indications for its use rather than expanding the relative indications. They turned to patients for their permission to perform the surgery and, more particularly, the sterilization which would ensure that surgery would never be needed again. However, the pressure to accept c-section was strong, especially when its alternative – embryotomy – was considered. To avoid embryotomy, particularly on a live child, the amount of acceptable risk increased. Fortunately, for both mothers and physicians, the mortality rates from c-sections were declining, making it a much clearer choice for women with absolute indications. At the same time, as physicians became more comfortable with the surgery, they expanded the relative indications for it. In doing so, they reconfigured the meaning of the term *risk* so that they claimed they were saving two individuals (mother and child) when in fact they were *saving* only one (the child) and not losing the other (the mother, who in many, if not most, cases could have survived childbirth without a c-section). The fact that physicians continued to see mothers being saved (in rhetoric) reflects the long-standing priority that Protestant physicians in particular had given to the life of the mother over that of her child. It also reflects a reality that all physicians lived with in their practices – fear of maternal mortality.

CHAPTER EIGHT

Maternal Mortality and Postnatal Care

The death or serious disablement of the mother has grave social implications. The records of any social agency, particularly of those agencies which have to do with juvenile delinquency, show very often that a broken home lies at the root of the delinquency or other social problems. A mother's care means more to a young child than does anything else in the world. Individual and national efficiency are dependent upon healthy mothers. The deaths of the mothers result in a much higher mortality rate among the infants who survive them.

Grant Fleming, 1933[1]

Grant Fleming's words capture the importance of the childbirth outcome. Maternal mortality or morbidity could have long-term consequences for the children left behind and for the well-being of society itself. Physicians never underestimated the dangers of mortality. Compared with many other Western countries, Canada had a high rate of maternal mortality, a fact that embarrassed physicians because it reflected poorly on the kind of care women received in childbirth. Within Canada, the rates varied from province to province and between home and hospital births, the former being statistically safer. Whatever the rates, at a personal level, losing a patient was a physician's greatest fear, and it was the ever-present context of his interaction with women who were pregnant or about to give birth. As a group, physicians speculated about the reasons for the high mortality rates. Not surprisingly, their assessment differed from that of recent feminist critics. The latter have stressed physician culpability.[2] The former focused on medical issues, blamed women, and at times acknowledged that practitioners were not providing the care women deserved. Their solution was to medicalize childbirth through continual prenatal supervision and care, and hospitalization for the birth. For the majority of women who survived childbirth, the postnatal period was medicalized as well. A period of relative non-intervention, it still had its own medical customs, many of which were similar to those practised by First Nations people and midwives. Physicians debated the benefits of the binder and early rising. The latter, in particular, became an issue, since it signalled the relative end of medical supervision.

Accurate statistics on maternal mortality are difficult to come by; until the 1930s, the figures were underreported by as much as 20 or 25 per cent. One physician of the time admitted, 'Some physicians prefer to report ... almost any other cause [of mortality] rather than puerperal sepsis or one of the other causes of maternal mortality.' Clearly, such an admission called into question a practitioner's expertise.[3] Even if we do not know what the true figures were, available statistics of the time indicate that maternal mortality rates were high. In 1901 almost 700 Canadian women lost their lives from childbirth causes. In 1921, 1,206 women did. For the year 1 July 1925 to 30 June 1926, Dr Helen MacMurchy undertook what was, for the time, a comprehensive survey of maternal mortality. In that year 1,532 women lost their lives as a result of childbirth, a rate of 6.4 per thousand live births. Four women died every day – women in their prime (average age thirty-one) who left behind grieving families (5,073 children). The MacMurchy report determined that for most of the first two decades of the century, the average rate of maternal mortality had been 5.5 per thousand live births, which made Canada's rate the fourth highest among countries collecting such statistics. The United States had an even poorer record: in 1915 maternal mortality rates were 6.1 per thousand live births; in 1918, 9.2; in 1921, 6.8; and they remained close to that figure throughout the 1920s.[4] Rates for other countries from 1911 to

1913 are as follows: Scotland, 5.70; Spain, 5.27; Switzerland, 5.21; France, 4.78; England and Wales, 3.94; Germany, 3.48; Norway, 2.90; Italy, 2.44; Sweden, 2.42; and Holland, 2.29.[5] In Canada, next to tuberculosis, childbirth was the greatest killer of women during their childbearing years, and the figures did not decline much until 1937. Even the 4.0 rate in 1940 was still high compared with that of other industrialized nations. By 1946, however, the maternal mortality rate had reached a low of 1.64 per thousand.[6]

Rates among Canadians varied greatly. Ignored by most commentators were ethnic differences. Based on the mother's ethnicity, maternal mortality rates in 1927–8 in Canada were 6.1 per thousand live births for English Canadian women, 8.4 for Russian Canadian, 4.9 for French Canadian, 3.9 for Italian Canadian, and 11.0 for Native women.[7] The latter statistic gives the lie to the perception that Native women had an easier birth experience than most other women in Canada. Of more interest to government officials were the regional differences, which indicated that some provinces were better able than others to decrease mortality rates. Manitoba and Saskatchewan did so even in the depths of the Depression. In 1929 Manitoba had a maternal mortality rate of 6.8 per thousand live births, which it appeared to have cut in half to 3.8 by 1934. Similarly, Saskatchewan's rate declined from a high of 7.1 in 1926 to 4.4 in 1934. In 1937 an article in *Saturday Night* that detailed the provincial rates pointed out that if the country as a whole could approach the rates of the province with the lowest maternal mortality, then Canada would have the sixth-lowest rate in an international comparison of maternal mortality – a vast improvement over its actual standing of twenty-first.[8] If one province could do it, all provinces could. By the late 1930s, rates in Ontario and British Columbia had declined. In 1939 Quebec's rate of 4.7 per thousand live births was the lowest since 1926 (see figure 3). The 1943 figures show the provincial range, with a high of 4.1 in Prince Edward Island and a low of 2.2 in Ontario.[9]

Individual physicians and hospitals gathered their own statistics to compare with the provincial and national rates. Canadian

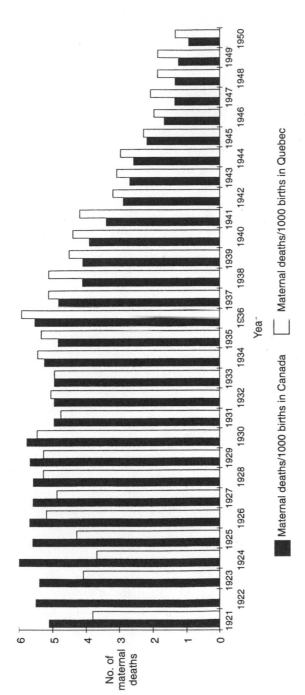

Figure 3 Comparative maternal death rate per 1000 live births in Quebec and Canada, 1921–1950

Source: Christine Payeur, 'Maternal Mortality in Quebec from the Medical Perspective and the Women's Point of View, 1890–1950 (MA thesis, Université de Montréal, 1998)

hospital officials were very aware of the reputation of hospitals as sites of danger. By making their mortality statistics better known, they fulfilled a public responsibility to be open about the care they provided to their patients – though the aim was also to assure potential patients that the institution was safe. In its annual reports, the Montreal Maternity Hospital always delineated its maternal mortality figures. Unlike the international, national, and provincial figures, its figures were not calculated on the basis of live births but simply on maternal deaths compared to the number of confinements. For 1901 the number of maternal deaths was one for the 229 confinements that took place in the hospital. If all 229 confinements had eventuated in live births, this would mean a rate of 4.3 per thousand live births, well below the national average. However, we cannot assume that all would have eventuated in live births, so the rate would have been higher. Since the hospital calculated mortality rates on the basis of death in relation to confinement, it claimed a maternal mortality rate of 0.43 per cent. The variation in rate over the years could be extreme, often being higher than the national average in the early decades and lower in the later ones.[10]

Many hospitals had both internal and external departments, and women could give birth through either. When in 1915 the maternal mortality rate in the Montreal Maternity Hospital was 0.64, the figure for births occurring in the home but supervised by the hospital was 0.54. In 1918 the hospital rate was 0.81 per cent and no mothers died in home confinements.[11] Of course, home births supervised by a hospital were by definition those expected to be uncomplicated. More difficult births were delivered in the hospital. Nor did hospital births show up well when compared with home births supervised by private practitioners. For example, H.J.G. Geggie, in looking at his pre-1919 practice in rural Quebec, noted that his maternal mortality rate had been one death out of 260, or four per thousand. His rate between 1920 and 1949, however, was six per thousand and was usually above the national average.[12] As Geggie's rate reveals, home births were not totally free of danger. Even when the best care was available, puerperal fever could develop. Herbert Bruce, himself a physician, told of his wife's confinement in which she had the professor of obstetrics at the University of Toronto deliver her at home and still developed fever.[13] Nevertheless, compared with hospital births, home birth mortality rates were lower and continued to be so. In 1928 only 30 per cent of women actually had their children in hospital, yet hospital births accounted for two-thirds of the maternal mortality rates.[14] In New York City a few years later, the situation was similar: studies revealed a hospital mortality rate twice that of home births.[15] Despite such figures, physicians persisted in supporting an increase in hospital births and comforted themselves that the higher mortality rates in hospitals reflected the higher-risk cases handled there.[16] Yet increased use of hospitals for maternity care and the inability of many institutions to keep up with the demand, especially during the Depression years, meant that conditions could be less than ideal. For example, the Vancouver General Hospital was so crowded that it placed women who had become septic in basement wards that were poorly ventilated and had inadequate facilities for nursing and food service.[17] Increasingly, however, commentators could extol the declining mortality rates in hospitals, comparing many of them favourably with the national average, and by the late 1940s physicians could argue that hospital births were now safer (in terms of mortality) than home births.[18]

The fact that during the first half of the century, mortality rates were lower when doctors or nurses were not even present was especially embarrassing for physicians. Dr M. Seymour, the medical officer of health for Saskatchewan, recalled his colleagues being upset when in 1919 he told them that women without medical care had lower rates of mortality than those with it. Throughout the 1920s and early 1930s, rural areas had lower maternal mortality rates than urban, even though fewer women in rural areas had access to a hospital or ongoing prenatal care. Even more demoralizing was a study done by the Ontario Red Cross in 1928 comparing its hospital mortality rates in isolated areas with the rates where no medical services were available at all. The latter were lower.[19]

One encouraging sign for those who believed in prenatal care

was that patients on public wards of hospitals who had partici-
pated in prenatal care programs had lower mortality rates than
patients who could afford private care but whose pregnancies
had been unsupervised. Winnipeg General Hospital had experienced a maternal mortality rate of 10.09 per thousand live births
for the period 1917–20, a figure in keeping with many other
hospitals but not particularly praiseworthy. After instituting a
prenatal clinic in 1921, the hospital saw a significant decline in its
mortality rate to 3.17 per thousand deliveries for the period 1923–
7, a rate half that of the country as a whole. But the hospital did
not factor in all maternal mortality deaths; it excluded women
who had entered with medical complications or were already in
grave distress. Thus, its low rate was only for a selected group of
women. The hospital's effort to reconfigure the statistics illustrates the embarrassment hospital authorities must have felt in
trying to explain the high rates in their institutions.[20]

Mortality rates did not tell the whole story. Many women
survived childbirth but were temporarily or permanently injured
by it. Morbidity rates were seldom kept, but some physicians
recognized that they could be worrisome. In 1930 C.B. Oliver of
Chatham, Ontario, concluded: 'Fifty per cent of women who
have borne children carry the marks of injury and many date a
life of permanent invalidism from the birth of their first baby.'[21]
Hospitals assessed morbidity by body temperature above normal. In the early years especially, when the fear of puerperal
sepsis was high, physicians kept a close watch on the temperature of their patients as an indication of well-being. For example,
the Montreal Maternity Hospital used any reading over 100.6° F
as an indication of morbidity. Using this measurement, in 1911–
12 the hospital had a morbidity rate of 15.8 per cent. The figure
increased to 21.8 per cent two years later and did not change
significantly until the end of the interwar period. The rate of the
external department, through which women were delivered in
their own homes, was considerably lower: in 1916 only 3.6 per
cent.[22] Other hospitals had similar morbidity rates, and while the
rates had generally declined by the early 1940s, owing to the
introduction of the sulphonamide drugs, some still remained

high, depending on the hospital and the circumstances.[23] Some physicians tried to explain the high rate of fever as physiological which, as James Goodall of McGill University pointed out in 1930, ignored the other 80 per cent of women who gave birth without running a fever of any kind. But he, too, had an explanation that focused attention away from the culpability of physicians and the hospital environment. He noted that in his experience the multiparous woman was more liable to fever than the primiparous. In the case of the former, the genital canal was more open to 'microbic invasions' and chronic endocervicitis (inflammation of the endocervix) from a previous birth, which subsequent birth trauma intensified. Thus, the design of a woman's body was the culprit. However, he did point out that the prone position in which doctors kept their patient after birth did not help, since it meant that 'she drains up-hill.'[24]

Physicians knew the major causes of maternal mortality: septicaemia associated with puerperal fever; toxaemias associated with vomiting of pregnancy and eclampsia; and haemorrhage. Estimates in the 1920s were that sepsis alone accounted for 27 to 33 per cent of deaths, haemorrhage 23 per cent, and toxaemias 22 per cent. A 1932 Canadian study estimated that of the 1,180 women who died from puerperal causes, sepsis was at fault in 23.9 per cent, toxaemias in 21.6 per cent, and haemorrhage and shock in 15.8 per cent. The 1942 statistics confirmed the primacy of these three causes, which accounted for 72.6 per cent of maternal deaths.[25] Although the three remained significant, puerperal deaths did fall. In 1944 Ernest Couture, director of the Division of Maternal and Child Hygiene, Ottawa, noted that between 1939 and 1942 the mortality rate from toxaemias of pregnancy had declined by 49 per cent, from haemorrhage 26 per cent, and from sepsis 19 per cent. Murray Blair of Vancouver General Hospital was not as sanguine, suggesting in 1945 that in the previous ten years, while improvement in sepsis deaths had been considerable, in toxaemia deaths the improvement had been only minor, and in haemorrhage-related deaths little had changed.[26]

The high maternal mortality rates and, to a lesser extent, the morbidity rates appalled most people. They represented a reality that most women had to face – potential death or injury in childbirth. Some women feared 'that journey into the valley of the shadow.' Others channelled fear into anger. Violet Mc-Naughton, in a paper submitted to the Canadian National Association of Graduate Nurses in the late teens, railed against such deaths: 'I am constantly crossing the tracks of dead babies and dead mothers who never ought to have died ... The state guards and protects our hogs and our forests and allows our children [and mothers] to die.'[27] Some popular commentators took the danger women faced and used it as an instructional tool. One who did so was Arthur W. Beall, who made a career of lecturing on sexual topics to young audiences. In his 1933 book, *The Living Temple: A Manual on Eugenics for Parents and Teachers*, he said that when telling young boys the facts of life, one should stress the sacrifices made by mothers, and in melodramatic language, he provided an example of what boys should hear: 'For, on the day that *you* were born, boys, *your* mother came up to the edge of the grave, then she slipped down, down, down, and into the grave. *Your* mother A-L-M-O-S-T went ... For on the day that you were born your mother went down into the Valley of the Shadow of Death so that you might live. Hands, now please, to the top storey and repeat: "On the day that I was born my mother went down into the Valley of the Shadow of Death, so that I might live."'[28]

Losing a patient in childbirth was probably the hardest loss a physician had to face. Childbirth was meant to bring joy, and instead maternal mortality brought tragedy. In some situations a physician could do little to stop the tragedy, and he would suffer feelings of professional inadequacy. The discussions of whether childbirth was physiological or pathological were part of physicians' efforts to come to terms with the high maternal mortality rates and the loss of some of their patients. For physicians who believed in the naturalness of childbirth, the death toll was perplexing. For those who saw childbirth as inherently pathological, especially for 'modern women,' the rates were not surprising, though they still represented the failure of modern medicine to respond to the problems modernity posed. Physicians expressed their concern in a number of ways: by representations to the government to support them in their prenatal educational efforts; through their various surveys of maternal mortality; by setting up maternal mortality committees; and with their efforts to keep track of trends in maternal mortality.[29] Like Violet McNaughton, some physicians became angry. In 1924 Joseph N. Nathanson of Ottawa called maternal mortality 'the greatest medical crime of to-day.'[30] Concerned about and embarrassed by the rates of maternal mortality, physicians were anxious to explain them. Some addressed the medical issues that complicated pregnancy; others focused on the lives women led; and still others discussed the possible culpability of physicians themselves in the care they provided (or did not provide) to women.[31]

Physicians were familiar with the complications of pregnancy – some of them unforseen, others linked to the health of the mother. Hospitals made a point of listing the number of births taking place and highlighting those with complications. As noted above, in 1901 the *Annual Report of the Montreal Maternity Hospital* listed 229 confinements. These included the use of forceps in seven, a craniotomy in one, a woman with eclampsia in four, birthing twins in two, placenta praevia in one, a breech presentation in two, and a face presentation in two.[32] Disproportion, placenta praevia, and eclampsia were conditions for which physicians early in the century could do little except to intervene in ways that potentially risked the mother's life. But in the interwar period in particular, physicians argued that with prenatal care they could help offset some of these conditions or at least intervene before the situation got out of hand. For his part, Ross Mitchell of Winnipeg puzzled over why some women developed sepsis and others did not under apparently similar conditions. His conclusion was that 'focal infections as of teeth, or tonsils, overwork, lack of rest, even mental depression and worry, predispose to infection. All these conditions are capable of being corrected if the patient is seen early in her pregnancy.'[33] Many physicians were eager to explain how maternal deaths were often the consequence of complicating factors for which they were not accountable. As already seen, many thought that childbirth itself was a complicating factor.

Some women had specific health problems which made it difficult for them to endure pregnancy and the complications attending it. Mrs Frances Patterson, age thirty and married for six years, entered the Royal Victoria Hospital, Montreal, on 4 October 1902. The previous day, she had experienced some bloody discharge, which stopped and then began again along with labour pains. On 4 October she had an early miscarriage. The complicating factor was that after the birth of her last child, three years earlier, she had developed acute diabetes. The doctors could do little, and on 9 October she died, although the records were unclear whether it was from complications resulting from her miscarriage or from the diabetes, or a combination of both.[34]

Studies done in the interwar period on maternal mortality emphasized both previous health problems and the perception that while pregnancy might be natural, it still placed extra burdens on a woman's system.[35] Even the declining birth rate became a factor, since it meant that a higher percentage of births were first births, and physicians believed that first births posed more danger to a woman than subsequent births (at least until the fifth birth). This belief remained popular after the interwar period, especially when doctors pointed out that not only did the declining birth rate create more first births, but more of those births were occurring in older women (who, they believed, experienced more complications than younger women).[36] Physicians also argued that complicated pregnancies helped explain the difference between rural and urban maternal mortality rates, the argument being that the complicated cases from the rural areas, whether from childbirth complications or previous health complications, were sent to city hospitals, thus increasing both hospital and urban maternal mortality rates.[37]

Recognizing the problems of pregnant women with poor health, Manitoba's minister of health and public welfare made a rather extreme suggestion in 1929: 'To improve the record in the case of patients whose general health is unsatisfactory might mean instructions on the delicate subject of birth-control, it might mean early interference in pregnancy already established, in any event it would mean exhaustive and repeated examinations of the potential mother until the cause of unsatisfactory health is determined and dealt with.'[38] A few even suggested that women with health problems should not marry or have children, and that if they did so, physicians should not be held accountable for the consequences.[39] The suggestion was also made that deaths linked to previous health complications should not be included in the maternal mortality statistics.[40] While there was a certain logic to this, it still would not explain why Canadian maternal mortality statistics were higher than those of many other countries. After all, the way of categorizing maternal deaths was common to several of them.

Physicians believed that they understood the medical needs of women in pregnancy and childbirth and that if, for whatever reason, women did not follow advice, responsibility lay with the individual woman not with the medical profession or the wider society. But many women, especially poor women, had limited choices, and as a result of their economic situation they might not have been able to take advantage of the maternal care resources offered. Doctors assumed that poorer women, who had less access to medical care, would have higher maternal mortality rates; but as seen, studies did not always support this assumption.[41] Perplexed but not daunted, physicians continually addressed the need for more women to have access to medical assistance. The famous 1925–6 study undertaken by Helen MacMurchy revealed that a high percentage of women who died were poor and in questionable health; but while acknowledging this, the study did not address the problem other than to urge that such women receive medical care.[42] That such studies did not address any underlying social and economic disparities is not surprising. Physicians as a group focused on what they knew best – medical care. Consequently, many hospitals set up maternal clinics in the interwar period to ensure that poor women had a full range of prenatal care. Women could either give birth at home or in the public ward of a hospital and, as seen, their maternal mortality rates in either case were lower than the national average. Women's organizations, too, supported access to medical services for all women.[43]

The focus of lay people and physicians in providing more services to the poor escalated in the Depression. Mrs Manifold of the Women's Navy League, Vancouver, spoke before the B.C. Royal Commission on State Health Insurance and Maternity Benefits in the early 1930s and told the commissioners: 'I am among the working-class a lot and as soon as a mother is pregnant the first thing she thinks of is the question, "How am I going to foot the bill?" And from the first month on it is continual dread and worry, a condition very bad for her.'[44] Toronto physician J.N.E. Brown also acknowledged that poverty stopped some of his indigent patients from getting in touch with him early in their pregnancies. But while Mrs Manifold seemed to understand their situation, Brown blamed the women.[45] However, his voice was atypical. During the Depression, most physicians in their public statements clearly understood that many women could not come to them because of financial concerns, and they tried to encourage governments to provide such women with monetary assistance.[46] From the physicians' point of view, it was a win-win situation: the women would benefit from the care physicians could provide, and the physicians would benefit through a guaranteed roster of paying patients.

In 1935 the Canadian Welfare Council completed a study on maternal mortality and found that 'impaired health' arising 'out of conditions of disease and malnourishment of the young mother in her own childhood and adolescence' was a significant cause of maternal mortality. The question was what to do. Proper nourishment was important, but some physicians argued that women were malnourished because they were overly concerned about their weight.[47] But while the middle and upper classes could afford to worry about body shape, many of the poor had to worry about keeping that body alive. A nutritional study done by Alan Brown in 1940 made a clear connection between low income and the inability of pregnant women to get enough to eat, and the linkage between poorly nourished women and complications of birth. Ernest Couture, director of the Division of Maternal and Child Hygiene, believed that there had been better nourishment among women during the war years, because of rationing and price-control regulations. In addition, the economic upswing during the war had meant that poorer women could afford to use the medical services available.[48]

Although some physicians were aware that many women either could not afford their services or lived in areas where medical services were few, others believed that too many women simply did not take advantage of medicine's assistance through ignorance. As a physician exclaimed at the thirty-sixth meeting of the Dominion Council of Health, in 1938, 'You cannot blame the medical profession. [Maternal mortality] is something that our efforts will not prevent, unless some drastic means are taken. It is particularly through ignorance of the women that these things occur.' One physician linked such ignorance with poverty (class).[49] Most physicians, however, assumed that the ignorance was widespread – most women did not know what was best for them. And, in general, society agreed. That was why the educational campaign that occurred in the interwar period was necessary. Physicians, governments, and women's organizations all focused on the need to educate women about pregnancy and childbirth, and the need for women (according to the campaign) to seek out medical direction throughout their pregnancies. Even Archbishop Williams, the Anglican metropolitan of Ontario, entered the fray and in 1928 blamed the death of so many women in childbirth on the poor education they received concerning motherhood.[50] Women had to be educated for their social role in life. But education was not always successful. As some commentators pointed out, some women simply ignored the advice given them or did not take advantage of the help available. In 1936 the author of an article in the *Canadian Medical Association Journal* specifically blamed the independence of the modern woman and her insistence on working in 'unsuitable occupations.'[51]

At times, doctors focused on race. The author of a 1913 editorial argued that the maternal mortality rates in Ontario should be lower in counties where Anglo-Ontarians lived, and he was quite perturbed to discover lower rates where Franco-Ontarians lived. Especially galling was the fact that physicians were not as numerous among Franco-Ontarians as among Anglo-Ontarians. The author was in a quandary to explain the results. If maternal mortality was race related, statistics suggested that Franco-Ontarians were a stronger 'race' than Anglo-Ontarians, a conclusion he did not wish to entertain. Consequently, he examined an equally repellent alternative – perhaps physicians were the cause of the difference! He raised it as a possibility only to reject it. Who or what was responsible remained unclear, though he asked, 'Are the parturient women themselves blamable for their own undoing?'[52] In the interwar years, too, some physicians focused on racial differences as an explanation of the high maternal mortality rates in Canada compared with elsewhere. Canada was becoming more racially diverse, and different racial groups experienced different rates of maternal mortality, which placed Canada and its physicians in a less than enviable position. Much of this discussion took place at the height of the eugenics movement and blamed birthing difficulties on intermarriage between races. A study done in Toronto by Toronto General Hospital and the University of Toronto, for example, focused on the 'varieties of foetal, maternal and paternal head and pelvic shapes as they were related to primary racial types, indicating the problems associated with racial admixtures as they might influence difficult labour in a new country such as Canada.'[53] By raising race, commentators did not have to address the social and economic situation in which various groups found themselves; rather, their explanation lay in the racial biology of the parents.

Another factor on which physicians focused to explain the high mortality rates (and for which they argued they were not responsible and thus should not be blamed) was death from abortion. Spontaneous abortion (miscarriage) was common, some estimates of it being 7 to 10 per cent of all pregnancies. At times, these abortions could lead to death. For example, if the abortion was not complete, some parts of the foetus might remain, resulting in sepsis. If the woman was aware of the abortion, she might go to a physician who could do a dilation and curettage (d & c), but risks accompanied every medical procedure, particularly if the physician did not secure a sterile field. Physicians argued that abortion deaths should not be attributed to them, which is what they felt maternal mortality statistics implied. Although they could more easily accept responsibility for the deaths resulting from d & c, many felt that these were not really maternal deaths but the result of a gynaecological procedure. Even more upsetting to physicians were abortion deaths from criminal action. As physicians liked to point out, the rates of mortality consequent on them were high and the incidence of such abortions was increasing.[54] The issue for physicians was that maternal mortality statistics included illegal abortion deaths (often categorized under puerperal sepsis and haemorrhage rather than under abortion) and these artificially inflated the mortality rate.[55] According to them, these deaths explained the increased maternal mortality rates in cities, as well as the difference between the low rates of maternal mortality in births directed by the VON, Red Cross, etc., compared with figures for the country as a whole, and the high maternal mortality rates for unwed women.[56]

By the late 1930s and the 1940s, physicians were more willing to meet the difficulties connected with abortion deaths head on. H.B. Van Wyck wrote in the *University of Toronto Medical Journal* that calculating maternal mortality based on live births underestimated the rate. All deaths associated with abortions (spontaneous and criminal) and all deaths connected to stillbirths were part of the maternal mortality picture.[57] Physicians were not on the defensive as much as they had been, probably because the official maternal mortality statistics were plummeting and physicians could begin to address the wider issue of deaths linked to pregnancy and birth, including abortion deaths. Indeed, with mortality rates declining, those linked to abortion loomed even larger.[58]

Because of their sensitivity about the high maternal mortality rates, physicians often engaged in a search for explanations that at times focused attention on aspects other than the actual care women received. By personalizing the causes to the situation of the individual patient – health, race, class, age – the physician absolved himself of responsibility. Nevertheless, physicians were willing to acknowledge that not all was well within the profession in terms of how doctors treated women. We have already seen that many who specialized in obstetrics considered that their training had been deficient. For some, the linkage between this and maternal mortality rates was clear. In 1905 A. Lapthorn Smith railed against practitioners who did not know how to care for the lacerations of the perineum, leaving it for a gynaecologist, such as himself, to undo what they had tried to do.[59] Dr W.B. Hendry, in examining the maternal mortality rates of the Burnside Lying-In Hospital from 1914 to 1922, found them 'appallingly high,' the result in many cases of 'lack of supervision during gestation, careless preliminary examinations or none at all, ill-timed and meddlesome interference, imperfect technique and an unrecognized disproportion between mother and child,' revealing a situation in which physicians had failed in what they were to do – protect the health and life of their patient.[60]

In the early decades of the century, accusations abounded that physicians were not practising aseptic techniques. The result was sepsis, causing puerperal fever and, too often, death. Physicians encouraged one another to treat patients in ways that would limit sepsis – using gloves, limiting vaginal examinations, sterilizing the genital area before birth.[61] The Halifax Medical College in the first decade of the century trained its students by insisting that 'no student attending the Practical Anatomy Room will be allowed to visit or attend patients.' The college was not going to take any chance of having infection introduced to patients. Its physicians had learned the lesson taught by Ignaz Semmelweiss, the Hungarian physician and medical pioneer of antisepsis in obstetrics, who in the nineteenth century had recognized that infection was carried by physicians from patient to patient. One notorious case of poor obstetric technique was that of Dr Harper Willson, which resulted in a 1909 inquiry by the Council of the College of Physicians and Surgeons of British Columbia into the death of his patient, Mrs R.H. Ley of Nelson. Testimony of a Dr Arthur revealed that on his way to see Mrs Ley he had met Willson, Mrs Ley's family physician. Arthur had been summoned when Willson could not be found. Despite the fact that Willson was apparently drunk, Arthur left him at Mrs Ley's and told the nurse to give him strong tea or coffee and he would be fine. Willson subsequently called in Arthur, asking him to bring his instruments and chloroform. The main charge against Willson was that he failed to sterilize the forceps used. The most intriguing aspect of the inquiry is the questioning of the practical nurse, Mrs Kenny. It was more an interrogation, as if the doctors and judge were seeking to blame her rather than Willson. They questioned her memory, asked leading questions, and seemed to encourage other witnesses to criticize her. Nonetheless, they had to find against Willson.[62]

It is difficult to know how many women died from sepsis in private practice in the early decades of the century, but the maternity hospitals kept careful records. In 1911 the Montreal Maternity Hospital reported that 37 per cent of maternal deaths were the result of infection. H.M. Little of McGill University took pains to rationalize the figures. Thirteen women had lost their lives to infection but, according to Little, only three deaths were a consequence of the treatment they had received in hospital. Seven of the women had entered hospital after having received treatment (and thus, supposedly, being infected at that point). One woman, who had had a sore throat, died of peritonitis, another died after a caesarian, and another died after a pubiotomy (surgical separation of pubic bone); the first was already suffering from a streptococcal infection, and the other two had died as a result of serious procedures which were intrinsically problematic. This left three dying from infection contracted as a result of birth in the hospital.[63] Little's explanation seemed rather forced, but it was understandable. He was trying to separate avoidable deaths, for which the hospital was responsible, from those for which they had little liability. Hospitals, especially those connected with teaching institutions, did seem to be very sensitive about decreasing the number of deaths from sepsis. Their staff were aware of the history of puerperal fever raging through hospitals. They too had learned the lessons of Semmelweiss. Teaching hospitals, in particular, were at pains to maintain aseptic techniques and an aseptic environment. Unfortunately, all hospitals were not teaching hospitals. Nor did all in private practice have the same concern. Some commentators pointed out that while sepsis in hospital maternity patients was declining, in private practice it was not.[64]

The call in the interwar period to treat obstetric cases with the same care as surgical cases was in part a call for better aseptic techniques. Colleagues warned one another that the naturalness of birth should not persuade physicians into thinking that they could avoid the same commitment to cleanliness. Critics claimed that sloppy obstetric technique was the major cause of sepsis and other causes of death.[65] In 1924 seven patients died at Toronto's Burnside Lying-In Hospital as a result of childbed fever. In 1936 seven women died of puerperal fever at Winnipeg General Hospital.[66] Yet, some physicians did not seem interested in improving. When in the early 1930s the Canadian Medical Association sent out a questionnaire suggesting to local associations the desirability of setting aside one meeting a year to focus on preventative obstetrics, the response was 'unsatisfactory.' To the ninety letters sent, only twenty-eight replies were received; and of the twenty-eight, only four societies held meetings on maternal welfare.[67] Obstetric specialists felt that the general practitioner simply did not take the issue seriously enough.[68]

Seen as a consequence of poor training and a cause of septic infection, the interventionist nature of obstetrics was said, by some physicians, to distort the naturalness of childbirth. Intervention could save a woman's life, but it could also place that life at risk. Although Western medicine was oriented toward intervention, the degree of intervention varied from country to country. A recent study of maternal mortality in the early twentieth century revealed significant differences between medicine as practised in the United States, for example, and elsewhere. In Holland the rate of obstetrical intervention was less than 1 per cent; in Sweden it was 3.2 per cent, but in New York it was 20 per cent, with sepsis deaths reaching 40 per 10,000 births (compared with only 4 when no intervention occurred). Who intervened also varied. In Britain the general practitioner did, but in the

United States both specialist and generalist were to blame.[69] In the early decades of the century, intervention could easily lead to sepsis if physicians did not take extreme care. The case of Mrs Stafford Healy, age thirty, was typical. On 14 June 1903 she delivered a child after a very long and instrumental birth. Subsequently she developed abdominal pain along with weakness and fever, a sure sign of puerperal fever, and entered the Royal Victoria Hospital, Montreal. She stayed in the hospital until 5 August and then left, against the wishes of her physicians.[70] The point is not to disagree with the use of forceps – in long labours they were indicated – but to suggest that their use could lead to other complications. The challenge of medicine was to know when to intervene and when not to. The fear of many physicians was that too many of their colleagues did not know where to draw the line either way.[71] To confuse the issue, the indications for intervention changed over time. Nevertheless, the concern about 'meddlesome' midwifery remained constant.

Looking at the maternal mortality rates in the mid-1920s, Helen MacMurchy castigated her colleagues for using forceps too much and not performing prenatal checkup enough. She was not the only critical voice. Looking at his own record and concerned about what his colleagues were doing, O.A. Cannon from Hamilton, Ontario, pointed out the flaws of much obstetrical practice: 'With little excuse men every day are rupturing the membranes too soon, forcibly dilating the cervix, applying forceps and doing version. All of these procedures potentially infect the uterus by conveying infection from below upwards.'[72] In 1928 Ross Mitchell of Winnipeg pointed out how the mortality rate at the Winnipeg General Hospital was half that of the country as a whole, and he claimed lack of intervention as a partial explanation. However, the conservative principles of the Winnipeg General's doctors consisted of replacing one form of intervention with another – specifically, replacing the use of forceps with the use of morphine and scopolamine.[73] The situation in the United States may have been more extreme. A 1933 study of maternal mortality in New York City discerned that 65.8 per cent of the deaths were preventable and that responsibility lay with the physician in 61.1 per cent of these and with the patient in only 36.7 per cent. Physician responsibility was almost equally divided between errors of technique (50.9 per cent) and judgment (49.1 per cent).[74] In England, almost half the deaths were avoidable, with 50 per cent of those being linked to deficiencies in facilities or in judgments by staff, 33 per cent due to lack of prenatal care, and 17 per cent due to negligence on the part of the patient.[75]

Despite the medical profession's self-criticism, the message given to women was the need for more medical attention, not less. How could this be, given the high rates of maternal mortality connected with physician-directed births for the first four decades of the century? Physicians were able to acknowledge the need for improvement on their part (or, more likely, that of their colleagues) and at the same time maintain their faith in medicine. The fault was not with medicine but with the way physicians practised it; anything that brought women closer to the medical *ideal* was desirable. By the 1940s, when it became clear that maternal mortality rates were decreasing, the emphasis on physician-related deaths also decreased. Not that physicians believed they had solved the problem. Far from it. But they did argue that they were heading in the right direction, something not possible in the earlier decades.[76] Murray Blair of Vancouver General Hospital, however, reminded his colleagues that errors in medicine would always occur: 'The man who makes no medical mistakes is the man with no practice.'[77]

The remedies that physicians advocated to reduce maternal mortality rates were associated with the perceived causes of maternal mortality. They looked to medical advances to treat some of the problems faced by women in pregnancy and childbirth. In some cases, these advances were not improvements in the actual care given to women but, rather, ways of offsetting the problems caused by the care provided. For example, in the late 1930s and the 1940s the introduction of the first sulphanilamides, and then antibiotic drugs, went a long way to control the problem of sepsis. These drugs did not prevent it, but they countered its virulence and thus lowered mortality from infection. In the same way, blood transfusions lessened the dangers posed by haemorrhage.[78] However, some physicians, such as W.G. Cosbie of Toronto General Hospital, were not willing to give exclusive credit to the new drug therapies; they pointed out that mortality had declined on the maternity wards before the introduction of the sulphanilamides.[79] More knowledge about nutrition and its role in a healthy pregnancy was also a factor in lowering the maternal mortality rate. Nutritional studies, especially in the Depression and afterwards, examined the nourishment women received and warned that pregnant women were among the least nourished members of a family.[80]

As already noted, many physicians thought that women were to blame for some of their own problems. The 'scientific motherhood' movement involved educating women about the needs of their bodies during pregnancy and childbirth, and instructed them on the crucial role that physicians could play in proffering advice and providing the care they needed. But the relationship between physician and patient was an unequal one. As Toronto physician W.B. Hendry told his colleagues, 'In maternal mortality the two main factors to be considered are the doctor and the mother. The work of the former and the education of the latter are of vital importance to the life of the community, and every doctor should be an educator.'[81] Women were to follow what the physician advised. Because the advice was scientific, women had to adjust their circumstances to meet its demands; any decisions made at odds with the advice would be deemed irrational. While this took away agency from women, at the same time the educational campaign raised the awareness of Canadians to the loss of maternal life, which the country could ill afford. Physicians such as Helen MacMurchy urged fellow physicians, husbands, and the public to value what a mother did.[82] MacMurchy noted the popularity of her series of advice books to women but commented that requests for no. 8, 'How to Take Care of Mother,' were not particularly high. 'The mother usually writes to ask for the books. She forgets herself. It is the mother who takes care of everybody. Who takes care of her? This is the duty of every nation and every citizen, especially every husband, every father, every boy, every girl, who reads this page. Take care of Mother. You will miss her when she is gone.'[83]

The educational campaign also informed physicians about what was necessary. Physicians' willingness to criticize the care being offered to women by other physicians and their concern about obstetric education meant that they knew they controlled some of the remedies. Understandably, these remedies were medical, not social. The whole thrust of the educational campaign was to convince women that they should use physicians, seek prenatal care, and give birth in hospital. Underlying these three aspects was the belief that if physicians gave the best care they could, maternal mortality would decrease significantly. Physicians offered the ideal even though the reality of what women received was sometimes much less.

Physicians believed in continual prenatal supervision. Even though many of the causes of mortality were connected to poor childbirth technique and could not be addressed by prenatal care, physicians could not give up their hope that continued medical supervision was the answer. And it was a factor. Deaths from toxaemias of pregnancy did decrease, in part because prenatal care allowed physicians to intervene and control the situation before full eclampsia developed. Perhaps as important, the emphasis on the necessity of prenatal care made physicians conscious of taking the pregnant woman seriously.[84] In turn, many hoped that medical supervision during pregnancy would culminate in a hospital birth. Strategically located hospitals were a practical answer for women who lived in isolated areas where the distances precluded personal medical care. The gradual decline in hospital maternal mortality encouraged physicians attached to hospitals, especially teaching hospitals, and allowed them to argue with conviction that they were safe places for women to be.[85] It is this perception that many feminist scholars have challenged.[86] But the spectre of maternal mortality never disappeared. It prompted physicians to intervene during both pregnancy and labour. Despite the high mortality rates for much of the first half of the twentieth century, physicians remained convinced that scientific medicine would ultimately come to the rescue of women.

While it is understandable why physicians felt compelled to believe in the medical system of which they were a part, it is more difficult to understand women's acceptance of medical science. And certainly they did accept it. Women's organizations supported the use of physicians and the increasing hospitalization of birthing. Individual women sought out medical assistance and went to hospital to deliver their children. Given the apparent higher mortality rates until the late 1930s in both physician-directed and hospital births, this would appear to be against their best interests. But although it is logical to assume that women knew the variation in the rates, there is little to suggest that in fact they did. Women's organizations knew that Canadian maternal mortality rates were high, but this did not necessarily translate into a condemnation of medicine. Indeed, their actions in support of increasing medicalization of birthing suggests the opposite. Women partook of the culture of science; they internalized it in their attempts to provide nutritious meals to their families. The North American orientation to a 'technological' fix may have been part of this, although much more research would be needed to substantiate it. The media, through advertising, bombarded women with the benefits of household appliances; belief in scientific or medical appliances was simply an extension of this. Lastly, in accepting medical science, Canadian women were not doing anything new. By the end of the nineteenth century, they had accepted the value of medical assistance, so what other choice did they have? Midwives were few and far between. In any case, death in childbirth was nothing new. The rates may have increased in the early twentieth century, but women had long accustomed themselves to the possibility of death. Doctors were their attempt to offset it, but in the end it would be God's will that prevailed.[87]

The question that most historians have addressed is the reason for the decline in Canadian maternal mortality rates. In general they have rejected hospitalization as a factor and focused on the introduction of sulpha drugs, better obstetric technique, and improved socio-economic conditions.[88] But what accounted for the high rates in the first place? We have seen that physicians had their own views. The statistics of other countries, especially those in Western Europe, suggest that a system in which trained midwives dominated seemed of benefit. Within Canada, Quebec consistently had lower maternal mortality rates than the national average in the 1920s, and one historian has suggested that prior to the mid-1930s Quebec's doctors were less interventionist than those elsewhere.[89] Whether it is possible to go beyond speculation is unclear.

What is clear is that maternal mortality was everpresent in physicians' consideration of childbirth. It coloured their view of birth, leading many to see childbirth as a potentially pathological process. Fear of maternal mortality prodded them to emphasize prenatal care and prepared them to intervene if there was any suggestion that the mother's life was at risk. Losing a woman in childbirth was such a horrendous outcome that the varying degrees of intervention did not loom as large as they might have done otherwise. As members of their profession, physicians worried that the high maternal mortality rates reflected badly on the efficacy of medical science and the way in which it was practised, although they could comfort themselves that American rates were higher. The focus on high maternal mortality rates was especially acute after the First World War, with its substantial loss of life and the subsequent and almost equally devastating loss of life in the influenza epidemic. Physicians in the interwar years queried and probed the causes of maternal mortality, focusing, as they had been trained to do, on the causes which medicine could respond to and control. In this way they could ignore the disturbing statistics that suggested that home and non-physician-directed births were safer than hospital and doctor-directed births. They argued that it was not medicine that was at fault but the nature of childbirth itself, the complications of pregnancy, and the existing health problems of many women. In addition, the lives some women led were culpable. While women were not responsible for the poverty in which some of them lived, they were responsible for ignoring medical advice and also for resorting to procedures such as abortion that could lead to death, thereby raising the rates of maternal mortality. Individual practitioners, too, were not blameless. Too often their training was deficient and they did not practise good medicine – for instance, by overlooking the problems of intervention and the importance of maintaining antiseptic conditions. The solution was more and better medical care. There was little wrong with medicine itself. Once doctors could practise the kind of medicine they should, other solutions would follow. Medical advances would show the way. Scientific motherhood would make it clear to women that if they would only consult a physician, follow a prescribed prenatal regimen, and give birth in a hospital, the lowering of maternal mortality rates would reflect the true value of medical care. Throughout the challenge posed by high mortality rates, doctors' faith in medical science remained unshaken.

Although maternal mortality rates haunted physicians, most women who gave birth did not die; and for those who did not, the story of childbirth was not over until after the immediate postnatal period. Physicians were not as involved in postnatal care as they believed they needed to be in prenatal care. Nonetheless, they continued to keep a watchful eye and gave advice on a variety of issues, among them the diet of the new mother, how to restore her figure to its prepregnant state, and, most contentious of all, how long she should remain in bed before rising and engaging in her usual activities. The irony is that in their views, many physicians did not differ significantly from the customs followed by First Nations people and midwives.

As we have already seen in the chapter on childbirth, many northern Aboriginal people provided a separate dwelling space or structure for a woman giving birth. Afterwards she would remain there for a specific period – among the Inuit until she stopped bleeding or, according to some, until the umbilical cord was no longer attached to the child. Before returning to her family she had to clean herself and dispose of her clothing and bedding. These customs were believed to ensure that the woman did not endanger her own health, that of her child, or the community. Of course, staying in a separate dwelling was only possible when the community was in a permanent or semi-permanent situation.[90] The Dene did not separate a birthing woman but insisted that she keep to her own side of the tent, relieve herself in a separate place, and not walk freely around the campsite until bleeding ceased. Among the Great Whale River people, the birthing mother remained supine for about a week with her head toward the tent door. The following week she avoided heavy work, often having a young girl help her.[91] Yet reports of some Native peoples in southern Saskatchewan suggest that their women did not stay lying down for any time at all after giving birth.[92]

Postnatal diets were generally limited, but the details of what the new mother could eat varied considerably from one group to another and also could vary depending on the sex of the child.[93] Reflecting the belief of the impurity of the postnatal period, many Native groups insisted that the woman drink and eat from her own pots.[94] Midwives in non-Native communities followed many similar customs. As seen in the chapter on midwives, they generally assisted the woman for a week to ten days after birth and insisted that new mother practise dietary restrictions. The focus of attention was the recuperation of the mother and her integration back into her family and community.

The patterns recommended by physicians were similar. They believed that proper and specific nourishment would help in recuperation. David James Evans of McGill, for example, in his 1900 textbook suggested 'milk, clear soup, gruel, cocoa, weak tea, toast, stale bread, and soft-boiled eggs' until the third day, after which there could be a gradual return to normal eating. He also stated that the woman could have a limited amount of malt liquor and wine if she was accustomed to them. Others agreed about the light diet immediately after birth, though they were not as willing as Evans to endorse alcoholic beverages.[95] The dietary advice did not change much over time. A 1930 American text advocated a light and largely liquid diet for about two days and 'substantial' food on the third. The author warned, however, that 'the giving of milk, cocoa and gruels between meals "to increase the supply of breast milk" should not be overdone,' since it could lessen the appetite for solid food.[96]

Like midwives in the early years of the century, many physicians advocated the abdominal binder, which they believed would allow the woman in bed to turn more easily and would give her support even after she began to sit up. Grace Hospital in St John's used binders well into the 1940s.[97] Other physicians, however, viewed binders as a holdover from the past. Evans believed that they could cause uterine displacement, though he advised some support and used what he referred to as a 'T' bandage. H.M. Little of McGill University tried to take a broader view of the binder. He recognized that its use was widespread in England and Canada, less common in Germany, and almost non-existent in France and the United States. He summarized its perceived advantages and disadvantages: it comforted the patient and preserved her figure, but it prevented involution of the uterus (the return of the uterus to its previous position) and was not clean. His own view was that the advantages were greatly exaggerated. Others agreed. A 1912 article in the *Canadian Practitioner and Review* asserted: 'A woman's "figure" is not preserved by wrapping about her a wrinkled, rolled up, hot, ill-fitting, unhygienic "binder"; the binder binds only in imagination, unless an insertion of elastic webbing is used.'[98]

Both Little and Evans continued to oppose the binder throughout the interwar period. In 1924 Little reported that he and Evans had run a series of tests and had determined that women who used the binder were more likely to develop backward displacements of the uterus than those who did not. Their conclusion: 'The binder has now been discredited.'[99] Others concurred. While P. Brooke Bland in his 1932 text recognized that some women found the binder of comfort, especially those 'with a fat or relaxed abdominal wall,' he argued that it was of little use in encouraging involution. Instead, he advised that when the patient finally left her bed, she should wear an elastic girdle. Why he saw a girdle as any different from a binder is unclear. Henricus J. Stander, the author of a 1941 text, also rejected the use of the binder. But he argued, as Bland did, that it was helpful for women with fat or pendulous abdomens. Despite his lukewarm endorsement, Stander stated that 'most authorities recommend ... a tightly fitting binder.'[100] Certainly, many women found it useful. A description of pioneer nursing in northern Alberta in the 1930s detailed the use of binders which the women made of flannel, or even salt bags if they could not afford the former. As well as providing a woman with support, the binder held sterile gauze over the navel area.[101] Percy Ryberg in his health manual was still advocating the binder in the early 1940s, telling women to wear it as long as they thought they needed it. Others simply observed that if a woman thought the binder helped, then she should use it.[102]

Like midwives, physicians advised women to stay in bed for approximately ten days after giving birth. Some even advised fourteen days.[103] While some women would have welcomed the rest, it was not without problems, depending on where the woman was and what regimen she had to follow. The Burnside Lying-In Hospital had extraordinarily specific directions for what a woman might do during this time. She could have her head and shoulders propped up 'for a few minutes' twelve hours after labour and after that three times a day for seven days. She could sit up in order to 'void urine' but otherwise should not sit until the fifth day, and then only in bed. She was not to leave her bed before the tenth day.[104] David James Evans in his 1900 textbook had his own regimen. He advised his student readers that it was not necessary to keep the patient on her back. She could turn herself gently from one side to the other, and after the first day could sit up for short periods.[105] Some saw such regimens as providing 'greater freedom' to the patient, since she no longer had to remain flat on her back. Thus the first challenge to tradition was allowing the woman to take more than the supine position.[106] In 1902 N. Preston Robinson of the County of Carleton General Hospital explained why he supported the new regimen: 'The practice of keeping a puerperal patient in bed, using bed-pan, etc., and almost motionless for ten days, I think has now become almost obsolete. I am a thorough believer in attending to nature's calls in the erect posture as soon as they occur, and I encourage the patient to sit erect in bed as soon as possible, because of the advantage of gravity in aiding the natural effort of the uterus to rid itself of the natural discharge.'[107] It would take several decades before this practice became customary. But even Robinson did not discuss getting out of bed on a permanent basis before the end of the ten-day period.

In 1909, Evans reported the findings about early rising from bed that were detailed in the *British Medical Journal*. In one hundred cases women had got up as soon as they wanted. The physician in charge reported no ill effects and responded to the four concerns about early rising that had kept the medical profession locked into the 'ten days in bed' recuperative period. First, he noted that drainage of any septic material was actually aided by the upright position, so fear of septic infection did not apply. Nor did he find involution delayed or hampered by early rising. Nor did uterine displacement occur. The last fear was pulmonary thrombosis and embolism in women who rose too early, but the author reported that such cases were rare. In addition to not fulfilling physicians' worst fears, early rising allowed women to maintain muscle tone and stimulated circulation and abdominal pressure, which lessened the constipation that so many women experienced during their lying-in period.[108] Those supporting early rising would repeat all these arguments throughout the subsequent years.

Herbert M. Little described the practical policy of the Montreal Maternity Hospital. He noted that not many women could afford to stay in bed during the ten days to three weeks that some physicians demanded. Their household responsibilities would not permit it. Recognizing this, the hospital instituted a modified early rising policy. Women were allowed to get out of bed earlier, but the hospital monitored their activities. It found that for most women, early rising was at the end of a week rather than after ten days. Despite the apparent success of the program, Little was not totally convinced. While uterine drainage was better, he asked whether perhaps uterine descent might be greater.[109]

David Berry Hart in his 1912 text also was not convinced. Like Little, he appealed to what *might* happen, though in his case it was in the unforseeable future. He acknowledged the debate that was occurring between supporters of early rising and those who held that a woman should have complete rest for ten days, followed by modified rest for an additional week. While he admitted that those who had instituted early rising, even after three days, had reported no ill effects, his response was one entrenched in custom: 'This ... is not enough. An untoward result of the early rising of the patient may not appear for years afterwards, in the shape of prolapsus uteri, major or minor.' He noted that if early rising was such a good thing, poor women would make a better recovery than wealthy women, since they were forced by poverty to return to their normal regimen very soon after birth. Yet 'it is the poor who overcrowd our hospitals with their slack pelvic floors and diseased tubal conditions.'[110] What he did not acknowledge was that there could be other reasons to account for the problems of the poor; also, hospitals might be crowded with the poor not because wealthy women did not have uterine difficulties but because they could afford to have physicians treat them at home. Nevertheless, Thomas Watts Eden in his 1915 text agreed with Hart that while 'primitive' or 'uncivilised' women did not stay in bed for ten days, there was no way of knowing what the 'remote ill-effects' of this had on them.[111] Civilized women did not need to emulate what was natural.

Although there may have been a debate in published medical circles, other sources suggest that the ten-day or more rule still held sway. Lucy Maud Montgomery reported not being able to leave the upper floor of her house for almost twenty days after the birth of her son in 1912.[112] Members of the National Council of Women worried that women in sparsely settled areas could not afford the luxury of staying in bed 'the requisite number of days,' and they feared that this would lead led to uterine displacement.[113] Toronto's Wellesley Hospital kept new mothers for nine days after the birth and did not allow them to have any visitors, which meant that husbands and wives could communicate only via notes carried by the nurses.[114] And while some at the Montreal Maternity Hospital may have been intrigued by early rising, the women who had their babies there stayed an average of 11.9 days after confinement.[115]

Once the woman was out of bed, some physicians in the early decades of the century stressed that care still needed to be taken: the woman should only *slowly* return to her normal activity. Of course, if she had been lying in bed for ten days, she would not have been capable of returning to her normal activity right away. J. Clarence Webster, in his 1903 textbook, suggested that she spend one hour or more a day 'in a half-recumbent posture' on a sofa and that she walk a bit each day, sit outside, or take a drive if the weather permits.' Adam H. Wright of the Burnside Lying-In Hospital also was very specific about what activity the woman could do. She 'may be allowed to walk in three weeks. She should be well in four weeks, but should not do much work for six weeks.' Others advised against using stairs for the same amount of time.[116] Physicians clearly aimed such advice at wealthy patients and emphasized the convalescent status of these women. Some also advised that resumption of sexual activity should not occur until after the second month.[117]

The interwar years saw an intensification of the early-rising debate. Some supported even longer stays in hospital, while others tried to encourage cutting back; thus the alternatives had become in some instances more extreme.[118] Hospital records indicate that in the interwar period the average stay for obstetric patients was almost two weeks, most of this time being after the birth of the child. In 1932 *Chatelaine* also reported an average two-week stay in hospital.[119] In private practice, the situation may have been much the same. Looking back on his career as a country doctor, William Victor Johnston claimed that the custom had been to keep women in bed two weeks after birth. In hindsight, he thought this was wrong: 'Many developed trouble walking and had pain in their feet from lack of exercise.'[120] But the stay varied depending on the patient. In 1928 the Royal Victoria Hospital, Montreal, found that public ward patients left the hospital sooner after rising from bed than private patients did. In British Columbia this was also true of Oriental patients.[121] If Johnston's patients stayed in bed for two weeks, it was only because they had a support network to help them. Many women did not. One young woman from rural Ontario gave birth to her first child in 1923. She and her husband were just starting out but had saved enough to have a physician attend the birth. After that a neighbour came for two days and then the young woman was on her own, with only the help that her husband could give. Organizations such as the National Council of Women worried about such women.[122]

Those supporting the ten-day (or more) rest in bed feared the repercussions of early rising. P. Brooke Bland in his 1931 text argued that early rising on the second or third day was 'unwise' and had led to several cases of fatal embolism.[123] R.W. Johnstone of the University of Edinburgh agreed that early rising could be dangerous, not only with respect to embolism but also because it resulted in uterine displacements. But recognizing that early rising did not allow the muscle tone to deteriorate, Johnstone encouraged the woman to do 'gentle exercise' while she remained in bed. He argued that most women enjoyed their time in bed and that poor women, especially, recognized that it was their only chance to rest.[124] This may have been true, but it is unclear how many poor women were able to take advantage of the recommended rest period. In 1935 a major British text worried about subinvolution and prolapse, and urged its readers to keep their patients in bed for two to three weeks, allowing women to get out of bed towards the end only to go to the bathroom. One can imagine what kind of clientele the authors envisioned and what condition the women would be in after such a prolonged period of inactivity. Clearly, it was a recommendation for a wealthy woman who could afford to have someone take care of both her new baby and her household while she remained in bed. Perhaps realizing that the shift to early rising was getting stronger, the authors of the text entertained the idea of some women being able to survive such a radical regimen – women of 'placid temperament' and of 'the heavy phlegmatic type.'[125]

Advocates of early rising in the interwar years and after believed that they were ahead of their time, perhaps not knowing the kind of sporadic support early rising had received from physicians earlier in the century. In 1930 C.B. Oliver described the regimen for his patients. On the second day after the birth, he let the woman sit in bed against a backrest and as 'early' as the eighth day she could sit in a chair for 'a few minutes.' He even admitted, 'I have no doubt many would make a speedier convalescence were they allowed out of bed even earlier.'[126] Others went a bit further and encouraged the woman to do exercises in bed to help with the involution of the uterus and to restore muscle tone around the uterus.[127] One of the strongest proponents of early rising was Harold Atlee, who had introduced it at the Grace Hospital, Halifax, in 1928 by 'encouraging ... patients to do mild exercises in bed, to get into a chair the day after delivery, and to walk about after that.' In his own inimitable way, he concluded: 'Not only did the *girls* feel better while they were in hospital, but they were able to go home and look after their families sooner, and with no ill effects.'[128] Until that time, the custom at the Grace had been to keep the women immobile in bed for twelve days, let them sit up for a couple more days, and then send them home. Atlee argued that early rising was worth a try simply because long rest seemed to result in women experiencing a psychological let-down and a lack of muscular tone when they returned home. Also, he pointed out that it was generally a good idea to question and investigate whether the arguments of the 'puerperal fundamentalists' were accurate. But although he believed in early rising, he still felt that women should remain in hospital for at least ten days.[129]

Elsewhere in the country other hospitals were introducing early rising. In the late 1940s the Royal Victoria Hospital, Montreal, instituted a physiotherapy program for women in which a physiotherapist came on a daily basis to supervise exercises by maternity patients.[130] Although the Grace Hospital in St John's followed a nine-day-in-bed rest rule, one of its physicians allowed his patients to walk from the birthing room to their beds. Needless to say, other physicians thought he was crazy. But medical literature increasingly supported the 'crazy' doctor. Early rising led to faster convalescence, a quick return to normal body functioning, less need for nursing care, and better morale among the mothers.[131]

Support for early rising came from an unexpected quarter – the pressures that an increased birth rate placed on hospital beds.[132] In the Lamont Clinic in Alberta, J.A. Alton pointed out that even with free hospitalization provided for maternity cases, the average length of time women were staying in 1947 was only 7.4 days. Similarly, a survey of thirty-five Nova Scotia hospitals reported an average stay of 7.6 days.[133] But we should not exaggerate the degree of early rising's adoption. Dorothy Atkinson re-called being allowed to dangle her legs over the bed nine days after giving birth and feeling 'dizzy' as a consequence of the exertion. Becki Crawford remembered that when she had her first child at Women's College Hospital, Toronto, in 1945, she was not even allowed to dangle her legs over the side of the bed. When she asked her physician, Marion Hilliard, if the inactivity was really necessary, Hilliard responded that Becki was to do as she was told and not worry about it. At the Royal Jubilee Hospi-tal in Victoria in 1949, patients still stayed an average of ten days after giving birth.[134] However, women did notice that with each subsequent birth the stay in hospital was shorter and certainly the time spent in bed was.[135] Those espousing traditional bed rest were perturbed by this development. In 1950, when told about the wonders of early rising, a patient in a Winnipeg hospital determined to try it for herself. She got up, and when her doctor found out he cried, 'You're going to *ruin* your insides, it's going to be a mess.'[136] Early rising, however, seemed here to stay. By 1993, Canadian hospitals reported an average stay of only 3.2 days after vaginal birth.[137]

Once the patient was out of bed, advice regarding activity was still at times very specific and class based. The British physician R.W. Johnstone, in his 1934 text, advised that by the end of the third week after leaving her bed, the woman may be allowed out for a drive and in the following week for short walks.'[138] It would be difficult to imagine most Canadian women following such a regimen. But even those who were familiar with the Canadian context were not always practical in their advice. Percy E. Ryberg, in a popular Canadian advice book, exhorted women: 'Stay in bed ten days if you can, and try to avoid all worries and cares of the household for about three weeks.'[139] The obligations of many women's lives made following such advice difficult. An Austro-Canadian woman living in Blake Township, near Fort William, Ontario, was up and cooking her husband's dinner four hours after a forceps delivery, and three days later she was working in the fields.[140]

In assessing the postnatal care provided by physicians, it is difficult not to compare it with that provided by midwives. Supporters of midwife care have emphasized the significant help that midwives gave women in the postnatal period, and this was certainly the case in the first half of the century. Often, however, it has been suggested that modern birthing practice did not offer similar care. But this really depended on where and under what conditions the birth took place. Women delivering in a hospital had daily care during their time in the institution. Women who birthed at home and were supervised by hospital personnel also had daily care. For example, at the turn of the century the Montreal Maternity Hospital ensured that nurses attended daily and that a resident physician examined the woman and child at the end of ten days.[141] Women covered by insurance through Metropolitan Life had up to eight postnatal visits from nurses.[142] Adam H. Wright described the regimen he advised in his 1908 text:

> After the first day the physician should see his patient at least once a day for a week, then every second or third day until the end of the third or fourth week. Such directions apply especially to attendance on patients in cities and towns. It happens in many country districts, that the physician in certain cases makes no subsequent visits after attending his patient in confinement. I do not think, however, that any physician should take the responsibility of conducting a case of labor without seeing his patient at least once or twice after the birth of the child.[143]

But this was an ideal that many urban and rural practitioners could not meet when there was no insurance, hospital, or public-health nursing support. Certainly, it was unaffordable for most Canadian families. Nonetheless, physicians did what they could and some went beyond medical care. In 1909 Thomas R. Ponton of MacGregor, Manitoba, described the first time he had to wash and dress a baby: 'The washing was easy but the dressing was hair raising. The mother was so grateful for not having to do it herself, as she had had to do in a previous labor.'[144]

In the interwar period and the following years, physicians continued to be aware of the need for postnatal care. The problems of cost and time were difficult to surmount, but as more women gave birth in hospital, they received fairly intensive supervision until they returned home. Medical literature warned that physicians (or nurses) should stay close to the patient for at least one or two hours immediately following the birth.[145] A 1936 text urged physicians to visit their patients at least twice a day for the first three days after the birth unless there was a nurse in attendance. If there was, only once a day was necessary. Until the patient left her bed, visits of once a day were to continue.[146] In hospitals, interns were to see their patients on the first, second, fourth, sixth and tenth days after confinement. Some hospitals even introduced postpartum clinics for non-hospital patients, and during the Depression they gave beds, bedding, and layettes to those in need.[147] While physicians and hospitals could not give the kind of personalized care midwives could, they certainly did not ignore the needs of the woman after birth, and some went out of their way to ensure their comfort and safety. Others, of course, did not. Many Montreal women in the interwar period recalled that their doctors did not even show up in time to deliver the baby and, when they did, certainly did not wash the baby, leaving it to whatever woman was there.[148] Unlike Dr Ponton in the earlier period, these doctors had a strong sense of the gendered division of labour.

Several conclusions emerge from an examination of the postnatal period. First was the aura of permission underlying the medical advice given to women; physicians phrased their descriptions in terms of what they would *allow* women to do, and this was often class-based. Second was the fact that the length of the immediate care period was perceived similarly by First Nations peoples, midwives, and physicians – approximately ten days. Third, the amount of care given to women did not vary significantly whether the birth was midwife or physician directed; even the nature of the care was at times similar, particularly the focus on diet and the use of the binder, although the details of each differed, with physicians losing confidence in the use of the binder over time. However, physicians, unlike midwives, emphasized the medical rather than social aspects of postnatal care. Fourth were the high expectations held for postnatal care and the difficulty that many practising physicians, and the families they treated, had in meeting them; the discrepancy between the ideal and reality has always been an underlying theme in medical practice. Last was the way in which change occurred in medicine – the willingness of some physicians to challenge accepted lore, such as the number of days spent in bed, and the unwillingness of others to do so regardless of evidence of its safety. Clinging to tradition provided many physicians with a comfort that originated in certainty, a rather scarce commodity in medicine. Given the threat of maternal mortality, comfort and certainty were values that practitioners regarded highly.

Conclusion

The themes of medical surveillance and the interventionist medical treatment of women throughout pregnancy, childbirth, and the immediate postnatal period are common strands in much of the historiography on childbirth. In *Giving Birth in Canada* I have argued that it is not the surveillance or intervention – but rather its nature – that is significant. All births, no matter where they occurred and in what kind of society, have been surrounded by customs that necessitated keeping track of what a pregnant or birthing woman did. The literature on the history of childbirth has been largely critical of its medicalization, but at the same time it has tended to romanticize the alternative – a woman-centred and midwife-directed birth. Yet midwives varied greatly both in their training and competency. Largely overlooked in the historical literature is the fact that midwives often aligned themselves with physicians and adopted aspects of the medical model. For example, in the first half of the twentieth century, many midwives tried to reduce the number of women in the birthing room, they adopted a supine position for the labouring women, and they were grateful for suggestions given to them by physicians. Looking to midwives in the first half of the twentieth century as a viable alternative to physician-directed birth is an exercise in a historical 'if.' By 1900, doctors already dominated birth in Canada – more so, indeed, than in the United States. For physicians, midwives were competitors, but only in a psychological sense.

Physicians in Canada, and the physician authors they read, comforted themselves that they had more to offer women in childbirth than midwives did. What they had to offer was medicalization. That physicians wanted to medicalize childbirth should not come as any great surprise. It was a way of applying their expertise. This book has traced the details of that process in the first half of the twentieth century, a period that has not been the primary focus of historians of childbirth. These were the years during which the medicalization of birth became complete, although its nature and efficacy were still open to debate. The medicalization of pregnancy, in particular, occurred during these years. Physicians increasingly privileged the signs of pregnancy over the embodied symptoms women experienced; they even medicalized maternal impressions. Physicians also wanted to maintain a regular surveillance of pregnant women. They may have disagreed with one another about what food, activities, and so on a pregnant woman should have or engage in, but all agreed that the woman should have a physician and should listen to that physician and to no one else. While such surveillance lessened the choices of women, it emphasized the significance and importance of the pregnant woman and the care she deserved. The act of childbirth itself increasingly took place in a hospital setting. But although the process of hospitalization was underway even at mid-century, many women still gave birth at home. This did not mean that these births were not medicalized. As I have pointed out, home birth could be just as interventionist as hospital births – indeed, even more so.

Intervention increased over time. In general, the intervention of Canadian practitioners was not as high as that in the United States, but neither was it as low as in some European countries. The intervention rates varied, depending on the intervention in question, the specific hospital, or the individual physician. My interest has been in trying to trace the patterns of intervention and the reasons for it. One aspect of the intervention was how one type gave way to another – for example, high forceps use gave way to c-section. A second was the way in which the indications for a specific intervention tended to widen over time. In some cases, the language of indication was generalized, making it more inclusive than exclusive of need. A third was the symbiotic relationship between varying interventions. At times, the parameters of a normative birth could widen, as when doctors seemed more willing, in the interwar years and beyond, to admit the safety of a first birth by an older woman than they had previously been willing to do. Nevertheless, they insisted that safety was a consequence of increased medical monitoring and advances.

The reasons for these patterns are less clear. The cynic would argue that intervention equalled money, and there is little doubt that more intervention occurred with paying than non-paying patients. Some physicians were themselves worried about this trend. The medical literature reveals a profession torn between warning against too much intervention and glorifying a physician's intervention when it saved the life of a patient. And intervention could do just that. In itself, intervention is not bad. Faced with a patient with severe pelvic disproportion, doctors gladly chose c-section over the alternative – death for the woman and child or dismemberment of the child. Intervention was the expression of a physician's skill (though the meaning of that term could vary). It was the focus of a physician's training. It was the reason for his presence – to intervene if necessary. 'If' was the operative word. In practice, it was difficult for physicians to know when to intervene. Losing a patient was an ever-present fear, especially in Canada, where maternal mortality rates were very high. This was the context in which interventionist decisions were made. Part of the context was the belief that modern women were simply not as capable as earlier women had been to deliver their children safely. Practitioners believed that women's bodies had a history. In the past, women had been able to give birth with little difficulty. Evidence of this, they argued, still existed in the bodies of First Nations and peasant women. Modern woman was at risk because her lifestyle interfered with the natural functioning of her body. As a result, practitioners believed that the percentage of non-problematic births had declined. However, they provided no proof of this; it was simply conventional wisdom and part of medical lore. They constructed a past utopia for women's bodies, but it was not a utopia to which they wanted to return. To do so would be to give up the progress that came with modernity. In the scenario constructed by physicians, women were in a bind. Their bodies no longer functioned as well as they once had, but in order to have them do so they would have to give up being modern, being civilized. Doctors saw themselves as the solution; they would be there to help women in their hour (actually months) of need. Such beliefs had become part of medical culture.

Central to medicalized childbirth was the relationship between the patient and her physician. Critics have focused on the lack of power that a woman had vis-à-vis her doctor. I agree. The expansion of prenatal care and the fact that women were visiting physicians more than ever before strengthened the power and influence of physicians over women. Interventionist births, too, lessened women's influence. In the early decades, physicians had consulted women about sterilization and performing c-sections, but by the interwar period this was no longer so true. The decisions taken had become medical and did not have the same moral overtones they had once had.

This is not to say that women were without agency. Physicians often complained about the non-compliance of women with respect to prenatal visits. While we do not always know the reasons for the non-compliance, a woman's health was only one part of her life. She had responsibilities to others, and at times she may have made decisions based on their needs or on what was feasible for her particular economic situation. Physicians complained that women too often sought information from sources other than their physicians. Especially galling was their willingness to listen to other women, who, after all, had only the experience of childbirth to inform them. Yet at times, women's agency allied itself with the medical profession. Women did seek out medical help and often viewed their doctors with considerable awe. They sought out physicians because they believed that medicine had something to offer – modernity. Women often insisted that the doctor do something to stop the pain of childbirth, even if that meant intervening with forceps. Some supported twilight sleep, although it was never as popular in Canada as it was in the United States. Women's organizations were among the most vociferous supporters of prenatal care and hospitalization for childbirth. That women endorsed the medicalization of childbirth should not come as a surprise. For many, medicalization meant safety; they, too, had faith in the objectivity of medical science and the physicians who possessed its knowledge. Nor is it surprising that they could believe this in the face of evidence to the contrary – the appalling maternal mortality rates of the first four decades of the century. People are often able to live with contradictions in their lives; women could focus on the ideal of birthing that medicine promised and could overlook the specific reality of their own birth experience. But while women may have accepted medicine, they did not necessarily jettison older beliefs. They continued to believe in maternal impressions, and although doctors focused on the signs of pregnancy, women still had confidence in the symptoms of their bodies.

If women were able to exert some semblance of agency, the flip side was the constraints experienced by physicians: legal, professional, institutional, moral, and personal. This is an area that historical researchers have ignored, at least when the focus has been on the treatment of women. The law constrained doctors. When there was severe disproportion or other health problems of the mother, physicians had to take care in deciding to abort the foetus, for abortion was illegal. The norms of their profession constrained them. Consensus on how to treat women in childbirth did not have the same authority as legal sanctions, but it was significant nevertheless. The discussion over indications for c-sections, the early-rising debates, and so on reflect physicians' desire to be in agreement with colleagues. Yet they were also in competition with those colleagues. The tension between specialists and family physicians, between surgeons and obstetricians, testifies to the ongoing jockeying for position within the profession. Doctors were not a monolith, and different groups within the profession disagreed with one another and at times expressed concern about the direction which their colleagues and medicine itself were taking. Doctors were also constrained by the medical institution in which they worked. Each hospital created its own mini-culture, and woe betide any physicians who did not conform. Also, their own personal morality constrained them. The sterilization issue was of particular moment for Roman Catholic physicians, but even Protestant physicians were uneasy about the procedure. And on an individual level, physicians were constrained by the mood they were in at the time. They might be impatient at how long a woman's labour was taking when they had other patients to see, or they might be frustrated by a patient's non-compliance.

Medicine and medical practitioners did have status and a certain amount of power, but the power of medicine was always greater than that of the individual practitioner. The science of medicine told physicians how things *should be*, but as front-line medical workers they faced how things *were*, day in and day out. The science of medicine, however, provided physicians with a specialized language, which served as a protective device that insulated them from the emotional world of patients, their friends, and relatives. Yet emotion, at times, underlay the language and metaphors of medicine. The image of medicine as the rescuer permeated the literature on pregnancy and childbirth. Physicians used apocalyptic images to describe what could happen to women if they did not follow the advice given them. They bolstered their uncertainty with a rhetorical confidence which, as some acknowledged, led their colleagues to react to situations too quickly. The dissonance between the science of medicine and its reality could be significant, leading to feelings of inadequacy, especially concerning the training they had received and the competition they faced. Those delivering babies believed that their status within the profession was low; furthermore, their patients did not always follow their advice or pay them. Uncertainty is integral to medicine simply because of the body's complexity. Much of the care that physicians wanted to provide to pregnant and birthing women was the ability to control what was happening within their bodies – not in functioning but in outcome. Control helped order the complexity of the body. It was part of a scientific or positivist approach and was a way that physicians had of lessening their uncertainty about what they did.

Integral to this was seeing the body as a machine. It was not the only possible view of the body (as witness the Inuit belief that the sex of the child could change during birthing), but it was the one that Western medicine and society had adopted. A machine, even a poorly working one, needs care, and it was the woman's responsibility to care for her machine. Women's bodies were problematic, but they could lessen the problems if they followed their mechanic's (doctor's) advice. If they did not do so, the physician was not to blame. The fact that physicians saw the body in such an essentializing fashion did not mean that they were oblivious of diversity among bodies. As has been seen, they differentiated between the modern and the premodern body, between the civilized and the savage body, between the young and the older body, between the middle-class and the working-class body. But at the same time, they saw women's bodies as something they could generalize. It was the latter view that provided certainty.

Because Western medicine saw the body as a machine, it favoured technological responses to it. Their medical education taught practitioners to look for problems and to fix them. Fixers don't wait, they act. The effectiveness of machines could be measured, and the history of childbirth reveals the increasing importance of measuring the body's functions. Bodies were similar enough that measurements of some bodies were a good reflection of all bodies. Measuring resulted in the creation of a norm – with respect to pregnancy and childbirth, and the way a normal (healthy) body should proceed. Anything outside the norm suggested problems or ill health. Measurements gave physicians something concrete by which to judge the progression of a pregnancy or labour; they were signposts agreed to by the wider profession, and while not always unanimously endorsed, they usually represented a consensus. The individual physician, faced with a specific patient, used these signposts in determining his response. His focus became the body and the measuring of its actions. As a result, the woman and her explanations of what her body was doing became of less value. Monitoring the body was something physicians did and felt confident doing. Depending on a patient's experience was not such a secure course of action; nor did it seem as objective or scientific. Depending on nature was not good enough either, for nature was too fickle. As an example of nature's failure, doctors pointed to the way that women's natural functioning in the modern day no longer gave them the ability to birth safely. Measurements became a way of determining the meaning of natural. Natural childbirth was a birth that fitted the measurement-created paradigm of a healthy birth. As long as the fit existed, intervention was unnecessary.

The induction of labour was an example of the measurement process. Physicians knew the average length of a pregnancy and assumed that all pregnancies should be that length. Shorter ones led to early and even premature births, and longer ones were those beyond term. Each had its own problems. At one level the scenario did not pose difficulties. But at another it did, for embedded in it was the assumption that physicians knew how to judge when conception occurred (which they did not). As well, physicians assumed that they knew where to draw the line between a short and long pregnancy. Because the measurement of length was predetermined, physicians responded to overterm pregnancies with induction. They took something uncertain and made it certain. Medical consensus worked in a similar way through dictums such as 'Once a caesarean always a caesarean.' Such beliefs made decision making easier and, as some feared, pro forma.

In order to deal with the numerous patients they saw, physicians generalized the experience of women. They created what became 'a woman's' experience. Working within the paradigm of science, they could have done little else. Generalizing women and treatment was a human response as well. If, in his experience, long drives during pregnancy had led to miscarriage in some patients, how could a physician not warn all his patients to avoid long drives? What made sense as medical care for one woman became medical care for all women. So care became less variable. But such directives looked at as a whole can appear controlling.

While some of the responses made by physicians enhanced their own status, other practitioners questioned the direction medicine was taking. The tension between the two was a reflection of medicine's energy and the incorporation of both science and art in its practice. Many within the profession worried that the technological fix overlooked the human needs of the patient. They reminded one another to be patient, to consider the consequences of their actions. They took pride in what they did and were dismayed when colleagues did not behave in a responsible or professional manner. There were few criticisms of the profession that could be made that physicians did not make themselves. And like their patients, they had to balance the ideal of what medicine offered against what was practical. The standards of ideal care kept increasing – more prenatal visits, the elimination of maternal mortality. Most practitioners were bound to assess the care they provided as wanting compared with the ideal; the divide between medical science and practice was difficult, if not impossible, to bridge.

Notes

Introduction

1 Molly Ladd-Taylor has defined maternalism as a 'specific ideology whose adherents hold (1) that there is a uniquely feminine value system based on care and nurturance; (2) that mothers perform a service to the state by raising citizen-workers; (3) that women are united across class, race, and nation by their common capacity for motherhood and therefore share a responsibility for all the world's children; and (4) that ideally men should earn a family wage to support their "dependent" wives and children at home.' Molly Ladd-Taylor, *Mother-Work, Women, Child Welfare and the State, 1890–1930* (Urbana: University of Illinois Press 1994), 3, cited in Seth Koven, 'The Ambivalence of Agency: Women, Families, and Social Policy in France, Britain, and the United States,' *Journal of Women's History* 9 (Spring 1997): 166.
2 Sharon Batt, *Patient No More: The Politics of Breast Cancer* (Halifax: Gynergy Books 1994); Leslie Doyal, *What Makes Women Sick? Gender and the Political Economy of Health* (New Brunswick, N.J.: Baywood Publishing 1994); Andrea L. Bonnicksen, *In Vitro Fertilization: Building Policy from Laboratories to Legislatures* (New York: Columbia University Press 1989); Suzanne Aims, *Immaculate Deception: A New Look at Women and Childbirth in America* (Boston: San Francisco Book Co./ Houghton Mifflin 1975); Nancy Stoller Shaw, *Forced Labour: Maternity Care in the United States* (London: Pergamon Press 1974); Doris B. Haire, *The Cultural Warping of Childbirth* (Milwaukee: International Childbirth Education Association 1972); Gena Corea, *The Mother Machine: Reproductive Technologies from Artificial Insemination to Artificial Wombs* (Markham, Ont.: Fitzhenry & Whiteside 1985); Ann Oakley, *Women Confined: Towards a Sociology of Childbirth* (London: Martin

Robertson 1980); Janice Raymond, *Women as Wombs: Reproductive Technologies and the Battle over Women's Freedom* (New York: Harper 1993); Robyn Rowland, *Living Laboratories: Women and Reproductive Technologies* (Bloomington: Indiana University Press 1992); Diana Scully, *Men Who Control Women's Health: The Miseducation of Obstetrician-Gynecologists* (Boston: Houghton Mifflin 1980); Sue Fisher, *In the Patients' Best Interest: Women and the Politics of Medical Decisions* (New Brunswick, N.J.: Rutgers University Press 1988); Judith Lorber, *Gender and the Social Construction of Illness* (Thousand Oaks, Calif.: Sage Publications 1997); Ruth Formanek, *The Meanings of Menopause: Historical, Medical, and Clinical Perspectives* (Hillsdale: Analytic Press 1990); Barbara Seaman and Gideon Seaman, *Women and the Crisis in Sex Hormones* (New York: Rawson Associates 1979); Kathy Davis, *Reshaping the Female Body: The Dilemma of Cosmetic Surgery* (New York: Routledge 1995); Nicole J. Grant, *The Selling of Contraception: The Dalkon Shield Case, Sexuality, and Women* (Columbus: Ohio State University Press 1992); Barbara Ehrenreich, *Complaints and Disorders: The Sexual Politics of Sickness* (Old Westbury, N.Y.: Feminist Press 1973); Emily Martin, *The Woman in the Body: A Cultural Analysis of Reproduction* (Boston: Beacon Press 1989); and Margarete Sandelowski, *Women, Health, and Choice* (Englewood Cliffs, N.J.: Prentice-Hall 1981). Some of the works were, of course, more nuanced than others. For example, in Martin's *The Woman in the Body*, the author was careful to point out that she was not criticizing individual physicians but rather the culture of medicine. She saw physicians as powerfully socialized. Nonetheless, she viewed medical technology as controlling women (13, 58).

3 Three examples are Helen Bequaert Holmes and Laura M. Purdy, eds., *Feminist Perspectives in Medical Ethics* (Bloomington: Indiana University Press 1992); Susan Sherwin, *No Longer Patient: Feminist Ethics and Health Care* (Philadelphia: Temple University Press 1992); and Susan Sherwin et al., *The Politics of Women's Health: Exploring Agency and Autonomy* (Philadelphia: Temple University Press 1998).

4 See Barbara Ehrenreich and Deirdre English, *For Her Own Good: 150 Years of Experts' Advice to Women* (New York: Anchor Press 1978); G. Barker-Benfield, *The Horrors of the Half-Known Life: Male Attitudes toward Women and Sexuality in Nineteenth-Century America* (New York: Harper 1977); Ann Oakley, *The Captured Womb: A History of Medical Care of Pregnant Women* (Oxford: Blackwell 1984); and Elizabeth Fee, ed., *Women and Health: The Politics of Sex in Medicine* (Farmingdale, N.Y.: Baywood Publishing 1983).

5 Edward Shorter, *A History of Women's Bodies* (New York: Basic Books 1982).

6 See Judith Walzer Leavitt, *Brought to Bed: Child-Bearing in America, 1750–*

1950 (New York: Oxford University Press 1986); Jane Lewis, *The Politics of Motherhood: Child and Maternal Welfare in England, 1900–1939* (London: Croom Helm 1980); Margarete Sandelowski, *Pain, Pleasure, and American Childbirth: From the Twilight Sleep to the Read Method, 1914–1960* (Westport, Conn.: Greenwood Press 1984); Richard W. Wertz and Dorothy C. Wertz, *Lying-In: A History of Childbirth in America* (New York: Free Press 1978); Marjorie Tew, *Safer Childbirth: A Critical History of Maternity Care* (London: Chapman & Hall 1990); and Barbara Rothman, *In Labour: Women and Power in the Birthplace* (London: Junction Books, 1982). The early studies did vary in how much they criticized medicine. Indeed, historical work was never as critical as those that focused on the contemporary period.

7 Holmes and Purdy, eds., *Feminist Perspectives*, xi.

8 For published Canadian literature that addresses some aspects of the history of childbirth, see Cynthia Abeele, '"The Mothers of the Land Must Suffer": Child and Maternal Welfare in Rural and Outpost Ontario, 1918–1940,' *Ontario History* 80 (Spring 1988): 183–206; Denyse Baillargeon, 'L'encadrement de la maternité au Québec entre les deux guerres: Les gardes de La Métropolitaine, les gouttes de lait et l'assistance maternelle,' *Bulletin du Regroupement des chercheurs-chercheuses en histoire des travailleurs et travailleuses du Québec* 47 & 48 (1990): 19–45; Cecilia Benoit, *Midwives in Passage* (St John's: Institute of Social and Economics Research Books 1991), and 'Traditional Midwifery Practice: The Limits of Occuptional Autonomy,' *Canadian Review of Sociology and Anthropology* 26 (August 1989): 633–49; C. Lesley Biggs, 'The Case of the Missing Midwives: A History of Midwifery in Ontario from 1795–1900,' *Ontario History* 75 (March 1983): 21–36; Suzann Buckley, 'Ladies or Midwives: Efforts to Reduce Infant and Maternal Mortality,' in Linda Kealey, ed., *A Not Unreasonable Claim: Women and Reform in Canada, 1880s–1920s* (Toronto: Women's Press 1979), 131–49; Brian Burtch, *Trials of Labour: The Re-emergence of Midwifery* (Montreal: McGill-Queen's University Press 1994); Cynthia Comacchio, 'Nations Are Built of Babies': Saving Ontario's Mothers and Children, 1900–1940 (Montreal: McGill-Queen's University Press 1993); Dianne Dodd, 'Advice to Parents: The Blue Books, Helen MacMurchy, M.D., and the Federal Department of Health, 1920–34,' *Canadian Bulletin of Medical History* 8, 2 (1991): 203–30; Rose Dufour, *Femme et enfantement: Sagesse dans la culture Inuit* (Quebec: Éditions Papyrus 1988); Patricia Kaufert and John O'Neil, 'Cooptation and Control: The Reconstruction of Inuit Birth,' *Medical Anthropology Quarterly* 4 (1990): 427–42; Hélène Laforce, *Histoire de la sage-femme dans la région de Québec* (Quebec: Institut québécois de recherche sur la culture 1985); Andrée Lévesque, 'Mères ou malades: Les québécoises de l'entre-deux-

guerres vues par les medecins,' *Revue d'histoire de l'Amérique française* 38, 1
(1984): 23–37; Norah Lewis, 'Reducing Maternal Mortality in British Columbia,' in B.K. Latham and R.J. Pazdro, eds., *Not Just Pin Money* (Victoria:
Camosun College 1984), 337–55; Jutta Mason, 'Midwifery in Canada,' in
Sheila Kitzinger, ed., *The Midwife Challenge* (London: Routledge 1988),
98–129; R. Marvin McGinnis, 'Women, Work and Childbearing: Ontario in
the Second Half of the Nineteenth Century,' *Histoire sociale* 24 (November
1991): 237–62; Jo Oppenheimer, 'Childbirth in Ontario: The Transition from
Home to Hospital in the Early Twentieth Century,' *Ontario History* 75
(March 1983): 36–61; Veronica Strong-Boag and Kathryn McPherson, 'The
Confinement of Women: Childbirth and Hospitalization in Vancouver,
1919–1939,' *BC Studies* 69–70 (Spring-Summer 1986): 142–75; and Katherine Arnup, Andrée Lévesque, and Ruth Roach Pierson, eds., *Delivering*
Motherhood: Maternal Ideologies and Practices in the Nineteenth and Twentieth
Centuries (London: Routledge, 1990).

9 The following are just a few of the studies available: Irvine Loudon, *Death*
in Childbirth: An International Study of Maternal Care and Maternal Mortality
1800–1950 (Oxford: Clarendon Press 1992); Alice E. Adams, *Reproducing the*
Womb: Images of Childbirth in Science, Feminist Theory, and Literature (Ithaca,
NY: Cornell University Press 1994); Jo Murphy-Lawless, *Reading Birth and*
Death: A History of Obstetric Thinking (Bloomington: Indiana University
Press 1998); Robbie Davis-Floyd, *Birth as an American Rite of Passage*
(Berkeley: University of California Press 1992); Robert Blank, *Mother and*
Fetus: Changing Notions of Maternal Responsibility (Westport, Conn.: Green-
wood Press 1992); Barbara Duden, *Disembodying Women: Perspectives on*
Pregnancy and the Unborn (Cambridge, Mass.: Harvard University Press
1993); Pamela Eakins, ed., *The American Way of Birth* (Philadelphia: Temple
University Press 1986); and Julia Stonehouse, *Idols to Incubators: Reproduc-*
tion Theory through the Ages (East Haven, Conn.: Scarlet Press, Inland Book
Co. 1995).

10 See Ludmilla Jordanova, *Sexual Visions: Images of Gender in Science and*
Medicine between the Eighteenth and Twentieth Centuries (Madison: University of Wisconsin 1989), and *Nature Displayed: Gender, Science and Medicine,*
1760–1820 (London: Longman 1999); Ruth Hubbard, Mary Sue Henifen,
and Barbara Fried, eds., *Biological Woman, the Convenient Myth: A Collection*
of Feminist Essays and a Comprehensive Bibliography (Cambridge, Mass.:
Schenkman 1982); Ruth Hubbard, *The Politics of Women's Biology* (New
Brunswick, N.J.: Rutgers University Press 1990); Cynthia Eagle Russett,
Sexual Science: The Victorian Construction of Womanhood (Cambridge, Mass.:
Harvard University Press 1989); Nelly Oudshoorn, *Beyond the Natural*

Body: An Archaeology of Sex Hormones (New York: Routledge 1994); Mariana Benjamin, ed., *Science and Sensibility: Gender and Scientific Enquiry 1780–1945* (Oxford: Blackwell 1991); Ruth Bleier, *Science and Gender: A Critique of Biology and Its Theories on Women* (New York: Pergamon Press 1984); Anne Fausto-Sterling, *Myths of Gender: Biological Theories about Women and Men* (New York: Basic Books 1985); Donna Haraway, *Primate Visions: Gender, Race, and Nature in the World of Modern Science* (New York: Routledge 1989); Sandra Harding, *Whose Science? Whose Knowledge? Thinking from Women's Lives* (Ithaca, N.Y.: Cornell University Press 1991); Sandra Harding and Jean F. O'Barr, eds., *Sex and Scientific Inquiry* (Chicago: University of Chicago Press 1987); Mary Jacobus, Evelyn Fox Keller, and Sally Shuttleworth, eds., *Body/Politics: Women and the Discoveries of Science* (New York: Routledge 1990); Evelyn Fox Keller, *Secrets of Life, Secrets of Death: Essays on Language, Gender, and Science* (New York: Routledge 1992); Helen Longino, *Science as Social Knowledge* (Princeton, N.J.: Princeton University Press, 1990); Nancy Tuana, *The Less Noble Sex: Scientific, Religious, and Philosophical Conceptions of Woman's Nature* (Bloomington: Indiana University Press 1993); Nancy Tuana, ed., *Feminism and Science* (Bloomington: Indiana University Press 1989); Lynda Birke and Ruth Hubbard, eds., *Re-Inventing Biology: Respect for Life and the Creation of Knowledge* (Bloomington: Indiana University Press 1985); Brian Easlea, *Science and Sexual Oppression: Patriarchy's Confrontation with Woman and Nature* (London: Weidenfeld and Nicolson 1981); Londa Schiebinger, *The Mind Has No Sex? Women in the Origins of Modern Science* (Cambridge, Mass.: Harvard University Press 1989), and *Nature's Body: Gender in the Making of Modern Science* (Boston: Beacon Press 1993); Bonnie Spanier *Im/Partial Science: Gender Ideology in Molecular Biology* (Bloomington: Indiana University Press 1995); Carol Tavris, *The Mismeasure of Women: Why Women Are Not the Better Sex, the Inferior Sex, or the Opposite Sex* (New York: Touchstone Books, 1992); Barbara Laslett, Sally Gregory Kohlstedt, Helen Longino, and Evelynn Hammonds, eds., *Gender and Scientific Authority: Essays Reprinted from Signs: Journal of Women in Culture and Society* (Chicago: University of Chicago Press 1996).

11 A fairly recent example is Murphy-Lawless, *Reading Birth and Death*, which seeks to understand how Western medicine gained control of childbirth (rather than simply demonizing medicine) in order that women might regain their agency. In so doing, Murphy-Lawless challenges the benefits of the medicalization of childbirth.

12 Joan Scott, *Gender and the Politics of History* (New York: Columbia University Press 1988), 2. Louise Newman has pointed out that 'gender is collec-

tively created and shared by a society or culture. It precedes and is what constructs the meaning given to both sexual and 'bodily' differences and the social experience of these differences. This does not mean that sexual differences would have no real existence apart from gender, only that sexual differences have no determinable meaning apart from gender.' Louise M. Newman, 'Critical Theory and the History of Women: What's at Stake in Deconstructing Women's History,' *Journal of Women's History* 2, 3 (1991): 62.

13 Susan Bordo, 'Feminism, Postmodernism, and Gender-Scepticism,' in Linda Nicholson, ed., *Feminism/Postmodernism* (New York: Routledge 1990), 139.

14 Hubbard, *The Politics of Women's Biology*, 137. See also Judith Butler, *Gender Trouble: Feminism and the Subversion of Identity* (New York: Routledge 1990).

15 Susan Bordo, *Unbearable Weight: Feminism, Western Culture, and the Body* (Berkeley: University of California Press 1993), 66–7, and Davis-Floyd, *Birth as an American Rite of Passage*, 45–6. The work by medical anthropologists has revealed that other ways of seeing the body are possible. First Nations peoples, for example, see body and person as one – spirit, body, mind, psyche are all interconnected and unable to be separated. Margaret Lock, in *Encounters with Aging: Mythologies of Menopause in Japan and America* (Berkeley: University of California Press 1992), has described the different perception that Japanese society has of the body. William Ray Arney has argued that since the Second World War an ecological metaphor of the body has come to dominate medicine and has led to a more complete surveillance and monitoring of the body. While true, I would argue that it is a matter of degree, for the monitoring and surveillance were certainly present in the prewar period, especially in prenatal care. William Ray Arney, *Power and the Profession of Obstetrics* (Chicago: University of Chicago Press 1982), 8–9.

16 The irony is that this may be even more true with respect to men, for the male body as the norm is very much essentialized.

17 Much of the literature on women and medicine is critical of the latter. Even the titles suggest the interpretive lens. In particular, see Sue V. Rosser, *Women's Health: Missing from U.S. Medicine* (Bloominton: Indiana University Press 1994); Dorothy H. Broom, *Damned If We Do: Contradiction in Women's Health Care* (North Sydney, Australia: Allen & Unwin 1994); Sandra Coney, *The Unfortunate Experiment: The Full Story Behind the Inquiry into Cervical Cancer Treatment* (Aukland, N.Z.: Penguin 1988); Gena Corea, *The Mother Machine: Reproductive Technologies from Artificial Insemination to Artificial Wombs* (Markham, Ont.: Fitzhenry & Whiteside 1985); Gena

Corea, *The Hidden Malpractice: How American Medicine Mistreats Women* (New York: Harper Colophon Books 1985); Claudia Dreifus, *Seizing Our Bodies: The Politics of Women's Health* (New York: Random House 1978); Leslie Laurence and Beth Weinhouse, *Outrageous Practices: The Alarming Truth about How Medicine Mistreats Women* (New York: Fawcett Columbine 1994); Mary Briody Mahowald, *Women and Children in Health Care: An Unequal Majority* (New York: Oxford University Press 1993); Robert Mendelsohn, *Male Practice: How Doctors Manipulate Women* (Chicago: Contemporary Books 1981); Eileen Nechas and Denise Foley, *Unequal Treatment: What You Don't Know about How Women Are Mistreated by the Medical Community* (New York: Simon and Schuster 1994); Janice G. Raymond, *Women as Wombs: Reproductive Technologies and the Battle over Women's Freedom* (New York: Harper 1993); Shelley Romalis, ed., *Childbirth: Alternatives to Medical Control* (Austin: University of Texas Press 1982); Diana Scully, *Men Who Control Women's Health: The Miseducation of Obstetrician-Gynecologists* (Boston: Houghton Mifflin 1980); Sandra Coney, *The Menopause Industry: How the Medical Establishment Exploits Women* (Alameda, Calif.: Hunter House 1994); Cesar A. Perales and Lauren S. Young, eds., *Too Little, Too Late: Dealing with the Healthy Needs of Women in Poverty* (New York: Harrington Park Press 1988).

18 Other factors such as race, age, ability, etc., play into this as well. Some women would have more power than other women, and indeed some women would have more power than some men patients.

19 For a discussion in accessing patient voices, see Eberhard Wolff, 'Perspectives on Patients' History: Methodological Considerations on the Example of Recent German-Speaking Literature,' *Canadian Bulletin of Medical History* 15, 1 (1998): 207–28. For a discussion of agency in women patients, see Wendy Mitchinson, 'Problematic Bodies and Agency: Women Patients in Canada, 1900–1950,' in Franca Iacovetta and Wendy Mitchinson, eds., *On the Case: Explorations in Social History* (Toronto: University of Toronto Press 1998), 266–86.

20 For an excellent study of the way in which aspects of pregnancy and birth are socially constructed, see Judy DeLoache and Alma Gottlieb, eds., *A World of Babies: Imagined Childcare Guides for Seven Societies* (Cambridge: Cambridge University Press 2000), and Brigette Jordan, *Birth in Four Cultures: A Cross-Cultural Investigation of Childbirth in Yucatan, Holland, Sweden, and the United States* (Montreal: Eden Press 1978).

21 In seeing medical birth as ritualistic, despite physicians' insistence that it was predominantly a physiological reality, I have been influenced by some of the anthropological literature on childbirth. I particularly found the

work of Robbie E. Davis-Floyd on contemporary American childbirth sympathetic. See her *Birth as an American Rite of Passage*.

22 Benjamin F. Miller and Claire Brackman Keane, *Encyclopedia and Dictionary of Medicine* (Philadelphia: W.B. Saunders 1978), 560.

23 For overviews of the historiography, see S.E.D. Shortt, 'Medical Professionalization: Pitfalls and Promise in the Historiography,' *Journal of the History of Science, Technology, and Medicine* 5 (September 1981): 210–19, and Wendy Mitchinson, 'Medical Historiography in English Canada,' *Health and Canadian Society* 1, 1 (1993): 205–28.

24 A prime example is Dianne Dodd and Deborah Gorham, eds., *Caring and Curing: Historical Perspectives on Women and Healing in Canada* (Ottawa: University of Ottawa Press 1994). The essays in this book examine women's involvement in health care, both as physicians and outside the traditional mainstream of medicine.

25 Gerald Grob, 'Presidential Address: Psychiatry's Holy Grail: The Search for the Mechanisms of Mental Diseases,' *Bulletin of Medical History* 72 (Summer 1998): 189.

26 Hospitals, too, varied in the care provided, depending on their size and whether they were teaching institutions or not. For a recent assessment of hospital variation in care, see Cheryl Levitt and Louise Hanvey, *Survey of Routine Maternity Care and Practices in Canadian Hospitals* (Ottawa: Health Canada and Canadian Institute of Child Health 1995).

27 Ehrenreich and English, *For Her Own Good*, and Oakley, *The Captured Womb*, are examples of books by scholars who viewed the medical profession as taking childbirth away from women. Others also have reacted against what they see as the medicalization of childbirth in its technologizing orientation in recent decades, and they compare and juxtapose it against a natural world, arguing that it ignores the social and psychological needs of women. As reflected in the literature of the women's health movement, the sense was that women had lost control of childbirth and wanted it back, so medicalization became a concept to criticize. See Raymond, *Women as Wombs*; Barbara Rothman, *In Labour: Women and Power in the Birthplace* (London: Junction Books 1982); and Judith Walzer Leavitt, *Brought to Bed: Child-Bearing in America, 1750–1950* (New York: Oxford University Press). Expressions of this in the Canadian literature can be found in Dominque Gaucher, France Laurendeau, and Louise-Hélène Trottier, 'Talking about Life: The Contribution of Women to the Sociology of Health,' in A.T. McLaren, ed., *Gender and Society: Creating a Canadian Women's Sociology* (Toronto: Copp Clark Pitman 1988), 80–96; Deborah Findlay, 'The Medical Gaze: Medical Models, Power, and Wom-

en's Health,' *Atlantis* 18, 1 & 2 (1992–3): 104–24; Arnup, Lévesque, and
Pierson, eds., *Delivering Motherhood*; and Dianne Dodd, 'Helen
MacMurchy: Popular Midwifery and Maternity Services for Canadian
Pioneer Women,' in Dodd and Gorham, eds., *Caring and Curing*, 135–62,
esp. 135.

28 Mary Rubio and Elizabeth Waterson, eds., *The Selected Journals of Lucy
Maud Montgomery*, vol. 2:, *1910–1921* (Toronto: Oxford University Press,
1987), 90–1; Nellie McClung believed that every woman desired children
and a home. Nellie McClung, *In Times like These*, ed. Veronica Strong-Boag
(Toronto: University of Toronto Press 1972), 86.

29 *Queen's Medical Quarterly* 5 (July 1908): 158; *University Magazine*, 1912, 689;
Winfield Scott Hall, *Sexual Knowledge* (Philadelphia: International Bible
House 1913), 209; *Report of the Royal Commission on a Dispute Respecting
Hours of Employment between the Bell Telephone Company of Canada, Ltd. and
Operators at Toronto, Ont.* (Ottawa: Government Printing Bureau 1907), 69;
Charles Harrington, *A Manual of Practical Hygiene for Students, Physicians,
and Health Officers*, 5th ed. (Philadelphia: Lea and Febiger 1914), 892; *Public
Health Journal* 7 (April 1916): 189.

30 *Dominion Medical Monthly* 23 (November 1904): 324

31 Carl Henry Davis, ed., *Gynecology and Obstetrics*, vol. 3 (Hagerstown, Md.:
W.F. Prior, 1935), chap. 8, 16.

32 Angus McLaren, *Our Master Race: Eugenics in Canada, 1885–1945* (Toronto:
McClelland and Stewart 1990), 82.

33 University of British Columbia, Vancouver School of Theology, Hugh
Dobson Papers box 10, file M1, 'A Statement on Christian Marriage.'

34 *Chatelaine*, April 1947, 14, 64; May 1947, 103; and June 1947, 6. For the
naturalness of the urge to mother, see also *Canadian Forum*, December
1936, 21–2. See also R.M. Franks, 'A Genetic and Comparative study of
Depressed Female Patients in the Toronto Psychiatric Hospital' (MA thesis,
University of Toronto, 1929); Andrée Lévesque, *La norme et les déviantes:
Des femmes au Québec pendant l'entre-deux-guerres* (Montreal: Éditions du
remue-menage 1989), 26, 28–9; Alfred Henry Tyrer, *Sex, Marriage and Birth
Control*, 10th ed. (Toronto: Marriage Welfare Bureau 1943), 48; *Chatelaine*,
December 1931, 13; *Canadian Home Journal*, October 1941: 96, and October
1945, 16; Sir Comyns Berkeley and Victor Bonney, *A Textbook of Gynaeco-
logical Surgery*, 4th ed. (London: Cassell 1942), 392; *Health* 17 (September–
October 1949): 10; Fred L. Adair, ed., *Obstetrics and Gynecology*, vol. 1
(Philadelphia: Lea & Febiger 1940), 539; *University of Toronto Medical
Journal* 25 (November 1947): 51.

35 Comacchio, '*Nations Are Built of Babies*,' 81. Canadians expressed few

concerns about what the total mothering role meant for women. One who did was a physician from Verdun, Quebec, who in 1932 worried about women identifying themselves only as mothers. What happened to these women when they reached their fifties and sixties and their children had left home and had lives of their own? *Canadian Medical Association Journal (CMAJ)*, 26 (January 1932): 60.

36 *Saturday Night*, 31 October 1942, 22.

37 Nelly Oudshoorn, 'The Decline of the One-Size-Fits-All Paradigm, or How Reproductive Scientists Try to Copy with Modernity' (paper presented to the conference 'Between Mothers, Goddesses, Monsters, and Cyborgs: Feminist Perspectives on Science, Technology and Health Care,' Odense University, Denmark, 2–5 November 1994), 6.

38 There were more than 25 French-language journals. For a complete listing of periodicals, see Charles G. Roland and Paul Potter, *An Annotated Bibliography of Canadian Medical Periodicals 1826–1975* (Toronto: Hannah Institute for the History of Medicine 1979).

39 Nancy Cott, *The Bonds of Womanhood: 'Woman's Sphere' in New England, 1780–1835* (New Haven, Conn.: Yale University Press 1977), 2.

40 Cynthia Abeele, '"Nations Are Built of Babies": Maternal and Child Welfare in Ontario, 1914–1940' (PhD thesis, University of Guelph, 1987), chap. 1, app. 1.1.

1: The Uncertain World of Medicine and Medical Practitioners

1 Queen's University Archives, A.Arch mc, F.B. Exner, 'The Nature of Medical Practice,' 1951, 4, address delivered to students in the medical faculty, senior class.

2 David Gollaher, 'From Ritual to Science: The Medical Transformation of Circumcision in America,' *Journal of Social History* 1 (Fall 1994): 20. By the end of the nineteenth century, medical practice had aligned itself to knowledge generated and validated by experimental science and characterized by universalized diagnostic and therapeutic categories. Treatment was no longer matched to the individual characteristics of the patient. See John Harley Warner, *The Therapeutic Perspective: Medical Practice, Knowledge, and Identity in America, 1820–1885* (Cambridge, Mass.: Harvard University Press 1986), 1.

3 D.W. Cathell, *The Physician Himself and Things That Concern His Reputation and Success*, 10th ed. (Philadelphia: F.A. Davis, 1898), 99.

4 *Maritime Medical News* 12 (July 1900): 222; Adam H. Wright, *A Textbook of Obstetrics* (New York: D. Appleton 1908), 428–9. Dr Murray Enkin has

referred to the 'flawed' nature of medicine as science or art. He prefers to use the word 'fashion': 'The fashion model would recognize that technologies can be introduced, become accepted as fashionable, then conventional, then be rejected, and decline or disappear, with little or no scientific justification.' See his foreword in Ian D. Graham, *Episiotomy: Challenging Obstetric Interventions* (Oxford: Blackwell Science 1997), x.

5 See *Nova Scotia Medical Bulletin* 5 (October 1926): 5; *Canadian Courier*, 19 June 1920, 25.

6 Mary Rubio and Elizabeth Waterson, eds., *The Selected Journals of Lucy Maud Montgomery*, vol. 3: 1921–1929 (Toronto: Oxford University Press 1992), 238; *Chatelaine*, January 1946, 56.

7 *Nova Scotia Medical Bulletin* 5 (April 1926): 21, 22.

8 Exner, 'The Nature of Medical Practice,' 4, 9.

9 Byron J. Good and Mary-Jo DelVecchio Good, '"Learning Medicine": The Construction of Medical Knowledge at Harvard Medical School,' in Shirley Lindenbaum and Margaret Lock, eds., *Knowledge, Power and Practice: The Anthropology of Medicine and Everyday Life* (Berkeley: University of California Press, 1993), 98. See also Susan Bordo, *Unbearable Weight: Feminism, Western Culture, and the Body* (Berkeley: University of California Press, 1993), 53. For an analysis of the way in which patients and doctors communicate with one another, see Sue Fisher, *In the Patients' Best Interest* (New Brunswick, N.J.: Rutgers University Press 1988), and Candace West, *Routine Complications: Troubles with Talk between Doctors and Patients* (Bloomington: Indiana University Press 1984). Few physicians objected to the language. It was what separated them from those 'not in the know.' Perhaps the one exception to this was the suspicion among physicians in the past about the jargon used by psychoanalysts. While recognizing the importance of psychology, there was a deep suspicion about its rigour and its use of uncommon language. Queen's University Archives, Faculty of Medicine, series 6, Notes and Lectures, box 5, John E. Plunkett, *The Book of the Post Graduate Course*, November 1945, 13. Plunkett was an Ottawa physician.

10 Ruth Hubbard, *The Politics of Women's Biology* (New Brunswick, N.J.: Rutgers University Press 1990), 12.

11 Janice Raymond, 'Medicine as Patriarchal Religion,' *Journal of Medicine and Philosophy* 7 (1982): 200–1.

12 Gwynne Basen, Margrit Eichler, and Abby Lippman, *Misconceptions: The Social Construction of Choice and the New Reproductive and Genetic Technologies* (Hull, Que.: Voyageur, 1993), 213.

13 David Gagan, *A Necessity among Us: The Owen Sound General and Marine Hospital, 1891–1985* (Toronto: University of Toronto Press 1990), 68–9.

14 Bordo, *Unbearable Weight*, 66–7.
15 Wilfred T. Grenfell, *Yourself and Your Body* (New York: Scribner's, 1924), 317. See also Barbara Rothman, *In Labour: Women and Power in the Birthplace* (London: Junction Books 1982), 34; Thomas McKeown, 'A Sociological Approach to the History of Medicine,' *Medical History* 14 (October 1970): 343; David Armstrong, 'The Doctor-Patient Relationship: 1930–1980,' in Peter Wright and Andrew Treacher, eds., *The Problem of Medical Knowledge: Examining the Social Construction of Medicine* (Edinburgh: Edinburgh University Press 1982), 110; and Stanley Joel Reiser, *Medicine and the Reign of Technology* (Cambridge: Cambridge University Press 1981), ix. The mechanistic view of the body is one with which most of us are familiar. But this is not the only way that one can look at the body. Studies in Japan have shown that 'health is understood as a state in which balance is maintained both between the body and its environment, physical and social, and among the various body parts; illness occurs when this balance is temporarily lost. There is no fragmentation of the body in this kind of representation, and boundaries are rather fluid.' Margaret Lock, *Encounters with Aging: Mythologies of Menopause in Japan and America* (Berkeley: University of California Press 1992), 228.
16 Lock, *Encounters with Aging*, 137.
17 *Canadian Practitioner and Review* 21 (March 1906): 148–9.
18 For a discussion of measurements and the mechanistic view of the body, see Alvin R. Feinstein, 'The Intellectual Crisis in Clinical Science: Medaled Models and Muddled Mettle,' *Perspectives in Biology and Medicine* 30 (Winter 1987): 223; Lock, *Encounters with Aging*, 137; and Margaret Lock and Gilles Bibeau, 'Healthy Disputes: Some Reflections on the Practice of Medical Anthropology in Canada,' *Health and Canadian Society* 1, 1 (1993): 151. For a discussion on the concept of 'normal,' see Mary Louise Adams, *The Trouble with Normal: Postwar Youth and the Making of Heterosexuality* (Toronto: University of Toronto Press 1997), 13–14, 85–6; Leonore Tiefer, *Sex Is Not a Natural Act and Other Essays* (Boulder, Colo.: Westview Press 1995), 12–13.
19 *Nova Scotia Medical Bulletin* 13 (October 1934): 513–14. See also William R. Houston, *The Art of Treatment* (New York: Macmillan 1936), 46. The interest in measurement has a long history. Alfred Crosby has been intrigued by the success of European imperialisms over others and has argued that the emergence of a quantitative model of reality as opposed to a qualitative model formed the basis of their success. See Alfred W. Crosby, *The Measure of Reality: Quantification and Western Society, 1250–1600* (Cambridge: Cambridge University Press 1997).
20 *Canadian Medical Association Journal (CMAJ)* 31 (August 1934): 191.

21 Margarete Sandelowski, *Women, Health, and Choice* (Englewood Cliffs, N.J.: Prentice-Hall 1981), 205, and Jo Murphy-Lawless, *Reading Birth and Death: A History of Obstetric Thinking* (Bloomington: Indiana University Press 1998), 12. See also Warner, *The Therapeutic Perspective*, 87–91. Warner argues that in the 1890s, doctors began to substitute normal for natural; that is, no longer were they comparing an individual's health by the natural state for the individual but rather to the norm of the population as defined through laboratory science based often on measurements. There was, then, a shift from qualitative to quantitative language.

22 Emily Martin, *The Woman in the Body: A Cultural Analysis of Reproduction* (Boston: Beacon Press 1987), 13; *CMAJ* 27 (October 1932): 397. As Howard Brody has pointed out, 'some of medicine works extremely well precisely because it treats people as being the same; and some of medicine works very well because it treats people as all being different.' Trisha Greenhalgh and Brian Hurwitz, eds., *Narrative-Based Medicine: Dialogue and Discourse in Clinical Practice* (London: BMJ Books 1998), xiii.

23 For Ontario hospitals, see Gagan, *A Necessity among Us*, 14, and 'The Report of the Inspector of Hospitals,' *Ontario Sessional Papers*, 1925, 8; 'Report of the Inspector of Hospitals and Sanatoria,' *Ontario Sessional Papers*, 1945, 6. For Saskatchewan, see Laurel Halladay, '"We'll See You Next Year": Maternity Homes in Southern Saskatchewan in the First Half of the Twentieth Century' (MA thesis, Carleton University, 1996), 120. For Canada, see G. Harvey Agnew, *Canadian Hospitals 1920 to 1970: A Dramatic Half Century* (Toronto: University of Toronto Press 1974), 4–5, and F.H. Lacey, ed., *Historical Statistics of Canada*, 2nd ed. (Ottawa: Statistics Canada 1983), B93–104.

24 Gagan, *A Necessity among Us*, 71.

25 Arlee D. McGee, *The Victoria Public Hospital (1888–1976)* (Fredericton, N.B.: Centennial Print and Litho 1984), 49.

26 McGill University Archives, *Annual Report of the Royal Victoria Hospital, Montreal*, 1901, 24; also the annual reports for 1905, 9; 1911, 9–10; 1915, 10; 1934, 27; 1935, 24; 1943, 20.

27 Morris Vogel, 'The Transformation of the American Hospital, 1850–1920,' in Susan Reverby and David Rosner, eds., *Health Care in America: Essays in Social History* (Philadelphia: Temple University Press 1979), 111.

28 Queen's University Archives, *Annual Report, Kingston General Hospital*, 1934, 5.

29 Figures from annual reports of Kingston General Hospital, 1906–47.

30 Ornella Moscucci, *The Science of Woman: Gynaecology and Gender in England* (Cambridge: Cambridge University Press 1990), 108–9.

31 'Victoria General Hospital: By-Laws and Regulations,' *Nova Scotia Journal*

of the House of Assembly, 17 June 1898, 4; *Annual Report, Victoria General Hospital,* 1920–1; *Nova Scotia Journal of the House of Assembly,* 1922, appendix 3B, 30; ibid., 1938–39, 27.

32 Thomas Watts Eden, 'Technique,' in Thomas Watts Eden and Cuthbert Lockyer, *The New System of Gynaecology,* vol. 3 (Toronto: Macmillan 1917), 283. Eden was still being quoted in 1935. See Carl Henry Davis, ed., *Gynecology and Obstetrics,* vol. 3 (Hagerstown, Md.: W.F. Prior, 1935), chap. 17, 12. Many general practitioners felt they could not keep up with the changes occurring, and in the early years of the century some took to 'ghosting' (by which an older physician hired a younger and better-trained physician to do the actual surgery on his patient). Eventually this system became illegal. A.I. Willinsky, *A Doctor's Memoirs* (Toronto: Macmillan 1960), 80.

33 See McGill University Archives, *Annual Report of the Montreal General Hospital 1901,* 83; 1920, 23; and 1940.

34 Marni Elizabeth Davis, 'Southern Kwakiutl Medicine' (MA thesis, University of Victoria, 1977), 51.

35 'History of Medical Services,' unpublished, sent to author by Ms Florence Cook, Otto Schaeffer Health Library, Government of Northwest Territories.

36 Memorial University of Newfoundland, Folklore and Language Archive, no. 79-319, Marjorie Hazel Lester, 'Traditional Lore, Proverbs and Sayings concerning Illness in Brigus and Brigus Gullies, CB,' p. 11. For a detailed look at folk treatment followed by women in the Canadian West, see Norah L. Lewis, 'Goose Grease and Turpentine: Mother Treats the Family's Illness,' *Prairie Forum* 15 (Spring 1990): 67–84.

37 Luc Lacourchière, 'A Survey of Folk Medicine in French Canada from Early Times to the Present,' in Wayland D. Hand, ed., *American Folk Medicine: A Symposium* (Berkeley: University of California Press 1976), 212.

38 Eliane Leslau Silverman, *The Last Best West: Women on the Alberta Frontier, 1880–1930* (Montreal: Eden Press 1984), 66. A revised and updated edition has recently been published (Calgary: Fifth House 1998).

39 *Chatelaine,* February 1932, 38. See also Linda Rasmussen, *A Harvest Yet to Reap: A History of Prairie Women* (Toronto: Women's Press 1976); the *Public Health Journal* was full of suggestions for care of the family and assumed that it would be the mother who would be responsible (e.g., March 1911, 113).

40 *Canadian Courier,* 13 April 1918, 6.

41 Dr Pierce, *Dr. Pierce's Neighbourhood Gossip Dream Book* (n.p., n.d.), 23. See also *Chatelaine,* April 1928, 42, and November 1928, 38; *Canadian Magazine,* May 1935, 55; *Canadian Home Journal,* March 1943, 57.

42 Victoria General Hospital Papers, Gordon Stiles, patient no. 101, register 94, Medical Department, admitted 18 December 1920, discharged 6 January 1921.

43 See *Saturday Night*, 8 January 1916, 23; *Canada Lancet* 42 (December 1908): 251–2; *Canadian Practitioner and Review* 33 (March 1908): 208; Jeff Warner, '"A Most Un-Christian Affair": The Maines, the Pincocks, and Spiritualism' (student paper, University of Waterloo, 1995), esp. 36–9; James William Opp, 'Religion, Medicine, and the Body: Protestant Faith Healing in Canada, 1880–1930' (PhD thesis, Carleton University, 2000).

44 British Columbia Archives, B.C. Royal Commission on State Health Insurance and Maternity Benefits, GR707, box 2, file 8, exhibit 65.

45 *CMAJ* 41 (July 1939): 75.

46 Vera Ernst McNichol, *Smiling through the Tears*, vol. 1 (Bloomington, Ont.: One M Printing 1970), 115.

47 Cynthia R. Comacchio, *'Nations Are Built of Babies': Saving Ontario's Mothers and Children, 1900–1940* (Montreal: McGill-Queen's University Press 1993), 200. See also Lewis, 'Goose Grease and Turpentine,' 69; *Saint John Globe*, 11 April 1914, 2; *Weekly Manitoba Liberal* (Portage La Prairie), 29 January 1914, 3; *Grain Growers' Guide*, 29 April 1914; *Canadian Courier*, 8 November 1919, 21.

48 Lee Stewart, *'It's Up to You': Women at UBC in the Early Years* (Vancouver: UBC Press 1990), 34. See also Colin Howell, 'Reform and the Monopolistic Impulse: the Professionalization of Medicine in the Maritimes,' *Acadiensis* 9 (1981): 20.

49 Meryn Elisabeth Stuart, '"Let Not the People Perish for Lack of Knowledge": Public Health Nursing and the Ontario Rural Child Welfare Project, 1916–1930' (PhD thesis, University of Pennsylvania, 1987), 27n37, 145, and esp. chap. 6. See also Meryn Stuart, 'Shifting Professional Boundaries: Gender Conflict in Public Health, 1920–1925,' in Dianne Dodd and Deborah Gorham, eds., *Caring and Curing: Historical Perspectives on Women and Healing in Canada* (Ottawa: University of Ottawa Press 1994), 49–70; Meryn Stuart, 'Ideology and Experience: Public Health Nursing and the Ontario Rural Child Welfare Project, 1920–1925,' *Canadian Bulletin of Medical History* 6 (Winter 1989): 111–32; and Meryn Stuart, '"Half a Loaf Is Better Than No Bread": Public Health Nurses and Physicians in Ontario, 1920–1925,' *Nursing Research* 41 (January–February 1992): 21–7. For other examples of tensions between physicians and nurses, see *Canadian Journal of Medicine and Surgery* 51 (April 1922): 159.

50 Houston, *The Art of Treatment*, 88.

51 Halladay, 'We'll See You Next Year,' 61.

52 Penelope Stewart, 'Infant Feeding in Canada: 1910–1940' (MA thesis, Concordia University, 1982), 99.
53 Barbara Keddy et al., 'The Nurse as Mother Surrogate: Oral Histories of Nova Scotia Nurses from the 1920s and 1930s,' *Health Care for Women International* 5 (1984): 189.
54 Stewart, 'Infant Feeding in Canada,' 98.
55 Mary Rubio and Elizabeth Waterson, eds., *The Selected Journals of L.M. Montgomery*, vol. 2: *1910–1921* (Toronto: Oxford University Press 1987), 100–1. See also Rubio and Waterson, eds., *The Selected Journals of L.M. Montgomery*, vol. 3, 23; *Chatelaine*, March 1928, 2; and November 1929, 41.
56 H.L. Burris, *Medical Saga: The Burris Clinics and Early Pioneers* (n.p., n.d.), 81.
57 Stewart, 'Infant Feeding in Canada,' 111.
58 *Nova Scotia Medical Bulletin* 13 (October 1934): 513–14; Dalhousie University Archives, Oxorn Papers, H.B. Atlee, *The Problem of Being a Woman* [post 1950], 158; *Canadian Journal of Medicine and Surgery* 35 (April 1914): 221.
59 *Public Health Journal* 9 (July 1918): 299. In 1912–13, a course in clinical paediatrics was added to the Dalhousie Medical School calendar.
60 *Dalhousie Medical Calendar*, 1919–20, 109; interview with Drs M and H, Halifax, 29 October 1993.
61 *Census of Canada, 1931*, vol. 7, table 40.
62 *Dalhousie Medical Journal* 4 (April 1939): 39.
63 *Saskatchewan Medical Journal* 2 (January 1910): 2.
64 *Canadian Public Health Journal* 21 (May 1930): 219.
65 William Victor Johnston, *Before the Age of Miracles: Memoirs of a Country Doctor* (Toronto: Fitzhenry & Whiteside Ltd., 1972), 4.
66 Jayne Elliott, '"Endormez-moi!" An Early Twentieth-Century Obstetrical Practice in the Gatineau Valley, Quebec' (MA thesis, Carleton University, 1997), 107.
67 *CMAJ* 25 (July 1931): 123. See also *Nova Scotia Medical Bulletin* 16 (February 1938): 140.
68 Juanne Nancarrow Clarke, *Health, Illness, and Medicine in Canada* (Toronto: McClelland and Stewart, 1990), 193.
69 Harry Oxorn, *Harold Benge Atlee M.D.: A Biography* (Hantsport, N.S.: Lancelot Press 1983), 103; Stewart, 'Infant Feeding in Canada,' 99.
70 T.F. Rose, *From Shaman to Modern Medicine: A Century of the Healing Arts in British Columbia* (Vancouver: Mitchell Press 1972), 106.
71 *Canada Lancet* 40 (January 1907): 395. See also Alexandria Dundas Todd, *Intimate Adversaries: Cultural Conflict between Doctors and Their Women Patients* (Philadelphia: University of Pennsylvania Press 1989), 12.

72 Carolyn E. Strange, *Toronto's Girl Problem: The Perils and Pleasures of the City, 1880–1930* (Toronto: University of Toronto Press 1995), 41.
73 *Canadian Home Journal*, November 1931, 8.
74 McGill University, Rare Books, Alton Goldbloom Papers, unpublished manuscript, 17.
75 *Canadian Doctor* 15 (July 1949): 32–3.
76 *Chatelaine*, March 1950, 61.
77 *Canadian Practitioner and Review* 27 (April 1902): 223.
78 Eva Mader Macdonald and Elizabeth M. Webb, 'A Survey of Women Physicians in Canada, 1883–1964,' *CMAJ*, 4 June 1966, 1224.
79 Ruth Brouwer, 'Home Lessons, Foreign Tests: The Background and First Missionary Term of Florence Murray, Maritime Doctor in Korea' (paper presented to the Canadian Historical Association, Montreal, 1995), 12–13; Enid Johnson MacLeod, *Petticoat Doctors: The First Forty years of Women in Medicine at Dalhousie University* (Lawrencetown Beach, N.S.: Pottersfield Press 1990), 62, 74, 78; interview with Drs M and H, Halifax, 29 October 1993.
80 *Canada Lancet* 52 (October 1918): 76.
81 In the first two decades of the century, University of Toronto was the only Ontario medical school that accepted women as a result of Toronto's policy of accepting all qualified applicants. R.D. Gidney and W.P.J. Millar, 'Medical Students at the University of Toronto, 1910–1940: A Profile,' *Canadian Bulletin of Medical History* 13 (1996): 29–52.
82 Marion O. Robinson, *Give My Heart: The Dr. Marion Hilliard Story* (Garden City, N.Y.: Doubleday 1964), 94, 131.
83 *Hospital World* 24 (June 1918): 166.
84 *Canadian Journal of Medicine and Surgery* 9 (May 1901): 366.
85 *Woman's Century*, August 1915, 3. The search for a supportive environment was a reason why many women physicians concentrated their practices on the care of women and children or became medical inspectors for schools. The most famous example of this pattern was Dr Helen MacMurchy, who in 1920 became chief of the Child Welfare Division of the new federal Department of Health. She had taught obstetrics and gynaecology at the University of Toronto, had examined the issue of feeble-minded children in the school systems of Ontario, and eventually became known as the author of the Blue Books, the federal government's effort to reach out to new mothers with the most up to date advice on maternal and child care. Dianne Dodd, 'Advice to Parents: The Blue Books, Helen MacMurchy, M.D. and the Federal Department of Health, 1920–1934,' *Canadian Bulletin of Medical History* 8 (1991): 207.

86 Good and DelVecchio Good, 'Learning Medicine, 90; and Susan Sherwin, *No Longer Patient: Feminist Ethics and Health Care* (Philadelphia: Temple University Press 1992), 192. See also Earl Shelp, *The Clinical Encounter: The Moral Fabric of the Patient-Physician Relationship* (Dordrecht: D. Reidel 1983); Armstrong, 'The Doctor-Patient Relationship,' 109–22.

87 Cathell, *The Physician Himself*, 98, 99.

88 Sandelowski, *Women, Health, and Choice*, 9. Sandelowski has pointed out that the decision is composed of personal readiness, social control, and situational factors. Among the former are a recognition of the seriousness of the problem, the acceptance of personal vulnerability, a predisposition to take action, the motivation to act, the ability to act, knowledge of desired action, and belief in it. Among the social control factors are social pressure to act and acceptability of the action. Among the latter are taking into account the effectiveness of the action, the pleasure of it, its effort, previous experience, favourable environment, and the attractiveness of action. While each negotiation is unique, there are nevertheless 'patterns of behaviour.' William Felstener and Austin Sarat, 'Enactments of Power: Negotiating Reality and Responsibility in Lawyer-Client Interactions,' *Cornell Law Review* 77 (1992): 1449–58. See also Greenhalgh and Hurwitz, eds., *Narrative-Based Medicine*. As Greenhalgh points out in her article 'Narrative-Based Medicine in an Evidence-Based World,' there are at least four different texts in a patient-doctor encounter. There is the experiential text, which is the patient's explanation of his or her illness; the narrative text, which is the physician's interpretation of the problem as given by the patient; the physical text, which is based on the physical exam of the patient; and the instrumental text, which is what medical test and technology reveal (258–9).

89 Silverman *The Last Best West*, 128; interviews with Eunice Jordan, 14 July 1993, and Esther Thomas, 21 July 1993; Dalhousie University Archives, Oxorn Papers, Correspondence A–M, Letter from Mrs Annie L. Atkinson to Harry Oxorn, 21 July 1980.

90 Mary Rubio and Elizabeth Waterson, eds., *The Selected Journals of L.M. Montgomery*, vol. 1: *1889–1910* (Toronto: Oxford University Press 1985), 342–3.

91 Margaret Andrews, 'Medical Attendance in Vancouver, 1886–1920,' in S.E.D. Shortt, *Medicine in Canadian Society: Historical Perspectives* (Montreal: McGill-Queen's University Press: 1981), 423.

92 McGill University, Rare Books, Alton Goldbloom, 'The Role of the Physician in the Rearing of Children,' 2.

93 Victoria General Hospital Papers, Sydney Thomas, patient no. 90, register 60, Medical Department, admitted 28 October 1930, discharged 12 November 1930.

94 Wright, *A Textbook of Obstetrics*, 428–9.

95 *CMAJ* 31 (August 1934): 191–2.

96 *Nova Scotia Medical Bulletin* 24 (May 1945): 226. See also Plunkett, *The Book of the Post-Graduate Course*, 13; and Exner, *The Nature of Medical Practice*, 3.

97 *CMAJ* 47, 5 (November 1942): 474.

98 British Columbia Archives, Walter Bapty Papers, Add. Mss. 1283, folder 3, 'Memoirs,' pt. 4, 13.

99 McGill University Archives, Royal Victoria Hospital, RG96, vol. 104, Gynaecology Case Charts, 1913, patient no. 6429, Mrs Letitia Danvers, admitted 24 November 1913. See also Armstrong, 'The Doctor-Patient Relationship,' 111.

100 Annette Scambler and Graham Scambler, *Menstrual Disorders* (London: Tavistock/Routledge 1993), 94.

101 *Canadian Journal of Medicine and Surgery* 27 (February 1910): 77.

102 *Everywoman's World*, November 1920, 42

103 *Nova Scotia Medical Bulletin* 12 (February 1933): 165. See also *Canadian Practitioner and Review* 36 (December 1911): 770; *Canadian Journal of Medicine and Surgery* 35 (April 1914): 221; *Nova Scotia Medical Bulletin* 5 (October 1926): 9; H.E. MacDermot, *History of the Canadian Medical Association*, vol. 2 (Toronto: Murray 1958), 139; McGill University Archives, *Annual Report of the Royal Victoria Hospital, Montreal*, 1942, 44; *Canadian Home Journal*, August 1943, 11; Plunkett, *The Book of the Post-Graduate Course*, 14; *Canadian Journal of Public Health* 36 (March 1945): 96; Helen Flanders Dunbar, *Emotions and Bodily Changes* (New York: Columbia University Press 1947), liv.

104 The literature on medicine and women is huge. See, for example, Elizabeth Fee, 'Women and Health Care: A Comparison of Theories,' *International Journal of Health Services* 5 (1975): 397–415; Thomas Laqueur, *Making Sex: Body and Gender from the Greeks to Freud* (Cambridge, Mass.: Harvard University Press 1990); Janet Golden, *A Social History of Wet Nursing in America: From Breast to Bottle* (Cambridge: Cambridge University Press 1996); Margaret Marsh and Wanda Ronner, *The Empty Cradle: Infertility in America from Colonial Times to the Present* (Baltimore: Johns Hopkins University Press 1996); Sharon Batt, *Patient No More: The Politics of Breast Cancer* (Halifax: Gynergy Books 1994); Gail Kellough, *Aborting Law: An Exploration of the Politics of Motherhood and Abortion* (Toronto: University

of Toronto Press 1996); Leslie Doyal, *What Makes Women Sick? Gender and the Political Economy of Health* (New Brunswick, N.J.: Rutgers University Press 1995); Elizabeth Fee and Nancy Krieger, eds., *Women's Health, Politics and Power: Essays on Sex/Gender, Medicine, and Public Policy* (Amityville, N.Y.: Baywood 1994); Fisher, *In the Patients' Best Interest;* Elizabeth Haiken, *Venus Envy: A History of Cosmetic Surgery* (Baltimore: Johns Hopkins University Press 1997); Judith Lorber, *Gender and the Social Construction of Illness* (Thousand Oaks, Calif.: Sage Publications 1997); Estelle Cohen, *Gender and the History of Gynecology: Constructing Biology as Social Knowledge* (New Brunswick, N.J.: Rutgers University Press 1995); Mary Spongberg, *Feminizing Venereal Disease: The Body of the Prostitute in Nineteenth-Century Medical Discourse* (London: Macmillan 1997); Evelyne Ender, *Sexing the Mind: Nineteeth-Century Fictions of Hysteria* (Ithaca, N.Y.: Cornell University Press 1995); Rima Apple, ed., *Women, Health and Medicine in America: A Historical Handbook* (New York: Garland 1990); Joan Jacobs Brumberg, *Fasting Girls: The Emergence of Anorexia Nervosa as a Modern Disease* (Cambridge, Mass.: Harvard University Press 1988); Janice Delaney, M.J. Lupton, and Emily Toth, *The Curse: A Cultural History of Menstruation* (New York: Mentor 1976); Barbara Ehrenreich and Deirdre English, *For Her Own Good: 150 Years of the Experts' Advice to Women* (Garden City, N.Y.: Anchor Press 1978); Elizabeth Fee, ed., *Women and Health: The Politics of Sex in Medicine* (Farmingdale, N.Y.: Baywood 1983); Ruth Formanek, *The Meanings of Menopause: Historical, Medical, and Clinical Perspectives* (Hillsdale: Analytic Press 1990); Diane Prince Herndl, *Invalid Women: Figuring Feminine Illness in American Fiction and Culture, 1840–1940* (Chapel Hill: University of North Carolina Press 1993); Wendy Mitchinson, *The Nature of Their Bodies: Women and Their Physicians in Victorian Canada* (Toronto: University of Toronto Press 1991); Moscucci, *The Science of Women;* Angus McLaren and Arlene Tigar McLaren, *The Bedroom and the State: The Changing Practices and Politics of Contraception and Abortion in Canada* (Toronto: McClelland and Stewart 1986); Nelly Oudshoorn, *Beyond the Natural Body: An Archeology of Sex Hormones* (New York: Routledge 1994); Barbara Seaman and Gideon Seaman, *Women and the Crisis in Sex Hormones* (New York: Rawson 1977); Sherwin, *No Longer Patient;* Elaine Showalter, *The Female Malady: Women, Madness, and English Culture, 1830–1980* (New York: Pantheon Books 1985); Susan M. Squier, *Babies in Bottles: Twentieth-Century Visions of Reproductive Technology* (New Brunswick, N.J.: Rutgers University Press 1994); Walter Vandereycken, *From Fasting Saints to Anorexic Girls: The History of Self-Starvation* (New York: New York University Press 1994); Patricia Anne Vertinsky, *The*

Eternally Wounded Woman: Women, Doctors, and Exercise in the Late Nine-teenth Century (Manchester, U.K.: Manchester University Press 1990); Phyllis Chesler, *Women and Madness* (Garden City, N.Y.: Doubleday 1972); Kathy Davis, *Reshaping the Female Body: The Dilemma of Cosmetic Surgery* (New York: Routledge 1995); Anita Clair Fellman and Michael Fellman, *Making Sense of the Self: Medical Advice Literature in Late Nineteenth-Century America* (Philadelphia: University of Pennsylvania Press 1981); Catherine Gallagher and Thomas Laqueur, eds., *The Making of the Modern Body* (Berkeley: University of California Press 1987); Linda Gordon, *Woman's Body, Woman's Right: A Social History of Birth Control in America* (New York: Penguin 1976); Nicole J. Grant, *The Selling of Contraception: The Dalkon Shield Case, Sexuality, and Women* (Columbus: Ohio State University Press 1992); John S. Haller Jr. and Robin Haller, *The Physician and Sexuality in Victorian America* (Chicago: University of Illinois Press 1974); Janice M. Irvine, *Disorders of Desire: Sex and Gender in Modern American Sexology* (Philadelphia: Temple University Press 1990); Lock, *Encounters with Aging;* Edward Shorter, *A History of Women's Bodies* (New York: Basic Books 1982); Todd, *Intimate Adversaries.*

105 Interview with Drs M and H, Halifax, 29 October 1993. See also Barton Cooke Hirst, *A Text-Book of Obstetrics,* 7th ed. (Philadelphia: W.B. Saunders 1912), 69.

106 Linda Gordon, *Heroes of Their Own Lives: The Politics and History of Family Violence: Boston, 1880–1960* (New York: Penguin 1988), 18.

107 http://medicine.ucsf.edu/housestaff/mrpn/august97/leader.html UCSF Medical Residents' Progress Notes, *Newsletter of the UCSF Medical Housestaff* 8 (August 1997), n.p. (checked 14 September 2000).

2: The Even More Uncertain World of Obstetrics

1 Barton Cooke Hirst, *A Text-Book of Obstetrics,* 7th ed. (Philadelphia: W.B. Saunders 1912), 170.

2 The following are just a few of the studies available. Judy Litoff, *American Midwives 1860 to the Present* (Westport, Conn.: Greenwood Press 1978); Barbara Rothman, *In Labour: Women and Power in the Birthplace* (London: Junction Books 1982); Katherine Arnup, Andrée Lévesque and Ruth Roach Pierson, eds., *Delivering Motherhood: Maternal Ideologies and Prac-tices in the Nineteenth and Twentieth Centuries* (London: Routledge 1990); Suzanne Aims, *Immaculate Deception: A New Look at Women and Childbirth in America* (Boston: San Francisco Book Co./Houghton Mifflin 1975); Nancy Stoller Shaw, *Forced Labour: Maternity Care in the United States*

(London: Pergamon Press 1974); Doris B. Haire, *The Cultural Warping of Childbirth* (Milwaukee: International Childbirth Education Association 1972); Gena Corea, *The Mother Machine: Reproductive Technologies from Artificial Insemination to Artificial Wombs* (Markham, Ont.: Fitzhenry & Whiteside 1985); Ann Oakley, *Women Confined: Towards a Sociology of Childbirth* (London: Martin Robertson 1980); Janice Raymond, *Women as Wombs: Reproductive Technologies and the Battle over Women's Freedom* (New York: Harper 1993); Robyn Rowland, *Living Laboratories: Women and Reproductive Technologies* (Bloomington: Indiana University Press 1992); Diana Scully, *Men Who Control Women's Health: The Miseducation of Obstetrician-Gynecologists* (Boston: Houghton Mifflin 1980); Marjorie Tew, *Safer Childbirth: A Critical History about Women and Power in the Birthplace* (London: Junction Books 1982).

3 Jo Murphy-Lawless, *Reading Birth and Death: A History of Obstetric Thinking* (Bloomington: University of Indiana Press 1998), 8.

4 *Canadian Practitioner and Review* 31 (October 1906): 548, 550. This kind of detail was reflected in cases reported to the medical press. See *Canadian Medical Association Journal (CMAJ)* 3 (September 1913): 750. The 'lust' for information was not limited to physicians: 'As Thomas Richards has remarked, the British Empire was united "not by force but by information."' Patrick A. Dunne, 'Making the 1891 Census in British Columbia,' *Histoire sociale* 31 (November 1998): 223–40.

5 Daniel Clark, *Mental Diseases: A Synopsis of Twelve Lectures Delivered at the Hospital for the Insane, Toronto, to the Graduating Medical Classes* (Toronto: William Briggs, n.d.), 90.

6 *Child and Family Welfare* 10, 2 (1934): 10; *CMAJ* 62 (February 1950): 109, 119. See also William Victor Johnston, *Before the Age of Miracles: Memoirs of a Country Doctor* (Toronto: Fitzhenry & Whiteside 1972), 40–1; Fred L. Adair, ed., *Obstetrics and Gynecology*, vol. 1 (Philadelphia: Lea & Febiger 1940), 27; *CMAJ* 50 (March 1944): 219; *Canadian Home Journal* 42 (December 1945): 42.

7 McGill University Archives, R 95, vol. 113, Obstetric Cases 23951–24000, 1921, forms in the case histories. See also Judith Walzer Leavitt, '"Science" Enters the Birthing Room: Obstetrics in America since the Eighteenth Century,' *Journal of American History* 70 (September 1983): 298. The emphasis on information is part of what John Harley Warner refers to as medical empiricism or the change in therapeutic epistemology that developed in the nineteenth century. John Harley Warner, *The Therapeutic Perspective: Medical Practice, Knowledge, and Identity in Ameican, 1820–1885* (Cambridge, Mass.: Harvard University Press 1986), 6.

8 Veronica Strong-Boag and Kathryn McPherson, 'The Confinement of Women: Childbirth and Hospitalization in Vancouver, 1919–1939,' in Arnup, Lévesque, and Pierson, eds., *Delivering Motherhood* 81.

9 *Canada Lancet* 47 (August 1914): 910; *Western Canadian Medical Journal* 1 (November 1907): 500. See also *Canadian Journal of Medicine and Surgery* 20 (September 1906): 179; *Saskatchewan Medical Journal* 2 (July 1910): 194; *Dominion Medical Monthly* 43 (October 1914): 115; *Canadian Practitioner and Review* 35 (February 1910): 86; *CMAJ* 1 (February 1911): 131; Joseph B. DeLee, *The Principles and Practice of Obstetrics* (Philadelphia: W.B. Saunders 1913), 273.

10 *CMAJ* 7 (May 1917): 413.

11 David Berry Hart, *Guide to Midwifery* (London: Rebman 1912), 202.

12 *Canada Lancet and Practitioner* 78 (April 1932): 111, 112; *CMAJ* 10 (October 1920): 902; *CMAJ* 17 (March 1927): 285; Jutta Mason, 'Midwifery in Canada,' in Sheila Kitzinger, ed., *The Midwife Challenge* (London: Pandora Press 1988), 115; Memorial University of Newfoundland, Folklore and Language Archive, no. 82-326, Barbara Doran, '"There Was No One but Myself": The Life of a Midwife in Outport Newfoundland,' 16; *Canada Lancet and Practitioner* 77 (December 1931): 160; *CMAJ* 22 (April 1930): 470; *Chatelaine*, March 1933, 63; *Canadian Nurse* 34 (September 1938): 475; *University of Toronto Medical Journal* 25 (November 1947): 51.

13 *Canadian Journal of Medicine and Surgery* 20 (1906): 179.

14 Queen's University, Queen's University Examination Papers, 1902, Faculty of Medicine. See also McGill University Archives, RG38; C12, C13, Examinations; Charles Jewett, ed., *The Practice of Obstetrics*, 2nd ed., (New York: Lea Brothers 1901), 249. Teaching hospitals and their teaching staff often had patients referred to them, which meant that students often saw especially rare and difficult cases, which gave them a sense that such cases were more common than they were. David M. Eddy, 'Clinical Policies and the Quality of Clinical Practice,' *New England Journal of Medicine* 307 (1922): 344.

15 Hirst, *A Text-Book of Obstetrics*, 158, 170.

16 Egbert H. Grandin and George W. Jarman, *A Textbook on Practical Obstetrics*, 3rd ed. (Philadelphia: F.A. Davis 1901), 245. See also *Western Canadian Medical Journal* 1 (November 1907): 500.

17 See Clark, *Mental Diseases*, 90; and Hirst, *A Text-Book of Obstetrics*, 9.

18 *Canadian Nurse* 26 (July 1930): 362, and (June 1930): 301–2; *CMAJ* 13 (June 1923): 379. See also *Nova Scotia Medical Bulletin* 10 (January 1931): 40; P. Brooke Bland, *Practical Obstetrics for Students and Practitioners* (Philadel-

phia: F.A. Saunders 1932), 543; *Canadian Nurse* 31 (November 1935): 487; *CMAJ* 34 (May 1936): 518 and (June 1936): 625; *CMAJ* 55 (September 1946): 294.

19 Cynthia Abeele, '"Nations Are Built of Babies": Maternal and Child Welfare in Ontario, 1914–1940' (PhD thesis, University of Guelph, 1987), 167. See also *Manitoba Medical Review* 14 (June 1934): 3, and Charles E. Rosenberg, 'Pathologies of Progress: The Idea of Civilization as Risk,' *Bulletin of the History of Medicine* 72 (Winter 1998): 714–30.

20 *CMAJ* 14 (August 1924): 698. See also *CMAJ* 20 (June 1929): 647–8; *Nova Scotia Medical Bulletin* 10 (January 1931): 40; *Canadian Nurse* 34 (September 1938): 475.

21 J.S. Fairbairn, *Gynaecology with Obstetrics: A Text-Book for Students and Practitioners* (London: Humphrey Milford, Oxford University Press 1924), 23. See also *Canadian Nurse* 24 (July 1928): 350; *Canadian Journal of Medicine and Surgery* 64 (1928): 133; *Canadian Nurse* 26 (June 1930): 301–2; Charles R. King, 'The New York Maternal Mortality Study: A Conflict of Professionalization,' *Bulletin of the History of Medicine* 65 (Winter 1991): 478; interview with Drs M and H, Halifax, 29 October 1993; *Nova Scotia Medical Bulletin* 19 (June 1940): 363. Elinor Black recalled that her professor, Dr Olafur Bjornson, also stressed and acted as if every pregnancy would be normal and she taught her own students the same. Julie Vandervoort, *Tell the Driver: A Biography of Elinor F.E. Black, M.D.* (Winnipeg: University of Manitoba Press 1992), 45, and information supplied by Dr Charles Roland; *Nova Scotia Medical Bulletin* 12 (September 1933): 528; J. Munro Kerr, with Donald McIntyre and D. Fyfe Anderson, *Operative Obstetrics: A Guide to the Difficulties and Complications of Obstetric Practice*, 4th ed. (London: Bailliere, Tindall, and Cox 1937), vii; *Canadian Nurse* 39 (September 1943): 582; *CMAJ* 62 (February 1950): 109.

22 *Canadian Journal of Medicine and Surgery* 20 (September 1906): 179. See also *Journal of the American Medical Association*, 6 January 1912, 1.

23 George M. White, 'The History of Obstetrical and Gynaecological Teaching in Canada,' *American Journal of Obstetrics and Gynecology* 77 (March 1959): 468.

24 Jayne Elliott in her thesis has postulated that the concern about education declined, and she linked it to the rise in hospital and laboratory training. See her '"Endormez-moi!": An Early Twentieth-Century Obstetrical Practice in the Gatineau Valley, Quebec' (MA thesis, Carleton University, 1997), 124.

25 *CMAJ* 13 (June 1923): 380. See also *CMAJ* 65 (May 1929): 130; and *CMAJ* 20 (February 1929): 181.

26 *Manitoba Medical Bulletin* 99 (November 1929): 7; *CMAJ* 62, supplement (September 1950): 233. See also Florence H.M. Emory, *Public Health Nursing in Canada* (Toronto: Macmillan, 1953), 285–6.

27 Irvine Loudon, *Death in Childbirth: An International Study of Maternal Care and Maternal Mortality 1800–1950* (Oxford: Clarendon Press 1992), 229.

28 White, 'The History of Obstetrical and Gynaecological Teaching in Canada,' 467.

29 H.L. Burris, *Medical Saga: The Burris Clinic and Early Pioneers* (np., nd.), 82.

30 *Dalhousie Medical Journal* 11, 1 (1958): 22.

31 For information on Dalhousie, see *Nova Scotia Medical Bulletin* 11 (April 1932): 460; *Dalhousie Medical Journal* 11, 1–3 (1937): 31; G. Enid MacLeod and Irene M.J. Szuler, 'Medical Missionairies of the Early Female Medical Graduates, 1894–1929,' *Nova Scotia Medical Journal* 69 (February 1990): 7–14; interview with Drs M and H, Halifax, 29 October 1993. For information on Manitoba, see *Manitoba Medical Bulletin* 99 (November 1929): 7. For information on Britain, see *Canada Lancet and Practitioner* 78 (April 1932): 114; and on Sweden, see *Hospital, Medical and Nursing World* 35 (April 1929): 115.

32 *Canada Lancet and Practitioner* 78 (April 1932): 112; *Manitoba Medical Bulletin* 81 (May 1928): 10; *Canadian Journal of Medicine and Surgery* 65 (May 1929): 131; *CMAJ* 20 (February 1929): 180; *Canada Lancet and Practitioner* 76 (April 1931): 93. While it was important for students to have practical experience before they graduated, the other side of the issue, and one seldom addressed by those proposing such changes, was the impact on the patients themselves. In teaching hospitals, the patients whom the students tended to see were the poorer ones, the non-paying patients. Private patients did not become the 'subjects' of medical training. For one woman's experience, see Denyse Baillargeon, 'L'encadrement de la maternité au Québec entre les deux guerres: Les gardes de La Métropolitaine, les gouttes de lait et l'assistance maternelle,' *Bulletin, RCHTQ* 47 & 8 (1990): 34–5.

33 Elliott, '"Endormez-moi!"' 2, 13, 46.

34 Letter from BR, 9 August 1993. During her internship, however, she felt that she had experienced an excellent apprenticeship system. The fainting episode was given to the author by Dr Robert Macbeth, 6 November 1999.

35 D. Sclater Lewis, *Royal Victoria Hospital, 1887–1947* (Montreal: McGill University Press 1969), 279; W.G. Cosbie, *The Toronto General Hospital, 1819–1965: A Chronicle* (Toronto: Macmillan 1975), 149. The Halifax Medical College calendar for 1911–12 had Obstetrics and Gynaecology listed

together, although not until 1922 was Harold Atlee appointed professor and Chairman of the first combined Department of Obstetrics and Gynaecology at Dalhousie. Harry Oxorn, *Harold Benge Atlee M.D.: A Biography* (Hantsport, N.S.: Lancelot Press 1983), 37. Not until 1926 did the Medical Faculty, University of Manitoba, combine the two. Ian Carr and Robert E. Beamish, *Manitoba Medicine: A Brief History* (Winnipeg: University of Manitoba Press 1999), 114. See also White, 'The History of Obstetrical and Gynaecological Teaching in Canada,' 468, 470.

36 *Canada Lancet* 47 (August 1914): 918; *CMAJ* 4 (June 1914): 470–1. See also Hart, *Guide to Midwifery*, 3; J. Munro Kerr, J. Haig Ferguson, James Young, and James Hendry, *Combined Textbook of Obstetrics and Gynaecology for Students and Medical Practitioners*, 2nd ed. (Edinburgh: E. & S. Livingstone 1933), 687.

37 Hirst, *A Text-Book of Obstetrics*, 9; *CMAJ* 4 (June 1914): 470–1.

38 See Fairbairn, *Gynaecology with Obstetrics*, 22–3; *Nova Scotia Medical Bulletin* 3 (1924): 6; *CMAJ* 20 (June 1929): 646; *Canadian Nurse* 39 (May 1943): 330; *University of Toronto Medical Journal* 25 (January 1948): 133.

39 *CMAJ*, 6 August 1977, 287. In recent years, similar arguments have been made. Lost in the technical advances that protect the life of the mother and her child is the concept of the mother as an individual with social as well as physical needs. Birth impinges on the life of the family, and thus physicians caring for pregnant women need to be encouraged to take a more family-centred approach.

40 Margaret Andrews, 'Medical Attendance in Vancouver, 1886–1920,' *BC Studies* 40 (Winter 1978–9): 32–56.

41 DeLee, *The Principles and Practice of Obstetrics*, 273, 320. See also *Canada Lancet* 47 (August 1914): 918; *Canadian Journal of Medicine and Surgery* 3 (June 1913): 404; *Canadian Practitioner and Review* 35 (February 1910): 86.

42 *Canada Lancet and Practitioner* 78 (April 1932): 112; Public Archives of Nova Scotia, Medical Archives Collection, file 318, 'Executive Meeting,' 6 July 1942, Nova Scotia Medical Society, 22.

43 *CMAJ* 20 (June 1929): 647–8.

44 McGill University, Rare Books, Alton Goldbloom Papers, draft of autobiography, 4–5. See also *CMAJ* 13 (June 1923): 379; *The Public Health Journal* 19 (December 1928): 578; *CMAJ* 22 (April 1930): 470; *Canadian Doctor* 4 (October 1938): 24.

45 *Canadian Journal of Medicine and Surgery* 65 (May 1929): 132; Joyce Antler and Daniel M. Fox, 'The Movement toward a Safe Maternity: Physician Accountability in New York City, 1915–1940,' *Bulletin of the History of Medicine* 50 (Winter 1976): 575.

46 Strong-Boag and McPherson,'The Confinement of Women,' 79; *Canadian Journal of Medicine and Surgery* 65 (May 1929): 132; *Chatelaine*, October 1931, 54; *Nova Scotia Medical Bulletin* 10 (January 1931): 40–1; *University of Toronto Medical Journal* 15 (March 1938): 225; *CMAJ* 42 (January 1940): 56; *Canadian Nurse* 46 (December 1950): 951.

47 Charlotte G. Best, 'Teaching Obstetrics at Home: Medical Schools and Home Delivery Services in the First Half of the Twentieth Century, *Bulletin of the History of Medicine* 72 (Summer 1998): 220–45

48 See Richard C. Norris, ed., *An American Text-Book of Obstetrics for Practitioners and Students* (Philadelphia: W.B. Saunders 1895), 718; *Dominion Medical Monthly* 15 (October 1900): 178; *Canada Lancet* 44 (September 1910): 33. For a description of the situation in which family doctors have found themselves, see Jacalyn Duffin, *History of Medicine: A Scandalously Short Introduction* (Toronto: University of Toronto Press 1999), chap. 14: 'A Many-Faceted Gem: Decline and Rebirth of Family Medicine,' 337–59.

49 DeLee, *The Principles and Practice of Obstetrics*, xii, 320.

50 Strong-Boag and McPherson, 'The Confinement of Women,' 79.

51 *Manitoba Medical Review* 21 (April 1941): 66.

52 Strong-Boag and McPherson, 'The Confinement of Women,' 79, 81. For an examination of this in the American context, see Dorothy C. Wertz, 'What Birth Has Done for Doctors: A Historical View,' *Women and Health* 8 (1983): 7–24.

53 *Canada Lancet and Practitioner* 76 (April, 1931): 95. One text suggested that only those with experience in anaesthesia in childbirth should be involved; being a graduate in medicine was not enough. Henricus J. Stander, *Williams Obstetrics: A Textbook for the Use of Students and Practitioner*, 8th ed. (New York: Appleton-Century 1941), 468.

54 Elliott, 'Endormez-moi!' 29, 107; Elliott has estimated that approximately one-sixth of H.J.G. Geggie's rural practice was obstetrical. Jacalyn Duffin has estimated that by the end of the nineteenth century, 12 per cent of James Langstaff's practice was obstetrical. Jacalyn Duffin, *Langstaff: A Nineteenth-Century Medical Life* (Toronto: University of Toronto Press 1993), 180.

55 *Chatelaine*, July 1928, 7. Of course this varied from region to region.

56 *Canadian Doctor* 4 (October 1938): 24; McGill University Archives, *Annual Report of the Royal Victoria Hospital, Montreal*, 1935, 56. Physicians approved of such schemes, certainly more so than cash bonuses paid directly to the mothers, fearing that the money would not be spent on medical care.

57 *Nova Scotia Medical Bulletin* 10 (May 1931): 322.

58 *Hospital, Medical and Nursing World* 30 (September 1926): 65. Some special-

ists acknowledged this as well. Harold Atlee told of how difficult it was to diagnose an ectopic pregnancy and how he had done so in many cases only to find it was a normal pregnancy, pelvic inflammatory disease, or uterine fibroids. *Nova Scotia Medical Bulletin* 20 (December 1941): 211.

59 D.W. Cathell, *The Physician Himself and Things That Concern His Reputation and Success*, 10th ed. (Philadelphia: F.A. Davis 1898), 115.

60 *Canadian Journal of Medicine and Surgery* 64 (1928): 133. See also Marion O. Robinson, *Give My Heart: The Dr. Marion Hilliard Story* (Garden City, N.Y.: Doubleday 1964), 158; *CMAJ* 20 (June 1929): 647; Stander, *Williams Obstetrics*, 410. *Canada Lancet* 34 (November 1900): 113; *Canadian Nurse* 26 (June 1930): 303.

61 Adair, ed., *Obstetrics and Gynecology*, 1:28; Robinson, *Give My Heart*, 91, 208–9; Marion Hilliard, *A Woman Doctor Looks at Love and Life* (Garden City, N.Y.: Doubleday 1957), 31. See also *Manitoba Medical Review* 21 (April 1941): 66; Oxorn, *Harold Benge Atlee M.D.*, 113.

62 For discussion of fees, see *Canada Lancet* 44 (September 1910): 36; *CMAJ* 1 (February 1911): 131; British Columbia Archives, *British Columbia Commission on Health Insurance 1919–21*, GR706, file 2 'Report,' 56; and file 1, 'Report on Maternity Insurance, 1921, 4; Strong-Boag and McPherson, 'The Confinement of Women,' 84. In 1927 the Manitoba Medical Association proposed a $25 fee for confinement cases. *Manitoba Medical Association Bulletin* 66 (February 1927): 3–4; *Chatelaine* 5 (May 1932): 24; *Maclean's*, 1 October 1945, 59.

63 *Canada Lancet and Practitioner* 78 (April 1932): 111–12. See also *Canada Lancet* 44 (September 1910): 36; *Canada Lancet and Practitioner* 77 (December 1931): 160; *CMAJ* 22 (April 1930): 470; *Canada Lancet and Practitioner* 76 (April 1931): 95; *CMAJ* 33 (December 1935): 672; Carl Henry Davis, ed., *Gynecology and Obstetrics* (Hagerstown, Md., 1935), 1:10.

64 See *Manitoba Medical Bulletin* 86 (October 1928): 8–9; *Canadian Journal of Medicine and Surgery* 64, 5 (1928): 133. Dianne Dodd, 'Helen MacMurchy, M.D. (1862–1953): Mothers and Doctors in the "Complete" Canadian Mother's Book' (paper presented to the Canadian Historical Association, Kingston, 1991), 18; *Chatelaine* March 1950, 14. From the patient's point of view, however, physicians were often deemed too expensive and too demanding of their fee. One French Canadian woman mentioned that calling a physician cost between $10 and $25, which represented more than a week's salary for many. Baillargeon, 'L'encadrement de la maternité au Québec entre les deux guerres,' 41.

65 *Montreal Medical Journal* 36 (June 1906): 400; Fairbairn, *Gynaecology with Obstetrics*, 256.

66 *Canada Lancet and Practitioner* 71 (August 1928): 46; this was the view of
   Harold Atlee. Interview with Drs M. and H., Halifax, 29 October 1993. See
   also *University of Toronto Medical Journal* 18 (November 1940): 47. A One
   Big Union member testifying before the British Columbia Commission on
   Health Insurance 1919–21 expressed similar sentiments. British Columbia
   Archives, *British Columbia Commission on Health Insurance 1919–21* GR706,
   file 3, 'Evidence,' 362.
67 Dianne Dodd, 'Helen MacMurchy: Popular Midwifery and Maternity
   Services for Canadian Pioneer Women,' in Dianne Dodd and Deborah
   Gorham, eds., *Caring and Curing: Historical Perspectives on Women and
   Healing in Canada* (Ottawa: University of Ottawa Press 1994), 152.
68 Provincial Archives of Nova Scotia, RT98, V645, Report of the Chief
   Superintendent, *VON Report, 1925*, 47. As Meryn Stuart points out, in
   isolated and rural areas public health nurses often substituted for physi-
   cians. Her thesis describes the power of these nurses and physicians'
   response in protecting their perceived territory. Meryn Elizabeth Stuart,
   '"Let Not the People Perish for Lack of Knowledge": Public Health Nursing and the Ontario Rural Child Welfare Project, 1916–1930' (PhD thesis,
   University of Pennsylvania, 1987), especially chap. 6; Meryn Stuart,
   'Shifting Professional Boundaries; Gender Conflict in Public Health, 1920–
   1925,' in Dodd and Gorham, eds., *Caring and Curing*, 49–70. Stuart empha-
   sizes the opposition of the physicians to public health nurse initiatives. In
   this book I recognize the fearfulness behind that opposition. When the
   VON was first contemplated, the National Council of Women (NCW) had
   a group of women with some training in mind, but the emphasis was on
   the caring and womanly aspects of nursing. However, due to opposition
   from physicians, the NCW helped create a much more professional group
   of nurses, the result being an end to the midwife task that the NCW had
   envisioned for the VON. Ironically, however, due to need, the VON often
   did some of the duties of midwives. Beverley Boutilier, 'Helpers or Hero-
   ines? The National Council of Women, Nursing, and "Woman's Work"
   in Late Victorian Canada,' in Dodd and Gorham, eds., *Caring and Curing*,
   17–48.
69 Laurel Halladay, '"We'll See You Next Year": Maternity Homes in Southern Saskatchewan in the First Half of the Twentieth Century' (MA thesis,
   Carleton University, 1996), 51, 58.
70 Kathryn Mae McPherson, 'Skilled Service and Women's Work: Canadian
   Nursing, 1920–39' (PhD thesis, Simon Fraser University, 1989), 275–6.
71 *Canadian Nurse* 77 (February 1981): 30.
72 *Canadian Journal of Public Health* 41 (May 1950): 180.

73 See *Hospital, Medical and Nursing World* 35 (April 1929): 115; *CMAJ* 20 (June 1929): 647; Mason, 'Midwifery in Canada,' 115; Harry Beckman, *Treatment in General Practice* (Philadelphia: W.B. Saunders 1931), 788; *Canadian Public Health Journal* 23 (December 1932): 562.

3: Midwives Did Not Disappear

1 Memorial University of Newfoundland Folklore and Language Archive (MUNFLA), no. 79-549, Debbie G. J. Hallett, 'Irene (Farwell) Bradley: The Art of Midwifery,' 11–12.
2 In the American context, the privileging of science is an important fact. Add to this the emphasis of many physicians that childbirth required intervention, the desire of doctors to increase their status, the isolation of midwives and lack of funding to train them, the dubious legal status midwives had, and the increase in hospitals and their willingness to take maternity cases – and the decline of midwifery becomes understandable. See Judy Litoff, *American Midwives, 1860 to the Present* (Westport, Conn.: Greenwood Press 1978), 139–41. Similar factors were at play in Canada. See C. Lesley Biggs, 'The Case of the Missing Midwives: A History of Midwifery in Ontario from 1795–1900,' *Ontario History* 75 (March 1983): 21–36, and Peter Ward, ed. *The Mysteries of Montreal: Memoirs of a Midwife by Charlotte Führer* (Vancouver: University of British Columbia Press 1984), 5. Beth Rushing has argued that market forces motivated physician an-tagonism and the decline of midwifery. 'Market Explanations for Occupa-tional Power: The Decline of Midwifery in Canada,' *American Review of Canadian Studies* 21 (1991): 7–27.

For an excellent discussion of midwifery in England in an earlier period, see Adrian Wilson, *The Making of Man-Midwifery: Childbirth in England, 1660–1770* (Cambridge, Mass.: Harvard University Press 1995). Wilson disagrees with the popular notion that midwifery declined as a result of changing fashions and the rise in medical technology. Wilson contends that woman's collective culture, which had once barred men from child-birth, began to break down. Women still continued to control birth, but the 'threshold of difficulty had fallen'; that is, more births were seen as problematic. This argument seems to follow that of William Arney, who speculates that men took over the control of birth not because of better education or the increasing use of technology but by reconceptualizing birth from being a natural act to using a rational or scientific approach: 'Rationalism freed birth from the constraints of nature and opened it to improvement, and the boundary between normal and abnormal births became a matter for dispute and contention.' It was the scientific or rational view of the body on which midwives' control of what was normal or abnormal could be challenged. William Ray Arney, *Power and the Profession of Obstetrics* (Chicago: University of Chicago Press 1982), 28, 49.

3 In fact, what subsequent chapters on physician-directed births reveal is that the overlap between physician and midwife care was greater than many scholars have been willing to acknowledge.

4 For a critique of the feminist view, see Gordon Jones's review of Litoff's *American Midwives* and Richard W. Wertz and Dorothy C. Wertz's *Lying-In: A History of Childbirth in America* in the *Journal of the History of Medicine and Allied Sciences* 34 (1979): 112–14, and Edward Shorter, *A History of Women's Bodies* (New York: Basic Books 1982).

5 J.T.H. Connor, '"Larger Fish to Catch Here than Midwives": Midwifery and the Medical Profession in Nineteenth-Century Ontario,' in Dianne Dodd and Deborah Gorham, eds., *Caring and Curing: Historical Perspectives on Women and Healing in Canada* (Ottawa: University of Ottawa Press 1994), 103–34, and Wendy Mitchinson, *The Nature of Their Bodies: Women and Their Doctors in Victorian Canada* (Toronto: University of Toronto Press 1991). Both Connor and I recognized the variety of factors that influenced the decline of midwives in central Canada by the end of the nineteenth century, although he is more sympathetic to the physicians' position than I perhaps was in my early work. Connor argued that medical practitioners were not uniform in their attitudes to midwives. Yet as Dianne Dodd and Deborah Gorham have made clear (and I agree), his argument does not lessen the feminist view of the midwife–doctor conflict. Dodd and Gorham, eds., *Caring and Curing*, 6. Physicians in the late nineteenth century were happy to see midwifery decline and were unwilling to support it. Like Connor, I argue that doctors' opposition to midwives is nuanced, but there is little doubt that as a group they were hostile. In his work, Connor seems (like the physicians) to accept skilled midwives but links their skill to formal training. Dianne Dodd, too, suggests the ambiguity of doctors' opposition to midwives. Dianne Dodd, 'Helen MacMurchy: Popular Midwifery and Maternity Services for Canadian Pioneer Women,' in Dodd and Gorham, eds., *Caring and Curing*, 135–62. Christine Payeur in her thesis notes the decline in midwife competence over a century. 'Maternal Mortality in Quebec from the Medical Perspective and the Women's Point of View, 1890–1950' (MA thesis, Université de Montréal, 1997), 42. Suzann Buckley focused on the opposition of nurses to midwives, thus reminding us that support did not divide along gender lines. Suzann Buckley, 'Ladies or Midwives? Efforts to Reduce Infant and Maternal Mortality,' in Linda

Kealey, ed., *A Not Unreasonable Claim: Women and Reform in Canada, 1880s–1920s* (Toronto: Women's Press 1976), 131–49.

6 Janet Elizabeth McNaughton, 'The Role of the Newfoundland Midwife in Traditional Health Care, 1900 to 1970' (PhD thesis, Memorial University of Newfoundland, 1989), 319.

7 See C. Lesley Biggs, 'Fragments from the History of Midwifery in Canada: A Reconsideration of the Historiographic Issues,' in Ivy Bourgeault, Cecilia Benoit, and Robbie Davis-Floyd, eds., *Reconceiving Midwifery: The New Canadian Model of Care* (Ann Arbor: University of Michigan Press, forthcoming).

8 See Biggs, ' The Case of the Missing Midwives: A History of Midwifery in Ontario from 1795–1900,' *Ontario History* 75 (March 1983): 36–60; Helen Laforce, *Histoire de la sage-femme dans la région de Québec* (Quebec: Institute québécois de recherche sur la culture, Collection: Edmond-de-Nevers no. 4, 1985).

9 Eliane Leslau Silverman, *The Last Best West: Women on the Alberta Frontier, 1880–1930* (Montreal: Eden Press 1984), 71; *Canadian Doctor* 6 (October 1940): 20.

10 Biggs, 'Fragments from the History of Midwifery in Canada,' 4 and 12 of draft.

11 Litoff, *American Midwives*, 27.

12 Joyce Antler and Daniel M. Fox, 'The Movement Toward a Safe Maternity: Physician Accountability in New York City, 1915–1940,' *Bulletin of Medical History* 50 (Winter 1976): 574.

13 For the Canadian figures, see *Canadian Journal of Medicine and Surgery* 33 (March 1913): 157; *Manitoba Medical Review* 26 (May 1946): 276; Jutta Mason, 'Midwifery in Canada,' in Sheila Kitzinger, ed., *The Midwife Challenge* (London: Pandora Press 1988), 116; John O'Neill and Patricia A. Kaufert, 'The Politics of Obstetric Care: The Inuit Experience' in W. Pen Handwerker, ed., *Births and Power: Social Change and the Politics of Reproduction* (San Francisco: Westview Press 1990), 59; Cynthia R. Comacchio, 'Nations Are Built of Babies': Saving Ontario's Mothers and Children 1900–1940* (Montreal: McGill-Queen's University Press 1993), 77; Cecilia Benoit and Dena Carroll, 'Aboriginal Midwifery in British Columbia: A Narrative Untold,' in Peter H. Stephenson, Susan J. Elliot, Leslie T. Foster, and Jill Harris, eds., *A Persistent Spirit: Towards Understanding Aboriginal Health in British Columbia* (Victoria: Canadian Western Geographical Series no. 31, 1995), 223–48.

14 See Cecilia Benoit, *Midwives in Passage: The Modernization of Maternity Care* (St John's: Social and Economic Studies no. 44, Institute of Social and Economic Research, Memorial University of Newfoundland 1999), 94.

15 MUNFLA, no. 78-401, Madonna Hickey, '[Aunt Annie Fizzard]: A 92-Year-Old Midwife from the Community of Grand Je Pierre, F.B.,' 6–7.

16 O'Neill and Kaufert, 'The Politics of Obstetric Care,' 58.

17 Laurel Halladay, '"We'll See You Next Year": Maternity Homes in Southern Saskatchewan in the First Half of the Twentieth Century' (MA thesis, Carleton University, 1996), 37.

18 MUNFLA, no. 75–285, Joyce Murphy, 'Olive Bishop: Midwife-Nurse of Pass Island, South Coast of Newfoundland, Hermitage Bay,' 14–18.

19 For a history of midwife training in Newfoundland, see Elizabeth Rosemary Summers, 'Historical Development of Public Health Nursing in Newfoundland, Canada, 1920–1950' (MSc thesis, Catholic University of America, 1967), 41; and Benoit, *Midwives in Passage*, 18–19.

20 McNaughton, 'The Role of the Newfoundland Midwife in Traditional Health Care,' 76–7, 86–8, 127, 136–7, 229.

21 *Woman's Century*, June 1919, 53; *Canadian Nurse* 20 (June 1924): 341.

22 See National Council of Women, *Yearbook 1924*, 72–3; *Public Health Journal* 16 (September 1925): 415.

23 Arney, *Power and the Profession of Obstetrics*, 20–4.

24 National Council of Women, *Report of the Annual Meeting 1906*, 36–8; Public Archives of Nova Scotia, RT98, V645, *VON Report, 1918*, 10, 30, and *VON Report, 1916*, 15.

25 Frances Swyripa, *Ukrainian-Canadian Women and Ethnic Identity, 1891–1991* (Toronto: University of Toronto Press 1993), 30, 32; *Woman's Century*, February 1917, 6; Halladay, 'We'll See You Next Year,' 36.

26 MUNFLA, no. 77–345, Wanda M. King, 'The Role of Midwife in the Community of N. Summerford Notre Dame Bay,' 6.

27 Dianne Dodd, 'Advice to Parents: The Blue Books, Helen MacMurchy, MD, and the Federal Department of Health, 1920–1934,' *Canadian Bulletin of Medical History* 8 (1991): 218.

28 MUNFLA, no. 77–65, Ruth Green, 'The Experiences and Role of Rhoda Maud Piercey as the midwife in the community of Winterton, Trinity Bay,' 6–7. See no. 73-160, M. Deanna Emberley, 'Folk Medicine of Newfoundland. Part 1. A Bay de Verde Midwife [Jane Ann Emberley]. Part 2. Folk Cures for Common Complaints,' 2; no. 77-345, Wanda King, 'The Role of the Midwife in the Community of N. Summerford Notre Dame Day,' 9.

29 MUNFLA, no. 77-139, Madonna Dove, 'Annie Andre: My Grandmother, a Midwife and a Newfoundlander,' 13–14.

30 McNaughton, 'The Role of the Newfoundland Midwife in Traditional Health Care,' 29, 40.

31 Halladay, 'We'll See You Next Year,' 404.

32 MUNFLA, no. 77-345, Wanda M. King, 'The Role of Midwife in the Com-
    munity of N. Summerford Notre Dame Bay,' 2; re payment, see also no.
    79-549, Debbie G.J. Hallett, 'Irene (Farwell) Bradley: The Art of Midwifery,'
    13; no. 77-65, Ruth Green, 'The Experiences and Role of Rhoda Maud
    Piercey as the Midwife in the Community of Winterton, Trinity Bay,' 24;
    no. 76-104, Kevin Paul Mark Saunders, 'Mrs. Freda Guinchard: Midwife
    on the Northern Peninsula and North-Western Section of Newfoundland,'
    25; no. 76-258, Lillian Joyce White. 'The Work of a Midwife in a Trinity Bay
    Community,' 10–11; no. 78-211, Carol Anne Ruby, 'Childbearing and
    Childbirth in Early Twentieth Century Newfoundland,' 103; no. 77-139,
    Madonna Dove, 'Annie Andre: My Grandmother, a Midwife, and a
    Newfoundlander,' 15–16. Others, too, were often paid in kind, especially
    early in the century. McNaughton, 'The Role of the Newfoundland Mid-
    wife in Traditional Health Care,' 24–5.
33 H.J.G. Geggie, *The Extra Mile: Medicine in Rural Quebec, 1885–1965* (Ottawa:
    National Library of Canada 1987), 106; MUNFLA, no. 73-44, Sandra
    Christine Janes, 'Elizabeth "Diddy" Day: Midwife and "Layer Away" of
    the Dead in Quidi Vidi village (St John's),' n.p.; no. 78-401, Madonna
    Hickey, '[Aunt Annie Fizzard]: A 92-Year-Old Midwife from the Commu-
    nity of Grand le Pierre, F.B.,' 8; no. 73-160, M. Deanna Emberley, 'Folk
    Medicine of Newfoundland. Part 1. A Bay de Verde Midwife [Jane Ann
    Emberley]. Part 2. Folk Cures for Common Complaints,' 3; no. 76-165,
    Gary Gale, 'Mrs. Susan Eveleigh, Midwife,' n.p.
34 See MUNFLA, no. 78-211, Carol Anne Ruby, 'Childbearing and Childbirth
    in Early Twentieth Century Newfoundland,' 63, 65; no. 75-21, Mary Har-
    riet Doyle, 'Midwifery in the Community of Calvert on the Southern Shore
    of Newfoundland,' 8; no. 84-307A, John Burke, 'Mrs. Annie LeMoine:
    A Profile of the Traditional Midwife in Port au Port,' 11. See also Janet
    McNaughton, 'Traditional Prenatal Care of Newfoundland Women' (paper
    presented to the Folklore Studies Association of Canada, McMaster Uni-
    versity, 1987), 5; and Joseph B. DeLee, *The Principles and Practice of Obstet-
    rics* (Philadelphia: W.B. Saunders 1913), 825.
35 MUNFLA, no. 76-104, Kevin Paul Mark Saunders, 'Mrs. Freda Guinchard:
    Midwife on the Northern Peninsula and North-Western Section of New-
    foundland,' 21–2. See also no. 77-139, Madonna Dove, 'Annie Andre: My
    Grandmother, a Midwife, and a Newfoundlander,' 15–16; no. 79-508, R.
    Douglas Wells, 'Aunt Lizzie Wells (1893–1977): Midwife,' 5.
36 McNaughton, in 'The Role of the Newfoundland Midwife in Traditional
    Health Care,' 240, told the story of Nora Ellsworth who, after having her
    leg amputated had women come to her for delivery.

37 McNaughton, 'The Role of the Newfoundland Midwife in Traditional Health Care,' 132; MUNFLA no. 70-15B, Marcus Hopkins, 'Some Observations of Midwifery as Practised in Three Newfoundland Communities from 1923 to 1966,' 23; Varpu Lindstrom-Best, *Defiant Sisters: A Social History of Finnish Immigrant Women in Canada* (Toronto: Multicultural History Society of Ontario 1988), 45.

38 MUNFLA, no. 73-160, M. Deanna Emberley, 'Folk Medicine of Newfoundland. Part 1. A Bay de Verde Midwife. Part 2. Folk Cures for Common Complaints,' 3, 5.

39 See MUNFLA, no. 77-237, Wilfred Thomas Rumbolt, 'Midwifery on the Coast of Labrador,' 5; no. 77-65, Ruth Green, 'The Experiences and Role of Rhoda Maud Piercey as the Midwife in the Community of Winterton, Trinity Bay,' 11; McNaughton, 'The Role of the Newfoundland Midwife in Traditional Health Care,' 240;

40 For position during birth, see MUNFLA, no. 78-211, Carol Anne Ruby, 'Childbearing and Childbirth in Early Twentieth Century Newfoundland,' 85; no. 75-21, Mary Harriet Doyle, 'Midwifery in the Community of Calvert on the Southern Shore of Newfoundland,' 14; no. 78-119, Larry Harvey, 'Life and Work of Aunt Nora (Lenora) Ellsworth, née Goodyear, 1877–1951: Her Work as a Healer and Midwife in Carmanville, N.D.B.,' 223–4; no. 79-549, Debbie G.J. Hallett, 'Irene (Farwell) Bradley: The Art of Midwifery,' 18; Janet McNaughton, 'Midwifery, Traditional Obstetric Care and Change in Newfoundland' (paper presented to the Ethnology/Ethnomedicine Group, Memorial University, December 1989), 6–7.

41 H. Gordon Green, *Don't Have Your Baby in the Dory: A Biography of Myra Bennett* (Montreal: Harvest House 1973), 98.

42 McNaughton, 'The Role of the Newfoundland Midwife in Traditional Health Care,' 146–7.

43 Marni Elizabeth Davis, 'Southern Kwakiutl Medicine' (MA thesis, University of Victoria, 1977), 26–7. See also Lesley Paulette, 'The Family Centred Maternity Care Project,' in Mary Crnkovich, ed., *'Gossip': A Spoken History of Women in the North* (Ottawa: Canadian Arctic Resources Committee 1990), 73–4.

44 Igloolik Oral History Project, Science Institute of the Northwest Territories, Government of the Northwest Territories, computer no. RU2, tape IE105, interview with Rachel Uyarsuk by Susan Avingaq, translated by Lucy Tapardjuk, 21 February 1990, transcript, 9–11.

45 *Alberta Medical Bulletin* 14 (July 1949): 12.

46 Davis, 'Southern Kwakiutl Medicine,' 26–7. See also Paulette, 'The Family Centred Maternity Care Project,' 73–4.

47 MUNFLA, no. 75-21, Mary Harriet Doyle, 'Midwifery in the Community of Calvert on the Southern Shore of Newfoundland,' 12–13. See also no. 76-142, Rex Piercey, 'Midwifery in Winterton, Trinity Bay,' 6.

48 MUNFLA, no. 77-65, Ruth Green, 'The Experiences and Role of Rhoda Maud Piercey as the Midwife in the Community of Winterton, Trinity Bay,' 11. See also no. 70—15B, Marcus Hopkins, 'Some Observations of Midwifery as Practised in Three Newfoundland Communities from 1923 to 1966,' 23; no. 78-401, Madonna Hickey, '[Aunt Annie Fizzard:] A 92-Year-Old Midwife from the Community of Grand le Pierre, F.B.' 13; no. 72-49, Ruthie Douglas Herder, 'Superstitions of Pregnancy and Infancy,' 11. Although men may not have been present in the birthing room in most cultures, they were close by. This was important in giving them an appreciation of what their wives had gone through and in allowing them to see and bond with their newborn child. One criticism of childbirth in the North in recent years is that by removing women to hospitals outside the communities, the family loses one of its most important experiences that ties it together – the cycle of life. Lesley Paulette (co-ordinator), *Report on Phase 1 of the Family Centered Maternity Care Project of the Native Women's Association of the NWT* (submitted to the Native Women's Association of the NWT Board of Directors, Yellowknife, NWT, 6 November 1987), 17.

49 *Canada Medical Record* 30 (July 1902): 293–4. See also Benoit, *Midwives in Passage*, 53.

50 MUNFLA, no. 76-165, Gary Gale, 'Mrs. Susan Eveleigh Midwife,' 22–3. See also McNaughton, 'The Role of the Newfoundland Midwife in Traditional Health Care,' 129–30.

51 See McNaughton, 'Midwifery, Traditional Obstetric Care and Change in Newfoundland,' 3–4; MUNFLA, no. 78-401, Madonna Hickey, '[Aunt Annie Fizzard:] A 92-Year-Old Midwife from the Community of Grand le Pierre, F.B.,' 10; no. 78-211, Carol Anne Ruby, 'Childbearing and Childbirth in Early Twentieth Century Newfoundland,' 91. Among the supplies that a 1936 text recommended for physicians to carry were a number of sterile goods, varying solutions and sutures, drugs, usual doctor-bag contents, and a list of 'other' supplies. For a complete list, see Frederick C. Irving, *A Textbook of Obstetrics for Students and Practitioners* (New York: Macmillan 1936), 152–3.

52 Geggie, *The Extra Mile*, 106; MUNFLA, no. 73-44, Sandra Christine Janes, 'Elizabeth "Diddy" Day: Midwife and "Layer Away" of the Dead in Quidi Vidi Village,' n.p.

53 Comacchio, *'Nations Are Built of Babies,'* 171.

54 See MUNFLA, no. 78-116, Mary Green, 'Midwifery in Outport Newfound-land,' 9. There was no explanation as to what the ergot was for.

55 Paulette, 'The Family Centred Maternity Care Project,' 73–4.

56 *Alberta Medical Bulletin* 14 (July 1949): 11–14.

57 Lindstrom-Best, *Defiant Sisters*, 45.

58 See MUNFLA, no. 78-211, Carol Anne Ruby, 'Childbearing and Childbirth in Early Twentieth Century Newfoundland,' 87–8, 94; no. 75-21, Mary Harriet Doyle, 'Midwifery in the Community of Calvert on the Southern Shore of Newfoundland,' 9–10; no. 76-165, Gary Gale, 'Mrs. Susan Eveleigh Midwife,' 12–13, 14–15; Geggie, *The Extra Mile*, 106

59 MUNFLA, no. 73-160, M. Deanna Emberley, 'Folkmedicine in Newfound-land. Part 1. A Pay de Verde Midwife [Jane Ann Emberley]. Part 2. Folk Cures for Common Complaints,' 4.

60 B.J. Banfill, *With the Indians of the Pacfic* (Toronto: Ryerson Press 1966), 96. See also MUNFLA, no. 76-258, Lillian Joyce White, 'The Work of a Mid-wife in a Trinity Bay Community,' 12–13; McNaughton, 'The Role of the Newfoundland Midwife in Traditional Health Care,' 134–5. Jutta Mason claimed that boiling instruments and preparing sterile cloths was not done much before the 1940s, but this research has revealed that not to be the case. Mason, 'Midwifery in Canada,' 102.

61 Edward Shorter is the historian most noted for his condemnation of midwife intervention. See his *A History of Women's Bodies*, chap. 3, 35–47. Most other studies of midwives view them in a more benevolent way. See, for example, McNaughton, 'The Role of the Newfoundland Midwife in Traditional Health Care.'

62 See McNaughton, 'The Role of the Newfoundland Midwives in Traditional Health Care,' 137.

63 MUNFLA, no. 75-285, Joyce Murphy, 'Olive Bishop: Midwife-Nurse of Pass Island, South Coast of Newfoundland, Hermitage Bay,' 17.

64 See MUNFLA, no. 78-211, Carol Anne Ruby, 'Childbearing and Childbirth in Early Twentieth Century Newfoundland,' 86; no. 75-21, Mary Harriet Doyle, 'Midwifery in the Community of Calvert on the Southern Shore of Newfoundland,' 17; no. 86-254, Gary Drover, 'The Life and Work of Mary Margaret Drover, Midwife, in the Community of Island Cove in the Early 20th Century,' 8.

65 MUNFLA, no. 84-307A, John Burke, 'Mrs. Annie LeMoine: A Profile of the Traditional Midwife in Port-au-Port,' 11; no. 75-285, Joyce Murphy, 'Olive Bishop: Midwife-Nurse of Pass Island, South Coast of Newfoundland, Hermitage Bay,' 2.

66 MUNFLA, no. 77-247, Linda Pauline Warford, 'Reminiscences of a Midwife of Upper Gullis in Conception Bay South,' 6–7.

67 Paulette, 'The Family Centred Maternity Care Project,' 75.

68 See Benoit, *Midwives in Passage*, 54; MUNFLA, no. 76-165, Gary Gale, 'Mrs. Susan Eveleigh Midwife,' 12–13, 14–15; no. 79-433, Joyce Sturge, 'A Look at Midwifery with One of Gambo's Midwives – Mrs. Bertha Feltham – from the Year 1931, Until Just After Confederation,' 13–14.

69 *Chatelaine*, October 1931, 53.

70 MUNFLA, no. 75-285, Joyce Murphy, 'Olive Bishop: Midwife-Nurse of Pass Island, South Coast of Newfoundland, Hermitage Bay,' 2. Midwives in England could not give chloroform either, and only after 1936 could they give gas and air analgesia, provided a physician had certified the patient. Very few midwives were qualified to give the analgesia. Ann Oakley, *The Captured Womb: A History of the Medical Care of Pregnant Women* (Oxford: Basil Blackwell 1984), 110.

71 MUNFLA, no. 86-254, Gary Drover, 'The Life and Work of Mary Margaret Drover, Midwives, in the Community of Island Cove in the Early 20th Century,' 8.

72 MUNFLA, no. 76-258, Lillian Joyce White, 'The Work of a Midwife in a Trinity Bay Community,' 16–17.

73 See MUNFLA, no. 78-211, Carol Anne Ruby, 'Childbearing and Childbirth in Early Twentieth Century Newfoundland,' 91–2; no. 73-44, Sandra Christine Janes, 'Elizabeth "Diddy" Day: Midwife and "Layer Away" of the Dead in Quidi Vidi Village,' n.p.; McNaughton, 'The Role of the Newfoundland Midwife in Traditional Health Care,' 142.

74 *Canadian Practitioner and Review* 31 (January 1906): 8; MUNFLA, no. 78-116, Mary Green, 'Midwifery in Outport Newfoundland,' 9; no. 77-65, Ruth Green, 'The Experiences and Role of Rhoda Maud Piercey as the Midwife in the Community of Winterton, Trinity Bay,' 9.

75 Amy V. Wilson, *No Man Stands Alone* (Sidney, B.C.: Gray's Publishing 1965), 48.

76 Wilfred Abram Bigelow, *Forceps, Fin and Feather* (Manitoba: D.W. Friesen, 1968), 51–2. For more information on Bigelow, see Ian Carr and Robert E. Beamish, *Manitoba Medicine: A Brief History* (Winnipeg: University of Manitoba Press 1999).

77 Samuel S. Peikoff, *Yesterday's Doctor: An Autobiography* (Winnipeg: Prairie Publishing 1980), 30–1.

78 Dianne Dodd, 'Helen MacMurchy, M.D. (1862–1953): Mothers and Doctors in the "Complete" Canadian Mother's Book' (paper presented to the Canadian Historical Association, Kingston, 1991), 6.

79 See MUNFLA, no. 76-258, Lillian Joyce White, 'The Work of a Midwife in a Trinity Bay Community,' 9–10; no. 78-211, Carol Anne Ruby, 'Childbearing and Childbirth in Early Twentieth Century Newfoundland,' 95.

80 See MUNFLA, no. 78-211, Carol Anne Ruby, 'Childbearing and Childbirth in Early Twentieth Century Newfoundland,' 96; no. 75-21, Mary Harriet Doyle, 'Midwifery in the Community of Calvert on the Southern Shore of Newfoundland,' 20.

81 Vilhjalmur Stefansson, *The Anthropological Papers of the American Museum of Natural History* 14, part 1: *The Stefansson-Anderson Arctic Expedition of the American Museum: Preliminary Ethnological Report* (New York 1914), 254. Sydney noted that in the present day the tendency seemed to be to burn it. Julie Cruickshank, *Life Lived Like a Story: Life Stories of Three Yukon Elders* (Vancouver: UBC Press 1992), 128–9; Davis, 'Southern Kwakiutl Medicine,' 17. The midwife in Aboriginal society was seldom referred to as a midwife. On the West Coast of British Columbia the Nuu-chah-nulth referred to the woman who helped in birth as 'she can do everything.' Often such a woman in various Aboriginal traditions had a close relationship akin to godparent with the child she helped deliver. Biggs, 'Fragments from the History of Midwifery,' 16 17 of draft

82 See McNaughton, 'The Role of the Newfoundland Midwife in Traditional Health Care,' 85, 88, 162–3; MUNFLA, no. 73-160, M. Deanna Emberley, 'Folkmedicine of Newfoundland. Part 1. A Bay de Verde Midwife. Part 2. Folk Cures for Common Complaints,' 8, 10; no. 73–44, Sandra Christine Janes, 'Elizabeth "Diddy" Day Midwife and "Layer Away" of the Dead in Quidi Vidi Village,' n.p.

83 See McNaughton, 'Midwifery, Traditional Obstetric Care and Change in Newfoundland,' 13–14; MUNFLA, no. 73-44, Sandra Christine Janes, 'Elizabeth "Diddy" Day: Midwife and "Layer Away" of the Dead in Quidi Vidi Village,' n.p.; Geggie, *The Extra Mile*, 41. For a description of the groaning cake, see MUNFLA, no. 78-211, Carol Anne Ruby, 'Childbearing and Childbirth in Early Twentieth Century Newfoundland,' 106–8.

84 See Benoit, *Midwives in Passage*, 53; Silverman, *The Last Best West*, 71; MUNFLA, no. 86-254, Gary Drover, 'The Life and Work of Mary Margaret Drover, Midwife, in the Community of Island Cover in the Early 20th Century,' 19; no. 73-160, M. Deanna Emberley, 'Folkmedicine of Newfoundland. Part 1. A Bay de Verde Midwife Part 2. Folk Cures for Common Complaints,' 3.

85 Silverman, *The Last Best West*, 68.

86 MUNFLA, no. 78-116, Mary Green, 'Midwifery in Outport Newfoundland,' 18. See also no. 82-326, Barbara Doran, '"There Was No One but

Myself": The Life of a Midwife in Outport Newfoundland,' 11; no. 79-508, R. Douglas Wells, 'Aunt Lizzie Wells (1893–1977): Midwife,' 6; no. 78-119, Larry Harvey, 'Life and Work of Aunt Nora (Lenora) Ellsworth, nee Goodyear, 1877–1951: Her Work as a Healer and Midwife in Carmanville, N.D.B.,' 24; no. 77-139, Madonna Dove, 'Annie Andre: My Grandmother, a Midwife, and a Newfoundlander,' 15–16.

87 Janet McNaughton, ed., *Outport Nurse: Margaret Giovannini* (St John's: Faculty of Medicine, Memorial University 1988), 19.

88 Geggie, *The Extra Mile*, 96, 106. See also MUNFLA no. 79-433, Joyce Sturge, 'A Look at Midwifery with One of Gambo's Midwives – Mrs. Bertha Feltham – from the Year 1931 Until Just After Confederation,' 17; no. 79-508, R. Douglas Wells, 'Aunt Lizzie Wells (1893–1977): Midwife,' 6.

89 See MUNFLA, no. 73-44, Sandra Christine Janes, 'Elizabeth "Diddy" Day: Midwife and "Layer Away" of the Dead in Quidi Vidi Village,' n.p.; no. 75-21, Mary Harriet Doyle, 'Midwifery in the Community of Calvert on the Southern Shore of Newfoundland,' 24; no. 76-165, Gary Gale, 'Mrs. Susan Eveleigh Midwife,' 22–3.

90 MUNFLA, no. 75-21, Mary Harriet Doyle, 'Midwifery in the Community of Calvert on the Southern Shore of Newfoundland,' 23.

91 MUNFLA, no. 77-65, Ruth Green, 'The Experiences and Role of Rhoda Maud Piercey as the Midwife in the Community of Winterton, Trinity Bay,' 24.

92 See MUNFLA, no. 78-211, Carol Anne Ruby, 'Childbearing and Childbirth in Early Twentieth Century Newfoundland,' 110–11; no. 75-21, Mary Harriet Doyle, 'Midwifery in the Community of Calvert on the Southern Shore of Newfoundland,' 34.

93 See MUNFLA, no. 75-21, Mary Harriet Doyle, 'Midwifery in the Community of Calvert on the Southern Shore of Newfoundland,' 34; no. 78-211, Carol Anne Ruby, 'Childbearing and Childbirth in Early Twentieth Century Newfoundland,' 110–11.

94 MUNFLA, no. 78-211, Carol Anne Ruby, 'Childbearing and Childbirth in Early Twentieth Century Newfoundland,' 116.

95 MUNFLA, no. 77-345, Wanda M. King, 'The Role of the Midwife in the Community of N. Summerford Notre Dame Bay,' 2. See also no. 73-44, Sandra Christine Janes, 'Elizabeth "Diddy" Day: Midwife and "Layer Away" of the Dead in Quidi Vidi Village,' n.p.; no. 73-160, M. Deanna Emberley, 'Folk Medicine of Newfoundland. Part 1. A Bay de Verde Midwife. Part 2. Folk Cures for Common Complaints,' 3; no. 77-87, Deborah Lee Ludlow, 'Doctoring by "Aunt Ida" in Harry's Harbour, Green Bay, Newfoundland,' 31; no. 77-237, Wilfrid Thomas Rumbolt, 'Midwifery on the Coast of Labrador,' 5.

96 MUNFLA, no. 78-401, Madonna Hickey, '[Aunt Annie Fizzard:] A 92-Year-Old Midwife from the Community of Grand le Pierre, F.B.,' 8.

97 MUNFLA, no. 77-65, Ruth Green, 'The Experiences and Role of Rhoda Maud Piercey as the Midwife in the Community of Winterton, Trinity Bay,' 27. See also no. 79-508, R. Douglas Wells, 'Aunt Lizzie Wells (1893–1977): Midwife,' 8.

98 Geggie, *The Extra Mile*, 106. The American situation in the first two decades of the century reveals that where midwife programs existed, infant mortality declined. Litoff, *American Midwives*, 96–7.

99 See MUNFLA, no. 73-160, M. Deanna Emberley, 'Folk Medicine of Newfoundland. Part 1. A Bay de Verde Midwife. Part 2. Folk Cures for Common Complaints,' 3; no. 84-307A, John Burke, 'Mrs. Annie LeMoine: A Profile of the Traditional Midwife in Port au Port,' 12; McNaughton, 'The Role of the Newfoundland Midwife in Traditional Health Care,' 60.

100 MUNFLA, no. 76-165, Gary Gale, 'Mrs. Susan Eveleigh,' 17.

101 Linda Rasmussen, *A Harvest Yet To Reap: A History of Prairie Women* (Toronto: The Women's Press 1976), n.p.

102 MUNFLA, no. 75-21, Mary Harriet Doyle, 'Midwifery in the Community of Calvert on the Southern Shore of Newfoundland,' 15.

103 See *Canadian Home Journal*, November 1940, 65; McNaughton, 'Midwifery, Traditional Obstetric Care and Change in Newfoundland,' 25; Dodd, 'Helen MacMurchy, M.D. (1862–1953),' 20.

104 Benoit, *Midwives in Passage*, 57, 96.

105 MUNFLA, no. 75-56, Christopher Albert Smith, 'Aunt Fanny: The Midwife of the Outport Community Southport from 1923–58,' 24–5.

106 McNaughton, 'Midwifery, Traditional Obstetric Care and Change in Newfoundland,' 25–6.

107 Biggs, 'Fragments from the History of Midwifery,' 20 of draft.

108 D.W. Cathell, *The Physician Himself and Things That Concern His Reputation and Success* (Philadelphia: F.A. Davis 1898), 116; *Canada Medical Record* 30 (August 1902): 379; *Canadian Practitioner and Review* 41 (May 1916): 209.

109 Adam H. Wright, *A Textbook of Obstetrics* (New York: D. Appleton 1908), vi, 85.

110 *Canada Medical Record* 30 (December 1902): 559.

111 Victoria General Hospital, Halifax, Patient Records, Mrs Ann Powell, 78/00, box 46; Mrs Mary Mott, 26/05, box 93.

112 McNaughton, 'The Role of the Newfoundland Midwife in Traditional Health Care,' 50–1.

113 Halladay, 'We'll See You Next Year,' 61.

114 Bigelow, *Forceps, Fin and Feather*, 52–3; *Canadian Practitioner and Review* 41 (October 1916): 439; Dodd, 'Advice to Parents,' 218. MacMurchy was

torn between her professional belief in the superiority of science and her recognition of the needs of women in rural Canada and the expertise of ordinary women in birthing. Dodd, 'Helen MacMurchy: Popular Midwifery and Maternity Services for Canadian Pioneer Women,' 135–62.

115 McNaughton, 'The Role of the Newfoundland Midwife in Traditional Health Care,' 49.

116 Mason, 'Midwifery in Canada,' 105–6; Irvine Loudon, *Death in Childbirth: An International Study of Maternal Care and Maternal Mortality* (Oxford: Clarendon Press 1992), 160–1. Loudon was looking back as far as the seventeenth century.

117 Comacchio, *'Nations Are Built of Babies,'* 78. See also Saskatchewan Archives Board, Violet McNaughton Papers, 'Infant Mortality' AIE31, 4–5. In Newfoundland, too, the concern of the doctors of St John's seemed to be the 'grannies.' Linda Cullum and Maeve Baird, '"A Woman's Lot": Women and Law in Newfoundland from Early Settlement to the Twentieth Century,' in Linda Kealey, ed., *Pursuing Equality: Historical Perspectives on Women in Newfoundland and Labrador* (St John's: Institute of Social and Economic Research, Memorial University 1993), 131; *Nova Scotia Medical Bulletin* 4 (May 1925): 5.

118 Comacchio, *'Nations Are Built of Babies,'* 78.

119 *Canadian Medical Association Journal (CMAJ)* 21 (October 1929): 449.

120 *CMAJ* 19 (August 1928): 230.

121 Buckley, 'Ladies or Midwives?' 131–49; Georgina Taylor, 'Ground for Common Action: Violet McNaughton's Agrarian Feminism and the Origins of the Farm Women's Movement in Canada' (PhD thesis, Carleton University, 1997), 428.

122 *CMAJ* 19 (August 1928): 232. See also *Hospital, Medical and Nursing World* 35 (April 1929): 115.

123 *Chatelaine*, October 1930, 28, and October 1931, 53.

124 *Canada Lancet and Practitioner* 77 (December 1931): 160–1.

125 See *CMAJ* 25, supplement (September 1931): xii; *CMAJ* 27, supplement (September 1932): xxv.

126 *CMAJ* 32 (March 1935): 352; Veronica Strong-Boag and Kathryn McPherson, 'The Confinement of Women: Childbirth and Hospitalization in Vancouver, 1919–1939,' in Katherine Arnup, Andrée Lévesque, and Ruth Roach Pierson, eds., *Delivering Motherhood: Maternal Ideologies and Practices in the Nineteenth and Twentieth Centuries* (London and New York: Routledge 1990), 82–3. See also *CMAJ* 29 (August 1933): 163.

127 James Robert Goodall, *Puerperal Infection* (Montreal: 1932), 26. See also

Canada Lancet and Practitioner 80 (April 1933): 111–12; *Nova Scotia Medical Bulletin* 10 (January 1931): 40–1; *Nova Scotia Medical Bulletin* 11 (April 1932): 461.

128 *Canadian Nurse* 34 (September 1938): 474–5.
129 Mason, 'Midwifery in Canada,' 106–7, 115.
130 *CMAJ* 33 (December 1935): 673.
131 *CMAJ* 38 (June 1938): 551.
132 British Columbia Archives, GR707, box 4, file 4, 'Digest of Evidence,' *B.C. Royal Commission State Health Insurance ... 1932*, 315.
133 William Victor Johnston, *Before the Age of Miracles: Memoirs of a Country Doctor* (Toronto: Fitzhenry & Whiteside 1972), 43.
134 MUNFLA, no. 76-165, Gary Gale, 'Mrs. Susan Eveleigh,' 22–3.
135 See McNaughton, 'The Role of the Newfoundland Midwives in Traditional Health Care,' 29, 40, 45; MUNFLA, no. 79–549, Debbie G.J. Hallett, 'Irene (Farwell) Bradley: The Art of Midwifery,' 11–12; no. 76-258, Lillian Joyce White, 'The Work of a Midwife in a Trinity Bay Community,' 5–7; no. 77-139, Madonna Dove, 'Annie Andre: My Grandmother, a Midwife, and a Newfoundlander,' 13–14.
136 See *Canadian Doctor* 8 (April 1941): 17, 19; *Canadian Nurse* 77 (February 1981): 30; Banfill, *With the Indians of the Pacific*, 96.
137 Mason, 'Midwifery in Canada,' 116.
138 *CMAJ* 48 (January 1943): 61.

4: The Expanding World of Prenatal Care

1 Parke, Davis and Co. advertisement, *Nova Scotia Medical Bulletin* 16 (March 1937): 171.
2 Ann Oakley, *The Captured Womb: A History of the Medical Care of Pregnant Women* (Oxford: Basil Blackwell 1984), 2. Katherine Arnup has also argued that medical advice to women takes away from women's traditional network. 'Educating Mothers: Government Advice for Women in the Inter-War Years,' in Katherine Arnup, Andrée Lévesque, and Ruth Roach Pierson, eds., *Delivering Motherhood: Maternal Ideologies and Practices in the Nineteenth and Twentieth Centuries* (London: Routledge 1990), 203. See also Abby Lippman, 'Prenatal Gender Testing and Screening: Constructing Needs and Reinforcing Inequities,' *American Journal of Medicine* 17 1 & 2 (1991): 15–50. True, but few people have asked what kind of agency the individual woman has within that network.
3 See Ellen Starr, 'The Role of the Midwife in rural Newfoundland' (unpublished paper for BA program, Middlebury College, 1981), 18; Barbara

Rothman, *In Labour: Women and Power in the Birth Place* (London: Junction Books 1982), 134

4 Vilhjalmur Stefansson, *Anthropological Papers of the American Museum of Natural History* 14, part 1: *The Stefansson-Anderson Arctic Expedition of the American Museum: Preliminary Ethnological Report* (New York 1914), 182, 329, 354–5. See also Betty Anne Daviss-Putt, 'Right of Passage in the North: From Evacuation to the Birth of a Culture,' in Mary Crnkovich, ed., *'Gossip': A Spoken History of Women in the North* (Ottawa: Canadian Arctic Resources Committee 1990), 93; Igloolik Oral History Project, Science Institute of the Northwest Territories, Government of the Northwest Territories, computer no. IE0005, tape IE005, interview with Rosie Iqalliyuq by Eugene Amarualik, translated by Louis Tapardjuk, 14 February 1990, transcript, 7.

5 Igloolik Oral History Project, computer no. HPU1, tape IE082, interview with Hanna Uyarak by Rhoda Uyarak, translated by Louis Tapardjuk, 15 January 1990, transcript, 3.

6 Lesley Paulette (coordinator) *Report on Phase 1 of the Family Centered Maternity Care Project of the Native Women's Association of the NWT* (Yellowknife: Native Women's Association of the NWT Board of Directors, 6 November 1987), 12. See also Marie Adele Rabesca, Diane Romie, Martha Johnson, and Joan Ryan, *Traditional Dene Medicine*, part 2: *Database* (Lac La Marie, NWT: Traditional Dene Medicine Project 1993), 296; Annie Okalik, 'A Good Life,' in Mary Crnkovich, ed., *'Gossip': A Spoken History of Women in the North*, 6–7; Daviss-Putt, 'Rights of Passage in the North,' 93; Stefansson, *The Stefansson-Anderson Arctic Expedition*, 354–5; Igloolik Oral History Project, computer no. SNA3, tape IE130, interview with Suzanne Aqatsiaq, by Therese Ukaliannuk, translated by Louis Tapardjuk, 7 March 1990, transcript, 16.

7 Igloolik Oral History Project, computer no. RU2, tape IE105, interview with Rachel Uyarasuk by Susan Avingaq, translated by Lucy Tapardjuk, 21 February 1990, transcript, 13.

8 Julie Cruickshank, *Life Lived like a Story: Life Stories of Three Yukon Elders* (Vancouver: University of British Columbia 1992), 246; Franz Boas, 'The Eskimo of Baffin Island and Hudson Bay,' American Museum of Natural History *Bulletin* 15 (1901): 143.

9 See Boas, 'The Eskimo of Baffin Island and Hudson Bay,' 143, 159; Laurie Lacey, *Micmac Indian Medicine: Traditional Way of Health* (Antigonish, N.S.: Formac 1977), 37.

10 Stefansson, *The Stefansson-Anderson Arctic Expedition*, 182, 329.

11 See conversation with JoAnn Lowell, translated by Lizzie Ippiak, 'Marie

Kilunik (Dogs Barking),' in Mary Crnkovich, ed., *'Gossip': A Spoken History of Women in the North* (Ottawa: Canadian Arctic Resources Committee 1990), 117; Daviss-Putt, 'Rights of Passage in the North,' 95; Igloolik Oral History Project, computer no. RU2, tape IE105, interview with Rachel Uyarasuk by Susan Avingaq, translated by Lucy Tapardjuk, 21 February 1990, transcript, 9.

12 See Igloolik Oral History Project, computer no. RU2, tape IE105, interview with Rachel Uyarasuk by Susan Avingaq, translated by Lucy Tapardjuk, 21 February 1990, transcript, 13.

13 See Roald Amundsen, *Roald Amundsen's 'The North West Passage': Being the Record of a Voyage of Exploration of the Ship Gjoa, 1903–1907*, vol. 2 (London: Constable 1908), 60–1; Memorial University of Newfoundland Folklore and Language Archive (MUNFLA), no. 78–211, Carol Anne Ruby, 'Childbearing and Childbirth in Early Twentieth Century Newfoundland,' 49–50.

14 *Grain Growers' Guide*, 21 August 1912, 14; National Council of Women, *Yearbook 1928*, 111. See also J. Clifton Edgar, *The Practice of Obstetrics ... for the Use of Students and Practitioners*, 3rd ed. (Philadelphia: Blakiston 1907), 185; Janet McNaughton, 'Traditional Prenatal Care of Newfoundland Women' (paper presented to the Folklore Studies Association of Canada, McMaster University, 1987), 5, and 'The Role of the Newfoundland Midwife in Traditional Health Care, 1900 to 1970' (PhD thesis, Memorial University, 1989), 111; MUNFLA, no. 75-21, Mary Harriet Doyle, 'Midwifery in the Community of Calvert on the Southern Shore of Newfoundland,' 2–3; *Public Health Journal* 19 (March 1928): 136; *Canadian Public Health Journal* 21 (May 1930): 223; Marion Hilliard, *A Woman Doctor Looks at Love and Life* (Garden City, N.Y.: Doubleday 1957), 26.

15 Mary Rubio and Elizabeth Waterson, eds., *The Selected Journals of Lucy Maud Montgomery*, vol. 2: *1910–1921* (Toronto: Oxford University Press 1987), 91, 97, 99, 148, 171. Other women, too, worried about what would happen to them and their children. Interview with Isme Southern, 24 August 1993.

16 Linda Rasmussen, *A Harvest Yet to Reap: A History of Prairie Women* (Toronto: Women's Press 1976), n.p.

17 See MUNFLA, no. 77-65, Ruth Green, 'The Experiences and Role of Rhoda Maud Piercey as the Midwife in the Community of Winterton, Trinity Bay,' 28–9; *Nova Scotia Medical Bulletin* 14 (March 1935): 170–1.

18 National Council of Women, *Yearbook 1928*, 111.

19 Interview with Becki Crawford, 9 July 1993; Marlene O'Brien, 'A History of Childbirth in Ontario' (student paper, University of Waterloo, 1994), 9;

interview with Wilma Hallman, 11 August 1993; *Public Health Journal* 17 (July 1926): 336.

20 Alice Stockham, *Tokology: A Book of Every Woman* (Toronto: McClelland, Goodchild, and Stewart 1916), 322.

21 MUNFLA, no. 75-21, Mary Harriet Doyle, 'Midwifery in the Community of Calvert on the Southern Shore of Newfoundland,' 7; no. 78-211, Carol Anne Ruby, 'Childbearing and Childbirth in Early Twentieth Century Newfoundland,' 76–7; *Health* 17 (September-October 1949): 18, 33.

22 H.J.G. Geggie, *The Extra Mile: Medicine in Rural Quebec, 1885–1965* (Ottawa: National Library of Canada 1987), 97.

23 Interview with Irma Avery, 15 June 1993. See also *Chatelaine*, October 1929, 53.

24 *Dalhousie Medical Journal* 1 (October 1936): 21; McNaughton, 'Traditional Prenatal Care of Newfoundland Women,' 13; *Canadian Home Journal*, November 1940, 9; MUNFLA, no. 77-139, Madonna Dove, 'Annie Andre: My Grandmother, a Midwife and a Newfoundlander,' 17–18; no. 75-21, Mary Harriet Doyle, 'Midwifery in the Community of Calvert on the Southern Shore of Newfoundland,' 6; no. 72-49, Ruthie Douglas Herder, 'Superstitions of Pregnancy and Infancy,' 7–9; no. 78-211, Carol Anne Ruby, 'Childbearing and Childbirth in Early Twentieth Century Newfoundland,' 61–2. We know most about maternal impressions in Newfoundland largely because medical science did not dominate pregnancy there as much as it did elsewhere in Canada. Where medical science dominated, the laity had more difficulty in publicly expressing such beliefs without being made to feel old-fashioned. Nevertheless, medical texts made clear the popular persistence of belief in maternal impressions; while many Canadians may have maintained a discrete public silence, they privately saw maternal impressions as part of conventional wisdom and common sense. Among the southern Kwakwa Ka'wakw (Kwakiutl) of British Columbia, a pregnant woman would make sure that she did not look on anything deformed or ugly in case her child was affected by this. Marni Elizabeth Davis, 'Southern Kwakiutl Medicine' (MA thesis, University of Victoria, 1977), 25–6. Even in the modern period, the allure of maternal impressions and external influences on the foetus is strong. See Carole H. Carpenter, '"Tales Women Tell": The Function of Birth Experience Narratives,' *Canadian Folklore* 7, 1–2 (1985): 221–34.

25 Stockham, *Tokology*, 92. See also MUNFLA, no. 75–21, Mary Harriet Doyle, 'Midwifery in the Community of Calvert on the Southern Shore of Newfoundland,' 7.

26 *Chatelaine*, March 1934, 51.

27 Ilka D. Dickman, *Appointment to Newfoundland* (Manhattan, Kans: Sun-flower University Press 1981), 27.

28 *Chatelaine*, October 1929, 53.

29 Cynthia R. Comacchio, *'Nations Are Built of Babies': Saving Ontario's Mothers and Children 1900–1940* (Montreal: McGill-Queen's University Press 1993), 211; and Denyse Baillargeon, 'Care of Mothers and Infants between the Wars: The Visiting Nurses of Metropolitan Life, les Gouttes de Lait, and Assistance Maternelle,' trans. Susan Jos, in Dianne Dodd and Deborah Gorham, eds., *Caring and Curing: Historical Perspectives on Women and Healing in Canada* (Ottawa: University of Ottawa Press 1994), 163–82; also 'Introduction,' in Dodd and Gorham, eds., *Caring and Curing*, 8–9.

30 *Canadian Doctor* 1 (November 1935): 10.

31 *Canadian Journal of Medicine and Surgery* 18 (August 1905): 115–17.

32 Ibid., 30 (December 1911): 368.

33 Ibid., 22 (August 1908): 79.

34 Francis H.A. Marshall, *The Physiology of Reproduction*, 2nd ed. (London: Longmans, Green 1922), 624–5, 659; *Canadian Home Journal*, November 1931, 80; *Saturday Night*, 5 June 1943, 18; *University of Toronto Medical Journal* 25 (November 1947). 50.

35 Adam H. Wright, *A Textbook of Obstetrics* (New York: D. Appleton 1908), 17; William Maddock Bayliss, *Principles of General Physiology* (London: Longmans, Green 1915), 291; Edgar, *The Practice of Obstetrics*, 24–5, 29; E.C. Dudley, *The Principles and Practice of Gynecology for Students and Practitioners*, 5th ed. (Philadelphia: Lea & Febiger 1908), 765. For estimates of sperm life, see Barton Cooke Hirst, *A Text-Book of Obstetrics*, 7th ed. (Philadelphia: W.B. Saunders 1912), 85, 89; E.E. Montgomery, *Practical Gynecology*, 4th ed. (Philadelphia: Blakiston 1912), 181; John J. Reese, *Text-Book of Medical Jurisprudence and Toxicology*, 8th ed. (Philadelphia: Blakiston 1912), 251; Ten Teachers, *Midwifery*, 5th ed. (London: Edward Arnold 1935), 57. Certainly other cultures were more generous in crediting women. Vilhjalmur Stefansson told of a belief among the people of Cape Perry where Inuit women gave birth to children without having had connection with a man. Stefansson, *The Stefansson-Anderson Arctic Expedition*, 213–14.

36 Emil Novak, *Textbook of Gynecology*, 2nd ed. (Baltimore: Williams & Wilkins, 1944), 512. In the 1930s a human ovum was viewed for the first time, and in the 1940s one physician paired human ova *in vitro* with sperm. Andrea L. Bonnicksen, *In Vitro Fertilization: Building Policy from Laboratories to Legislatures* (New York: Columbia University Press 1989), 12.

37 Fred L. Adair, ed., *Obstetrics and Gynecology* (Philadelphia: Lea & Febiger 1940), 33; Charles Herbert Best and Norman Burke Taylor, *The Living Body:*

A Text in Human Physiology, 4th ed. (New York: Henry Holt, 1948), 537. See also Henricus J. Stander, *Williams Obstetrics: A Textbook for the Use of Students and Practitioner*, 8th ed. (New York: Appleton-Century 1941), 176.

38 *Alberta Medical Bulletin* 14 (October 1949): 13. For the classic description of egg and sperm, see Emily Martin, 'The Egg and the Sperm: How Science Has Constructed a Romance Based on Stereotypical Male-Female Roles,' *Signs: Journal of Women and Culture and Society* 16 (Spring 1991): 485–501.

39 Richard C. Norris, ed., *An American Text-Book of Obstetrics for Practitioners and Students* (Philadelphia: W.B. Saunders 1895), 176.

40 See Edgar, *The Practice of Obstetrics*, 26–7; Dudley, *The Principles and Practice of Gynecology*, 769; Hirst, *A Text-Book of Obstetrics*, 86, 91.

41 Carl Henry Davis, ed., *Gynecology and Obstetrics*, vol. 3 (Hagerstown, Md: W.F. Prior 1935), chap. 8, 17, and chap. 9, 33. See also J.M. Munro Kerr, J. Haig Ferguson, James Young, and James Hendry, *Combined Textbook of Obstetrics and Gynaecology for Students and Medical Practitioners*, 2nd ed. (Edinburgh: E. & S. Livingstone 1933), 731.

42 *Canadian Practitioner and Review* 41 (June 1916): 236–7. See also Joseph B. DeLee, *The Principles and Practice of Obstetrics* (Philadelphia: W.B. Saunders 1913), 69; Marshall, *The Physiology of Reproduction*, 669.

43 Thomas Clifford Allbutt, W.S. Playfair and Thomas Watts Eden, eds., *A System of Gynaecology*, 2nd ed. (London: Macmillan 1906), 893.

44 *Canadian Nurse* 27 (June 1932): 289; for additional discussion on sex determination, see *Canadian Medical Association Journal* (*CMAJ*) 22 (June 1930): 878; Alfred Henry Tyrer, *Sex, Marriage and Birth Control*, 10th ed. (Toronto: Marriage Welfare Bureau 1943), 237–8; Stander, *Williams Obstetrics*, 176.

45 *The Journal of Preventive Medicine and Sociology* 16 (March 1914): 105–6.

46 *Canadian Practitioner and Review* 31 (December 1906): 670.

47 See National Council of Women, *Yearbook 1921*, 410–11; Comacchio, '*Nations Are Built of Babies*,' 74, 84–5; Veronica Strong-Boag and Kathryn McPherson, 'The Confinement of Women: Childbirth and Hospitalization in Vancouver, 1919–1939,' in Arnup, Lévesque, and Pierson, eds., *Delivering Motherhood*, 75–107; British Columbia Archives, GR707, box 4, file 4, B.C. Royal Commission State Health Insurance 1932, 'Digest of Evidence,' 365; Saskatchewan Archives Board, Violet McNaughton Papers, 'Infant Mortality,' AIE31, 4–5.

48 *Manitoba Medical Bulletin* 81 (May 1928): 11. Cynthia Comacchio has argued that physicians supported an educational campaign to inform women even though they understood that better distribution of health care would meet the needs of the poor because 'state provision for health care threatened their professional and class interest.' '*Nations Are Built of*

Babies,' 13–14. I would agree only in part. It wasn't state involvement per se that physicians objected to but a specific kind of state involvement.

49 *Canadian Child* 7 (August 1926): 2. See also *CMAJ* 14 (June 1924): 495; *Canada Lancet and Practitioner* 68 (January 1927): 26; *Canadian Nurse* 22 (June 1926): 301; *Manitoba Medical Bulletin* 81 (May 1928): 11.

50 *University of Western Ontario Quarterly* 6 (1936): 46. See also National Council of Women, *Yearbook 1930*, 124; P. Brooke Bland, *Practical Obstetrics for Students and Practitioners* (Philadelphia: F.A. Saunders 1932), 126; Ten Teachers, *Midwifery*, 79.

51 Kitchener-Waterloo Hospital, patient no. 97, Mrs. William Dietrich, entered 2 January 1943.

52 Comacchio, *'Nations Are Built of Babies,'* 233.

53 *Montreal Medical Journal* 29 (September 1900): 652; Wright, *A Textbook of Obstetrics*, 38. See also J. Bland-Sutton and Arthur E. Giles, *The Diseases of Women: A Handbook for Students and Practitioners*, 5th ed. (London: Rebman 1906), 226; Hirst, *A Text-Book of Obstetrics*, 142.

54 *Montreal Medical Journal* 29 (September 1900): 652; *Canada Medical Record* 28 (November 1900): 475; Egbert H. Grandin and George W. Jarman, *A Textbook on Practical Obstetrics* (Philadelphia: F.A. Davis 1901), 70. See also *Canadian Practitioner and Review* 36 (October 1911): 614; Hirst, *A Text-Book of Obstetrics*, 144, 158; *Canada Lancet* 48 (October 1914): 76–7; DeLee, *The Principles and Practice of Obstetrics*, 250, 257.

55 Victoria General Hospital Patient Records, Mrs Sally Torrence, box 35, 374/00, admitted 21 May 1900, discharged 24 May 1900.

56 See *Montreal Medical Journal* 29 (September 1900): 652; *Canadian Journal of Medicine and Surgery* 8 (October 1900): 239; *Canada Medical Record* 28 (November 1900): 475.

57 Bland-Sutton and Giles, *The Diseases of Women*, 227. See also Grandin and Jarman, *A Textbook on Practical Obstetrics*, 65, 70.

58 David Berry Hart, *Guide to Midwifery* (London: Rebman 1912), 125. See also Barton Cooke Hirst, *A Text-Book of Obstetrics*, 144.

59 Interview with Wilma Hallman, 11 August 1993.

60 J.S. Fairbairn, *Gynaecology with Obstetrics: A Text-Book for Students and Practitioners* (London: Humphrey Milford, Oxford University Press 1924), 93. See also *CMAJ* 17 (December 1927): 1469.

61 Victoria General Hospital, patient no. 412, register no. 143, patient Mrs Lillian Cowper Curry, admitted 12 October 1930, discharged 3 November 1930. See also Aleck William Bourne, *Synopsis of Midwifery and Gynaecology*, 3rd ed. (Toronto: Macmillan 1925), 17; Bland, *Practical Obstetrics*, 128; Stander, *Williams Obstetrics*, 254.

62 *CMAJ* 22 (February 1930): 253.

63 *University of Toronto Medical Journal* 8 (March 1931): 183; *CMAJ* 24 (April 1931): 491.

64 *McGill Medical Undergraduate Journal* 2 (April 1933): 210–13. See also *Nova Scotia Medical Bulletin* 12 (May 1933): 300–2; *CMAJ* 28 (June 1933): 599; *CMAJ* 34 (April 1936): 431; Julie Vandervoort, *Tell the Driver: A Biography of Elinor F.E. Black* (Winnipeg: University of Manitoba Press 1992), 153.

65 *Nova Scotia Medical Bulletin* 28 (October 1949): 238.

66 *Canadian Journal of Medical Technology* 11 (June 1949): 72.

67 See Grandin and Jarman, *A Textbook on Practical Obstetrics*, 81; Hirst, *A Text-Book of Obstetrics*, 158; DeLee, *The Principles and Practice of Obstetrics*, 231; Charles Jewett, ed., *The Practice of Obstetrics*, 2nd ed. (New York: Lea Brothers 1901), 122–3; Edgar, *The Practice of Obstetrics*, 185; *Montreal Medical Journal* 31 (October 1902): 771; Henry Jellett, *A Manual of Midwifery for Students and Practitioners*, 2nd ed. (London: Bailliere, Tindall and Cox 1910), 253.

68 'Saving the Babies,' *Health Bulletin*, 1919.

69 David James Evans, *Obstetrics: A Manual for Students and Practitioners* (Philadelphia: Lea Brothers 1900), 43. See also Thomas Watts Eden, *A Manual of Midwifery* (Toronto: Macmillan, 1915), 77; J. Clarence Webster, *A Text-Book of Diseases of Women* (Philadelphia: W.B. Saunders 1907), 111; Stefansson, *The Stefansson-Anderson Arctic Expedition*, 208; *Canadian Practitioner and Review* 27 (April 1902): 214; Hart, *Guide to Midwifery*, 52, 141, 143.

70 See Norris, ed., *An American Text-Book of Obstetrics*, 221; Eden, *A Manual of Midwifery*, 77; Evans, *Obstetrics*, 43, 186; Jewett, ed., *The Practice of Obstetrics*, 125; DeLee, *The Principles and Practice of Obstetrics*, 111; Thomas Watts Eden and Cuthbert Lockyer, eds., *The New System of Gynaecology*, vol. 1 (Toronto: Macmillan 1917), 742; Edgar, *The Practice of Obstetrics*, 188; J. Clarence Webster, *A Textbook of Obstetrics* (Philadelphia: W.B. Saunders 1903), 142.

71 *Canadian Journal of Medicine and Surgery* 38 (October 1915): 110.

72 See Davis, ed., *Gynecology and Obstetrics*, vol. 1, chap. 9, 39; *Canadian Public Health Journal* 25 (July 1934): 349–50; Ten Teachers, *Midwifery*, 54–5; *Manitoba Medical Review* 18 (August 1938): 148; Stander, *Williams Obstetrics*, 205; *CMAJ* 55 (September 1946): 294; *Chatelaine*, October 1950, 76.

73 *University of Toronto Medical Journal* 25 (November 1947): 52. See also *Canadian Journal of Public Health* 39 (September 1948): 352.

74 British Columbia Archives, GR707, box 4, file 4, B.C. Royal Commission on State Health Insurance and Maternity Benefits, 1932, 'Digest of Evidence,' 166, 292.

75 *CMAJ* 13 (July 1923): 493; *Nova Scotia Medical Bulletin* 9 (1930): 239; McGill University Archives, Montreal General Hospital, patient no. 1049, Mrs George Cunningham, admitted 13 February 1946, discharged 23 February 1946. See also Andrée Lévesque, 'Mères ou malades: Les québécoises de l'entre-deux-guerres vues par les medecins,' *Revue d'histoire de l'Amérique Française* 38 (1984), 28; *Canada Lancet and Practitioner* 68 (January 1927): 26; *Canadian Nurse* 22 (June 1926): 301; *Public Health Journal* 17 (July 1926): 336.

76 *CMAJ* 14 (October 1924): 908. See also *Canadian Public Health Journal* 28 (December 1937): 592–3; *Canadian Nurse* 34 (September 1938): 474.

77 *Canadian Practitioner and Review* 34 (January, 1909): 46. See also Wright, *A Textbook of Obstetrics*, 55; Evans, *Obstetrics*, 56; *Canadian Practitioner and Review* 31 (March 1906): 144; *Canadian Journal of Medicine and Surgery* 38 (September 1915): 84.

78 Jellett, *A Manual of Midwifery for Students and Practitioners*, 167.

79 See Jewett, ed., *The Practice of Obstetrics*, 211; Webster, *A Textbook of Obstetrics*, 142; Edgar, *The Practice of Obstetrics*, 188; *Canadian Journal of Medicine and Surgery* 24 (August 1908): 65; *CMAJ* 13 (April 1923): 253.

80 See *CMAJ* 1 (October 1911): 1072; DeLee, *The Principles and Practice of Obstetrics*, 231; *Canadian Journal of Medicine and Surgery* 38 (September 1915): 84; *Canadian Journal of Medicine and Surgery* 30 (December 1911): 333.

81 Baillargeon, 'Care of Mothers and Infants in Montreal between the Wars,' 165.

82 *CMAJ* 13 (April 1923): 253. See Public Archives of Nova Scotia, RT98, V645, *VON Report, 1913*, 21; W.G. Cosbie, *The Toronto General Hospital, 1819–1965: A Chronicle* (Toronto: Macmillan 1975), 150.

83 *CMAJ* 1 (February 1911): 131.

84 *CMAJ* 14 (June 1924): 496.

85 For advice, see McGill University, Rare Books, Montreal Diet Dispensary Collection, Metropolitan Life Insurance Co., 'The Baby' (Ottawa, n.d.), 1; *CMAJ* 14 (May 1924) 372, and (June 1924): 497; *CMAJ* (October 1924): 908; *Canada Lancet and Practitioner* 64 (March 1925): 101; J.G. Fitzgerald, *An Introduction to the Practice of Preventive Medicine*, 2nd ed. (St Louis: C.V. Mosby 1926), 522; *Canadian Journal of Medicine and Surgery* 75 (February 1934): 42–3; T.R. Nichols, *Instructions for Expectant Mothers and the Care of Infants* (Stratford 1932), 5–6; *Child and Family Welfare* 10 (1934): 11; Davis, *Gynecology and Obstetrics*, vol. 1, chap. 5, 29; *Child and Family Welfare* 11 (January 1936): 23; Stander, *Williams Obstetrics*, 282; *University of Western Ontario Quarterly* 6 (1936): 47; *Nova Scotia Medical Bulletin* 15 (July 1936): 444; Frederick C. Irving, *A Textbook of Obstetrics: For Students and Practition-*

ers (New York: Macmillan, 1936), 83; *CMAJ* 37, supplement (1937): 64; McGill University Archives, Montreal General Hospital, RG96 vol. 0421, file 00635, 'Notes on Nursing Obstetrics,' n.p.; *CMAJ* 49, supplement (September 1943): 19; *CMAJ* 52 (June 1945): 564; Paul T. Harper, *Clinical Obstetrics* (Philadelphia: F.A. Davis 1930), 462; *Health* 16 (November–December 1948): 9. Variations on all these recommendations occurred. In England the ideal prenatal care recommended in 1929 was a first visit at four months and then another at six months, seven months, and thereafter every two weeks until the thirty-sixth week, when weekly visits should occur. Oakley, *The Captured Womb*, 79–80.

86 F.L. Adair, ed., *Maternal Care and Some Complications* (Chicago: University of Chicago Press 1939), 9. See also *CMAJ* 48 (April 1943): 314.

87 Interview with Dorothy Atkinson, 15 June 1993; also interviews with Faith Matthews, 21 October 1994, and Ruth Howard, 25 August 1993.

88 See *CMAJ* 14 (June 1924): 496; McGill University Archives, Montreal General Hospital, RG96 0421, file 00635, 'Notes on Obstetric Nursing,' n.p.; Stander, *Williams Obstetrics*, 291; *CMAJ* 49, supplement (September 1943): 19; Alfred C. Beck, *Obstetrical Practice*, 4th ed. (Baltimore: Williams & Wilkins 1947), 161; *Health* 16 (November–December 1948): 9. Percy E. Ryberg, *Health, Sex and Birth Control* (Toronto: Anchor Press 1942), 174. A Winnipeg physician in 1937 even suggested that women should come to their physicians before pregnancy to ensure that they were 'fit to conceive,' and his was not the only voice advocating this. *CMAJ* 36 (April 1937): 378.

89 Oakley, *The Captured Womb*, 72.

90 Baillargeon, 'Care of Mothers and Infants in Montreal between the Wars,' 165; Penelope Stewart, 'Infant Feeding in Canada: 1910–1940' (MA thesis, Concordia University, 1982), 86–7.

91 Public Archives of Nova Scotia, RT98, V645, *VON Report 1929*, 46. See also *American Journal of Public Health* 29 (1939): 250; Florence H.M. Emory, *Public Health Nursing in Canada* (Toronto: Macmillan 1953), 289.

92 *The CMAJ* 37 (1937): 547.

93 *Canadian Nurse* 46 (December 1950): 953, 962.

94 Public Archives of Nova Scotia, RT98, V645, *VON Report, 1922*, 67, 69. See also *VON Report, 1923*, 67; *Public Health Journal* 17 (July 1926): 335.

95 Janice Raymond, 'Medicine as a Patriarchal Religion,' *Journal of Medicine and Philosophy* 7 (1982): 200.

96 Canada, Department of Health, *The Canadian Mother's Book* (Ottawa: King's Printer 1921). See also Katherine Arnup, 'Educating Mothers: Government Advice for Women in the Inter-war Years,' in Arnup,

Lévesque, and Pierson, eds., *Delivering Motherhood*, 195; *Dalhousie Medical Journal* 2 (April 1937): 40; *Manitoba Medical Review* 17 (July 1937): 130; *Chatelaine*, July 1928, 6; *CMAJ* 31 (November 1934): 517; *CMAJ* 36 (April 1937): 378.

97 *Canada Lancet and Practitioner* 68 (January 1927): 29; *CMAJ* 31 (November 1934): 517. See also *Canadian Nurse* 23 (October 1927): 537; Fitzgerald, *An Introduction to the Practice of Preventive Medicine*, 522.

98 See Stewart, 'Infant Feeding in Canada,' 128; *Canadian Nurse* 20 (June 1924): 340; *Public Health Journal* 18 (June 1927): 253.

99 Interview with Betty McKenzie, 19 July 1993; also interviews with Geraldine Mitchell, 8 June 1993; Janice Youmans, 3 June 1993; and Joan Carr, 22 July 1993. Joan remembered reading a book but could not remember which one. E.M. Robertson of Queen's University recommended the following advice books: *Expectant Motherhood* by N.J. Eastman; *Getting Ready to Be a Mother (Father)* by Hazel Corbin; *Mother and Baby Care in Pictures* by Louise Zabriskie; *Canadian Mother and Child* by the Department of Health, Canada; and *Childbirth without Fear* by Grantly Dick Read. *Alberta Medical Bulletin* 12 (July 1947): 17.

100 *Modern Medicine of Canada* 1 (November 1946): 38–9; *Canadian Journal of Public Health* 39 (September 1948): 353. See also *Canadian Nurse* 43 (May 1947): 345; *Health* 16 (Nov.–Dec. 1948): 9.

101 This was certainly true of Dr Ernest Couture in *The Canadian Mother and Child* (Ottawa, 1949). Beth Light and Ruth Roach Pierson, eds., *No Easy Road: Women in Canada 1920s to 1960s* (Toronto: New Hogtown Press 1990), 194.

102 Janet Elizabeth McNaughton, 'The Role of the Newfoundland Midwife in Traditional Health Care, 1900 to 1970' (PhD thesis, Memorial University, 1989), 108.

103 *Canada Lancet and Practitioner* 78 (April 1932):110; *American Journal of Public Health* 29 (1939): 251; *CMAJ* 17 (December 1927): 1468. See also *Chatelaine*, July 1928, 6; Denyse Baillargeon, 'L'encadrement de la maternité au Québec entre les deux guerres: Les gardes de La Metropolitaine, les gouttes de lait et l'assistance maternelle,' *Bulletin RCHTQ* 47 & 48 (1990): 33; *CMAJ* 31 (August 1934): 175. For Manitoba rates, see *CMAJ* 45 (August 1941): 138–9; for concern about unmarried women, see *Canada Lancet and Practitioner* 78 (April 1932): 110; McGill University Archives, *Annual Report of the Royal Victoria Hospital*, 1940, 45. In England the percentage of women having prenatal care was 33.89 per cent in 1931 and 38.89 in 1932. Oakley, *The Captured Womb*, 80.

104 Jo Oppenheimer, 'Childbirth in Ontario: The Transition from Home to Hospital in the Early Twentieth Century,' in Arnup, Lévesque, and Pierson, eds., *Delivering Motherhood*, 67. See also *Canadian Journal of Public Health* 35 (May 1944): 180; Dominion Bureau of Statistics, Department of National Health and Welfare, *A Study in Maternal, Infant and Neo-Natal Mortality in Canada* (Ottawa 1945), 16. In H.J.G. Geggie's rural Quebec practice, 50 per cent of his patients received some prenatal care in the 1930s and 1940s. In Dr Walmsley's practice in Prince Edward County, Ontario, the figure was between 56 and 93 per cent between 1941 and 1943. Jayne Elliott, '"Endormez-moi!": An Early Twentieth-Century Obstetrical Practice in the Gatineau Valley, Quebec' (MA thesis, Carleton University, 1997), 139, 143.

105 Light and Pierson, eds., *No Easy Road*, 193.

106 Emory, *Public Health Nursing in Canada*, 286.

107 William Victor Johnston, *Before the Age of Miracles: Memoirs of a Country Doctor* (Toronto: Fitzhenry & Whiteside 1972), 40–1; *Canadian Welfare* 16 (January 1941): 13; *Public Health Journal* 19 (March 1928): 136; Kitchener-Waterloo Hospital, patient no. 97, Mrs Frank Dinnie, admitted 2 January 1943.

108 *Canadian Home Journal*, November 1940, 65.

109 Interview with Geraldine Mitchell, 9 June 1993; Meryn Elisabeth Stuart, '"Let Not the People Perish for Lack of Knowledge": Public Health Nursing and the Ontario Rural Child Welfare Project, 1916–1930' (PhD thesis, University of Pennsylvania, 1987), 196.

110 Comacchio, 'Nations Are Built of Babies,' 242.

111 For advice on activities, see Norris, ed., *An American Text-Book of Obstetrics*, 180; DeLee, *The Principles and Practice of Obstetrics*, 227; Evans, *Obstetrics: A Manual for Students and Practitioners*, 55; Jewett, ed., *The Practice of Obstetrics*, 153; Jellett, *A Manual of Midwifery*, 255; Hart, *Guide to Midwifery*, 143.

112 Jewett, ed., *The Practice of Obstetrics*, 153. See also Evans, *Obstetrics*, 55; Wright, *A Textbook of Obstetrics*, 61.

113 Jellett, *A Manual of Midwifery*, 253; Stockham, *Tokology*, 91–2.

114 *The Canada Lancet* 44 (October 1910): 127; Jellett, *A Manual of Midwifery*, 256.

115 See Evans, *Obstetrics*, 55; Jewett, ed., *The Practice of Obstetrics*, 153; Edgar, *The Practice of Obstetrics*, 185; *Montreal Medical Journal* 37 (January 1908): 24; Wright, *A Textbook of Obstetrics*, 61; Hart, *Guide to Midwifery*, 143; DeLee, *The Principles and Practice of Obstetrics*, 227.

116 *Canadian Journal of Medicine and Surgery* 38 (October 1915): 111; and

Provincial Board of Health, Ontario, *A Little Talk about the Baby* (Toronto: King's Printer 1913), 3.

117 See Grandin and Jarman, *A Textbook on Practical Obstetrics*, 77; *Montreal Medical Journal* 37 (January 1908): 24; DeLee, *The Principles and Practice of Obstetrics*, 228; *Montreal Medical Journal* 32 (February 1903): 101–2. Bathing has a diuretic effect which may make the kidneys feel relieved.

118 *Canadian Nurse* 14 (March 1918): 905.

119 Grandin and Jarman, *A Textbook on Practical Obstetrics*, 77; see *Canada Lancet and Practitioner* 78 (April 1932): 110; Harper, *Clinical Obstetrics*, 459; *CMAJ* 37 (December 1937): 551; Davis, ed., *Gynecology and Obstetrics*, vol. 1, chap. 5, 26; Adair, ed., *Maternal Care and Some Complications*, 22; Stander, *Williams Obstetrics*, 292.

120 See Fairbairn, *Gynaecology with Obstetrics*, 107; *Chatelaine*, October 1928, 56; Irving, *A Textbook of Obstetrics*, 87; *Saturday Night*, 1 October 1942, 22. The prohibition against putting hands above the head has a long history but is usually cited as an 'old wives' tale.'

121 Elliott, 'Endormez-moi!' 139.

122 *Chatelaine*, October 1931, 53; Irving, *A Textbook of Obstetrics*, 87; Hilliard, *A Woman Doctor Looks at Love and Life*, 26, 52; Marion Hilliard, *Women and Fatigue: A Woman's Doctor's Answer* (Garden City, N.Y.: Doubleday 1960), 48.

123 *Canada Lancet and Practitioner* 78 (April 1932): 110. See also *Chatelaine*, October 1928, 56.

124 Nichols, *Instructions for Expectant Mothers and the Care of Infants*, 9. See also Davis, ed., *Gynecology and Obstetrics*, vol. 1, chap. 5, 26; Ten Teachers, *Midwifery*, 78.

125 Light and Pierson, eds., *No Easy Road*, 195.

126 See Bland, *Practical Obstetrics for Students and Practitioners*, 134; *University of Western Ontario Quarterly* 6 (1936): 47; *Nova Scotia Medical Bulletin* 15 (July 1936): 447; Beck, *Obstetric Practice*, 182.

127 *CMAJ* 37 (December 1937): 550; *Halifax Herald*, 1 September 1936. See also Adair, ed., *Maternal Care and Some Complications*, 21; Beck, *Obstetric Practice* 182; *Nova Scotia Medical Bulletin* 15 (July 1936): 447; Dalhousie University Archives, Oxorn Papers, H.B. Atlee, 'The Problem of Being a Woman,' 90.

128 *Canadian Nurse* 29 (February 1933): 81. See also Stander, *Williams Obstetrics*, 278; *Health* 16 (Nov.–Dec. 1948): 26.

129 William Thompson Lusk, *The Science and Art of Midwifery* (New York: D. Appleton 1889), 121; Wright, *A Textbook of Obstetrics*, 61; Evans, *Obstetrics*, 55; Jewett, ed., *The Practice of Obstetrics*, 154; Edgar, *The Practice of Obstetrics*, 188.

130 Norris, ed., *An American Text-Book of Obstetrics*, 181; Jellett, *A Manual of Midwifery for Students and Practitioners*, 255; Jewett, ed., *The Practice of Obstetrics*, 154. See also *Canada Lancet* 44 (October 1910): 127; Edgar, *The Practice of Obstetrics*, 188. DeLee, *The Principles and Practice of Obstetrics*, 227–8; Stockham, *Tokology*, 159.

131 DeLee, *The Principles and Practice of Obstetrics*, 825.

132 Bland, *Practical Obstetrics for Students and Practitioners*, 136;. Kerr et al., *Combined Textbook of Obstetrics and Gynaecology*, 161; R. W. Johnstone, *A Text-Book of Midwifery: For Students and Practitioners*, 6th ed. (London: A. & C. Black 1934), 93; Davis, ed., *Gynecology and Obstetrics*, vol. 1, chap. 5, 28;. Stander, *Williams Obstetrics*, 282, 295; Adair, ed., *Maternal Care and Some Complications*, 25; Ryberg, *Health, Sex and Birth Control*, 178.

133 Dalhousie University Archives, Oxorn Papers, H.B. Atlee, 'The Problem of Being a Woman,' 100.

134 *Canadian Child* 4 (September–October 1923): 2; *Canadian Child* 7 (August 1926): 3; *Chatelaine*, March 1933, 59; Adair, ed., *Maternal Care and Some Complications*, 27; *Canada Lancet and Practitioner* 64 (March 1925): 101–2; Ryberg, *Health, Sex and Birth Control*, 177; Beck, *Obstetric Practice*, 181.

135 *Nova Scotia Medical Bulletin* 4 (May 1925): 4; 'Traces,' GRP25, 'First Baby' interview, 21 August 1991.

136 *Canadian Practitioner and Review* 27 (April 1902): 214.

137 *Montreal Medical Journal* 37 (January 1908): 24; Edgar, *The Practice of Obstetrics*, 186; Jellett, *A Manual of Midwifery for Students and Practitioners*, 254.

138 *Canada Lancet and National Hygiene* 63 (July 1924): 2. See also *Canada Lancet and Practitioner* 64 (March 1925): 102; Stander, *Williams Obstetrics*, 292–3; Beck, *Obstetrical Practice*, 178; 'Traces,' GRP25, 'First Baby' interview, 21 August 1991; *Nova Scotia Medical Bulletin* 3 (1924): 10; *CMAJ* 14 (June 1924): 496; *CMAJ* 17 (December 1927): 1436. Harper, *Clinical Obstetrics*, 459; *CMAJ* 38 (June 1938): 550; *Chatelaine*, March 1945, 12.

139 Interviews with Dorothy Atkinson, 15 June 1993, and Irma Avery, 15 June 1993.

140 *CMAJ* 37 (December 1937): 547; Adair, ed., *Maternal Care and Some Complications*, 18; *CMAJ* 46 (January 1942): 4; *CMAJ* 30 (January 1934): 15; Ten Teachers, *Midwifery*, 78; *CMAJ* 37 (December 1937): 547; *CMAJ* 59 (November 1948): 431.

141 *Canadian Public Health Journal* 30 (January 1939): 6. Certain food supplements were being advertised during this period and studies were being done that revealed the importance of vitamin supplements. *Chatelaine*, October 1929, 53; *CMAJ* 26 (June 1932): 740.

142 *CMAJ* 42 (April 1940): 362; interview with Joan Carr, 22 July 1993; *CMAJ* 44 (May 1941): 541: *CMAJ* 49 (November 1943): 378; *McGill Medical Journal* 14 (April 1945): 192.

143 McGill University Archives, Rare Books, Montreal Diet Dispensary Collection, *National Health Review*, January 1940, reprint.

144 *Chatelaine*, March 1945; 13; *CMAJ* 53 (November 1945): 435; *Canadian Home Journal*, December 1945, 68; Archibald Donald Campbell and Mabel A. Shannon, *Gynaecology for Nurses* (Philadelphia: F.A. Davis 1946), 243; *Health* 18 (Jan.–Feb. 1950): 12.

145 Marlene O'Brien, 'A History of Childbirth in Ontario' (student paper, University of Waterloo, 1994), 10.

146 Comacchio, *'Nations Are Built of Babies,'* 86.

147 Heather MacDougall, *Activists and Advocates: Toronto's Health Department 1883–1983* (Toronto: Dundurn Press 1990), 205.

148 Fairbairn, *Gynaecology with Obstetrics*, 108; Harper, *Clinical Obstetrics*, 459; Bland, *Practical Obstetrics*, 88, 135; Ten Teachers, *Midwifery*, 78; Stander, *Williams Obstetrics*, 813.

149 Nichols, *Instructions for Expectant Mothers and the Care of Infants*, 9–10. See also Ten Teachers, *Midwifery*, 78; *CMAJ* 37 (December 1937): 551.

150 Ryberg, *Health, Sex and Birth Control*, 176; *Maclean's*, 1 October 1945, 58; interviews with Jane Rutherford, 28 July 1993, and Betsy Lawrence, 30 August 1993.

151 *Nova Scotia Medical Bulletin* 14 (March 1935): 171. See also Adair, ed., *Obstetrics and Gynecology volume 1*, 169.

152 *Canadian Home Journal*, December 1945, 42. See also *Nova Scotia Medical Bulletin* 3 (January 1924): 10; *CMAJ* 14 (June 1924): 496; *CMAJ* 17 (December 1927): 1436; Harper, *Clinical Obstetrics*, 459; *CMAJ* 38 (June 1938): 550; *Chatelaine*, March 1945, 12.

153 *CMAJ* 53 (November 1945): 434.

154 Jewett, ed., *The Practice of Obstetrics*, 155. Some late-nineteenth-century texts that continued to be used well into the twentieth century reflect acceptance of maternal impressions. Norris, ed., *An American Text-Book of Obstetrics for Practitioners and Students*, 213.

155 Edgar, *The Practice of Obstetrics*, 188; *Canada Lancet* 44 (October 1910): 126, 128. See also Winfield Scott Hall, *Sexual Knowledge* (Philadelphia: International Bible House 1913), 215; DeLee, *The Principles and Practice of Obstetrics*, 229; *Canadian Journal of Medicine and Surgery* 35 (April 1914): 212.

156 Amanda Leathem, 'The Orillia Asylum for Idiots: Custodial Care for the Mentally Handicapped of Ontario, 1876–1910' (student paper, University of Waterloo, 1987), 24; Department of Labour, *Report of the Royal Commis-*

sion on a Dispute Respecting Hours of Employment between the Bell Telephone Company of Canada, Ltd. and Operators at Toronto, Ont. (Ottawa: Government Printing Bureau 1907), 72; *Public Health Journal* 3 (June 1912): 308; *CMAJ* 28 (April 1933): 395; *Dalhousie Medical Journal* 1 (April 1936): 25.

157 Grandin and Jarman, *A Textbook on Practical Obstetrics*, 79. See also *Canada Lancet* 38 (March 1905): 657.

158 Hall, *Sexual Knowledge*, 215, 230. See also *Canada Lancet* 44 (October 1910): 126. Hall, of course, was only looking at one type of 'cause.' Aristotle discerned four kinds of causation: the material cause, the efficient cause, the formal cause, and the final cause. The usual example to explain the nature of the causes is building a house. The bricks, stones, wood, etc., are the material cause; the builder is the efficient cause; the blueprints are the formal cause, and the purpose of the house is the final cause. See Stephen Jay Gould, *Hen's Teeth and Horses's Toes: Further Reflections in Natural History* (New York: W.W. Norton 1983), 79–80.

159 DeLee, *The Principles and Practice of Obstetrics*, 228–9.

160 *Canada Lancet* 38 (March 1905): 658. See also *Canada Lancet* 44 (October 1910): 126.

161 *Chatelaine*, November 1928, 19; *Canada Lancet and Practitioner* 64 (March 1925): 102. See also *Chatelaine*, March 1934, 51; Davis, ed., *Gynecology and Obstetrics*, vol. 1, chap. 5, 28.

162 *Canadian Nurse* 27 (June 1932): 286–7.

163 *CMAJ* 34 (April 1936): 469.

164 *Canadian Nurse* 29 (February 1933): 81.

165 *Canadian Journal of Public Health* 39 (September 1948): 352.

166 Eden, *A Manual of Midwifery*, 221; Adair, ed., *Obstetrics and Gynecology*, 1:648–9; Hilliard, *Women and Fatigue*, 49; *Canadian Journal of Public Health* 35 (May 1941): 175; *University of Toronto Medical Journal* 26 (February 1949): 200.

167 Margaret Blackman, *During My Time: Florence Edenshaw Davidson, a Haida Woman* (Vancouver: Douglas and McIntyre 1982), 105.

168 Lusk, *The Science and Art of Midwifery*, 121; Norris, ed., *An American Text-Book of Obstetrics*, 181; Berry, *Obstetrics*, 55; Jewett, ed., *The Practice of Obstetrics*, 154; Edgar, *The Practice of Obstetrics*, 188; Jellett, *A Manual of Midwifery for Students and Practitioners*, 155; Davis, ed., *Gynecology and Obstetrics*, vol. 1, chap. 5, 28; Irving, *A Textbook of Obstetrics*, 83; Adair, ed., *Maternal Care and Some Complications*, 25; *CMAJ* 46 (January 1942): 5; *Chatelaine*, March 1945, 13; Campbell and Shannon, *Gynaecology for Nurses*, 243.

169 *Montreal Medical Journal* 32 (February 1903): 101–2. See also Stander,

Williams Obstetrics, 813. This text also mentioned the influence of industrial poisons on the sperm of the father leading to problems with foetal development. See also *Saturday Night*, 31 October 1942, 22; *Canadian Journal of Public Health* 39 (September 1948): 352; *Alberta Medical Bulletin* 14 (April 1949): 28. The same pattern existed with respect to stillbirths. *CMAJ* 11 (September 1921): 616.

170 *American Journal of Obstetrics and Gynecology* (1922): 40–1.

171 Hart, *Guide to Midwifery*, 341, 343.

172 *Public Health Journal* 15 (October 1924): 453. See also *Canadian Journal of Medicine and Surgery* 75 (February 1934): 42–3; *Nova Scotia Medical Bulletin* 15 (July 1936): 444; *Chatelaine*, February 1944, 32; *CMAJ* 53, supplement (September 1945): 21; Russell L. Cecil and Robert F. Loeb, eds., *A Textbook of Medicine*, 9th ed. (Philadelphia: W.B. Saunders, 1959), 331; *CMAJ* 23 (July 1930): 51.

173 *CMAJ* 38 (May 1938): 448.

174 *CMAJ* 14 (October 1924): 908.

175 Bland, *Practical Obstetrics for Students and Practitioners*, 133.

176 *University of Toronto Medical Journal* 10 (February 1933): 117; Harriet Simand, '1938–1988: Fifty Years of DES – Fifty Years Too Many,' in Christine Overall, ed., *The Future of Human Reproduction* (Toronto: The Women's Press 1989), 95–6; *CMAJ* 41 (July 1939): 99; *Alberta Medical Bulletin* 13 (January 1948): 58, 67; *University of Toronto Medical Journal* 26 (February 1949): 204; *Alberta Medical Bulletin* 14 (April 1949): 27.

177 Edgar, *The Practice of Obstetrics*, 186.

178 *University of Toronto Medical Journal* 8 (March 1931): 155, 162; Bland, *Practical Obstetrics for Students and Practitioners*, 88.

179 Harry Oxorn, *Harold Benge Atlee M.D.: A Biography* (Hantsport, N.S.: Lancelot Press 1983), 115; and *CMAJ* 15 (1925): 388–9.

180 *University of Toronto Medical Journal* 3 (November 1925): 6. See also *Nova Scotia Medical Bulletin* 9 (1930): 240; *CMAJ* 28 (May 1933): 513.

181 *CMAJ* 28 (May 1933): 513–14.

182 *CMAJ* 21 (December 1929): 658–9.

183 *University of Western Ontario Quarterly* 13 (March 1943): 23–4. See also *University of Toronto Medical Journal* 8 (March 1931): 156, 160; *CMAJ* 28 (January 1933): 48; Ten Teachers, *Midwifery*, 54–5; *Canadian Nurse* 31 (November 1935): 487; Charles Herbert Best and Norman Burke Taylor, *The Physiological Basis of Medical Practice: A University of Toronto Text in Applied Physiology* (Baltimore: W. Wood 1937), 786–7.

184 *Journal of Obstetrics and Gynaecology of the British Empire* 41 (1934): 753. See

also *New England Journal of Medicine*, 8 February 1973, 289; Iris Marion Young, *Throwing Like a Girl and Other Essays in Feminist Philosophy and Social Theory* (Bloomington: Indiana University Press 1990), 169.

185 *Manitoba Medical Review* 30 (January 1950): 40. Barbara Clow argues that in the 1950s doctors saw vomiting of pregnancy as psychosomatic. Because they didn't have the time to deal with this, they treated women with drugs to calm them. This set the stage for the administration of thalidomide (Presentation by Barbara Clow, Women, Science, and Health Conference, York University, 5 March 1999). In the 1970s, the psychogenic interpretation still held sway. See K. Jean Lennane and R. John Lennane, 'Alleged Psychogenic Disorder in Women: A Possible Manifestation of Sexual Prejudice,' *New England Journal of Medicine*, 8 February 1973, 289.

186 *Canadian Journal of Medicine and Surgery* 38 (September 1915): 85–6; *CMAJ* 6 (February 1916): 116–17; Norris, ed., *An American Text-Book of Obstetrics*, 635; *Canada Lancet* 33 (March 1900): 386.

187 Johnston, *Before the Age of Miracles*, 40–2; *CMAJ* 14 (October 1924): 908.

188 See Cosbie, *The Toronto General Hospital*, 203; *CMAJ* 31 (November 1934): 517.

189 Victoria General Hospital, Halifax, patient Mrs Alice Kellaher, patient no. 1170, admitted 29 May 1921, discharged 15 June 1921.

190 *Nova Scotia Medical Bulletin* 3 (1924): 10; *CMAJ* 52 (June 1945): 563.

191 *CMAJ* 17 (December 1927): 1436; *Alberta Medical Bulletin* 13 (January 1948): 58; *CMAJ* 24 (April 1931): 618.

192 *Manitoba Medical Review* 14 (May 1934): 7. See also *CMAJ* 36 (April 1937): 378; Dominion Bureau of Statistics *A Study in Maternal, Infant and Neo-Natal Mortality in Canada* (Ottawa: Department of National Health and Welfare 1916), 16; *CMAJ* 52 (June 1945): 564.

193 'Traces,' GRP25, 'First Baby' interview 21 August 1991.

194 Kitchener-Waterloo Hospital, patient Mrs Loewen, patient no. 1378, admitted 17 April 1945.

195 Queen's University Archives, F.B. Exner, *The Nature of Medical Practice*, 1951, 6.

196 David M. Eddy, 'Variations in Physician Practice: The Role of Uncertainty,' *Health Affairs* 3 (1984): 77.

5: Childbirth

1 Henry Jellett, *A Manual of Midwifery for Students and Practitioners*, 2nd ed. (London: Bailliere, Tindall and Cox 1910), 349.

2 In the introduction to their book, Katherine Arnup, Andrée Lévesque, and Ruth Roach Pierson acknowledge women's agency in going to the hospital, but they also emphasize the negative aspects of hospital births; see *Delivering Motherhood: Maternal Ideologies and Practices in the Nineteenth and Twentieth Centuries* (London: Routledge 1990), xvii, xxi. Robbie E. Davis-Floyd, in *Birth as an American Rite of Passage* (Berkeley: University of California Press 1992), argues that women who follow the standardized way of birth are not succumbing to 'false-consciousness' as some feminist critics have suggested but, rather, their choices are 'embedded in the hegemonic cultural model of reality' as reflected in the cultural models in existence (5). While this view does not blame women for making the choices they do, it suggests almost a cultural determinism that lessens recognition of women's agency.

3 *Maritime Medical News* 15 (June 1903): 200. See also *Maritime Medical News* 18 (April 1906): 123; Barton Cooke Hirst, *A Text-Book of Obstetrics*, 7th ed. (Philadelphia: W.B. Saunders 1912), 170.

4 J. Clifton Edgar, *The Practice of Obstetrics ... for the Use of Students and Practitioners*, 3rd ed. (Philadelphia: Blakiston's, 1907), 463.

5 Joseph B. DeLee, *The Principles and Practice of Obstetrics* (Philadelphia: W.B. Saunders, 1913), xii–xiii.

6 Charles A.L. Reed, ed., *A Text-Book of Gynecology* (New York: D. Appleton 1901), 6.

7 See Ann Oakley, 'Wisewoman and Medicine Man: Changes in the Management of Childbirth,' in Juliet Mitchell and Ann Oakley, eds., *The Rights and Wrongs of Women* (Harmondsworth, Middlesex: Penguin Books 1976), 18.

8 *Queen's Medical Quarterly* 3 (October 1905): 25–6. See also Patricia Jasen, 'Race Culture, and the Colonization of Childbirth in Northern Canada,' *Social History of Medicine* 10 (December 1997): 386.

9 J. Clarence Webster, *A Textbook of Obstetrics* (Philadelphia: W.B. Saunders 1903), 145. See also *Canadian Medical Association Journal (CMAJ)* 7 (May 1917): 405. The use of animal analogies in birthing was quite common. In 1911 R.J. Ewart argued that women generally gave birth at night because this was a holdover from earlier times when nighttime birth would be safest and also because it ensured the woman less chance of being disturbed. *Public Health Journal* 2 (October 1911): 467. See also C. Henry Davis, *Painless Childbirth Eutocia and Nitrous Oxid-Oxygen Analgesia* (Chicago: Forbes 1917), 13; *Dominion Medical Monthly* 28 (March 1907): 116.

10 *Dominion Medical Monthly* 23 (November 1904): 324, 326.

11 *Dominion Medical Monthly* 28 (March 1907): 116.

12 *Western Canadian Medical Journal* 3 (July 1909): 313.
13 He also felt that a woman under the age of sixteen posed problems. Thomas Watts Eden, *A Manual of Midwifery*, 4th ed. (Toronto: Macmillan 1915), 241. Other commentators felt that any woman under the age of eighteen, at least in northern countries, was too young to have a child. *Woman's Century*, October 1917, 9.
14 *Canadian Practioner and Review* 21 (October 1906): 550.
15 *CMAJ* 3 (October 1913): 844.
16 For discussion of physician practices, see *Nova Scotia Medical Bulletin* 4 (May 1925): 3; *CMAJ* 14 (August 1924): 704; *CMAJ* 23 (October 1930): 597; *CMAJ* 31 (August 1934): 175; *CMAJ* 48 (January 1943): 49. For discussion of age, see Percy E. Ryberg, *Health, Sex and Birth Control* (Toronto: Anchor Press 1942), 174; *Health* 17 (Sept.–Oct. 1949): 33. See also Frederick C. Irving, *A Textbook of Obstetrics: For Students and Practitioners* (New York: Macmillan 1936), 358–9; William Albert Scott and H. Brookfield Van Wyck, *The Essentials of Obstetrics and Gynecology* (Philadelphia: Lea & Febiger 1946), 32.
17 *CMAJ* 42 (March 1940): 240, 243. See also *CMAJ* 49 (July 1943): 63; *CMAJ* 48 (April 1943): 313; *Modern Medicine of Canada* 1 (December 1946): 34; *Modern Medicine of Canada* 2 (October 1947): 32; *CMAJ* 59 (September 1948): 271; *Modern Medicine of Canada* 4 (July 1949): 23; *Health* 17 (Sept.–Oct. 1949): 10; *Alberta Medical Bulletin* 15 (April 1950): 17. For others, the focus was not the age but the diet of the woman; those who had poor diets experienced more complications. *CMAJ* 46 (January 1942): 5; *Saturday Night*, 1 February 1949, 16.
18 See Dalhousie University Archives, Harry Oxorn Papers, H.B. Atlee, 'Grace Maternity Hospital, 1922–1972,' n.d., 5; Harry Oxorn, *Harold Benge Atlee M.D.: A Biography* (Hantsport, N.S.: Lancelot Press 1983), 154, 116, 113; *Canadian Hospital* 26 (September 1949): 40.
19 *CMAJ* 36 (April 1937): 377.
20 For Chipman's views, see *CMAJ* 13 (June 1923): 381, and (July 1923): 493; *CMAJ* 14 (August 1924): 704–5. See also Paul T. Harper, *Clinical Obstetrics* (Philadelphia: F.A. Davis 1930), 128. In 1957 the Dominion Bureau of Statistics defined illnesses as including 'injuries and confinements as well as diagnoses of disease and undiagnosed symptoms.' Dominion Bureau of Statistics, Department of National Health and Welfare, *Canadian Sickness Survey, 1950–51*, no. 11, `Illness Frequency by Class of Illness, Age and Sex' (Ottawa, July 1957), 6.
21 See *CMAJ* 14 (August 1924): 698. See also *CMAJ* 20 (June 1929): 647. Nurses saw a similar problem in that women either felt that birthing was

dangerous and so feared it to extremes or felt it was a natural process and did not take precautions. *Public Health Journal* 17 (July 1926): 336. See also *CMAJ* 22 (January 1930): 64; *CMAJ* 26 (March 1932): 279; *CMAJ* 28 (January 1933): 42; J.M. Munro Kerr, J. Haig Ferguson, James Young, and James Hendry, *Combined Textbook of Obstetrics and Gynaeoclogy for Students and Medical Practitioners*, 2nd ed. (Edinburgh: E. & E. Livingstone 1933), 360; *Nova Scotia Medical Bulletin* 14 (March 1935): 170; J.M. Munro Kerr, with Donald McIntyre and D. Fyfe Anderson, *Operative Obstetrics: A Guide to the Difficulties and Complications of Obstetric Practice*, 4th ed. (London: Bailliere, Tindall and Cox 1937) vii; Fred. L. Adair, ed., *Obstetrics and Gynecology*, vol. 1 (Philadelphia: Lea & Febiger 1940), 35; *CMAJ* 62 (February 1950): 109.

22　*Canada Lancet and National Hygiene* 63 (July 1924): 1–2. See also *CMAJ* 45 (December 1941): 539; Ryberg, *Health, Sex and Birth Control*, 41–2.

23　Cynthia R. Comacchio, *'Nations Are Built of Babies': Saving Ontario's Mothers and Children 1900–1940* (Montreal: McGill-Queen's University Press 1993), 107. See also *Canada Lancet and Practitioner* 71 (October 1928): 123.

24　*Canadian Home Journal* 37 (November 1940): 9. See also *Health* 17 (Sept.– Oct. 1949): 10.

25　For discussion of active versus sedentary existence, see J.S. Fairbairn, *Gynaecology with Obstetrics: A Text-Book for Students and Practitioners* (London: Humphrey Milford, Oxford University Press 1924), 735; R.W. Johnstone, *A Text-Book of Midwifery: For Students and Practitioners*, 6th ed. (London: A. & C. Black, 1934), 92; Ryberg, *Health, Sex and Birth Control*, 41– 2; *Canadian Home Journal*, November 1931, 83; *CMAJ* 26 (February 1932): 178; *Canadian Journal of Medicine and Surgery* 77 (March 1935): 70; Carl Henry Davis, ed., *Gynecology and Obstetrics*, vol. 1 (Hagerstown, Md: W.F. Prior 1935), 1; *Canadian Journal of Public Health* 41 (May 1950): 177–8. Edgar, *The Practice of Obstetrics*, 463. For influence of hair colour, see P. Brooke Bland, *Practical Obstetrics for Students and Practitioners* (Philadelphia: F.A. Saunders 1932), 433. For discussion of nationality, see *Canadian Public Health Journal* 31 (July 1940): 320.

26　*Canadian Journal of Medicine and Surgery* 77 (March 1935): 70–2. In the United States as well, doctors believed that intermarriage led to an increase in obstetric complication. Irvine Loudon, *Death in Childbirth: An International Study of Maternal Care and Maternal Mortality, 1800–1950* (Oxford: Clarendon Press 1992), 342.

27　C. Lesley Biggs, 'Fragments from the History of Midwifery in Canada: A Reconsidertion of the Historiographic Issues,' in Ivy Bourgeault, Cecilia Benoit, and Robbie Davis-Floyd, eds., *Reconceiving Midwifery: The New Canadian Model of Care* (Ann Arbor: University of Michigan Press, forthcoming), 8–9 of draft. In the 1970s a similar argument was put forward to explain why Inuit women needed to be evacuated to hospitals for birthing – they had been corrupted by contact with civilization. John O'Neill and Patricia Leyland Kaufert, 'Inriktakpunga! Sex Determination and Inuit Struggle for Birthing Rights in Northern Canada,' in Faye D. Ginsburg and Rayna Rapp, eds., *Conceiving the New World Order: The Global Politics of Reproduction* (Berkeley: University of California Press 1995), 59–73.

28 *CMAJ* 21 (December 1929): 656; *Nova Scotia Medical Bulletin* 4 (May 1925): 3; *CMAJ* 14 (August 1924): 704; *CMAJ* 17 (November 1927): 1289; *CMAJ* 28 (January 1933): 46; *CMAJ* 50 (March 1944): 219.

29 On the importance of the mother's life, see *Canadian Practitioner and Review* 33 (June 1908): 372; Harry Oxorn, *Harold Benge Atlee M.D.*, 86; Janet Elizabeth McNaughton, 'The Role of the Newfoundland Midwife in Traditional Health Care, 1900 to 1970' (PhD thesis, Memorial University of Newfoundland, 1989), 152–3; *CMAJ* 31 (October 1934): 437.

30 See *Canada Medical Record* 31 (August 1903): 368; Thomas Watts Eden and Cuthbert Lockyer, eds., *The New System of Gynaecology*, vol. 1 (Toronto: Macmillan 1917), 742; *Bulletin of Ontario Hospitals for the Insane* 5 (October 1911): 29. One study of British Columbia's Provincial Hospital for the Insane between 1905 and 1915 revealed that it was the male committal agents who focused on reproductive issues much more than female ones. Mary-Ellen Kelm, '"The Only Place Likely to Do Her Any Good": The Admission of Women to British Columbia's Provincial Hospital for the Insane,' *BC Studies* 96 (Winter 1992–3): 82–3; *Bulletin of Ontario Hospitals for the Insane* 4 (July 1911): 37; *CMAJ* 19 (September 1928): 294–5; Ten Teachers, *Midwifery*, 5th ed. (London: Edward Arnold 1935), 215.

31 See Julie Cruickshank, *Life Lived Like a Story: Life Stories of Three Yukon Elders* (Vancouver: University of British Columbia Press 1992), 128; Vilhjalmur Stefansson, *Anthropological Papers of the American Museum of Natural History*, 14, part 1: *The Stefansson-Anderson Arctic Expedition of the American Museum: Preliminary Ethnological Report* (New York 1914), 162; Marni Elizabeth Davis, 'Southern Kwakiutl Medicine' (MA thesis, University of Victoria, 1977), 26–7; Irma Honigmann and John Honigmann, 'Child Rearing Patterns among the Great Whale River Eskimo,' *University of Alaska Anthropological Papers* 2 (1953): 32; Igloolik Oral History Project, Science Institute of the Northwest Territories, Government of the Northwest Territories, computer no. IE085, tape IE085, interview with Sarah Amakllak Haulli by Rhoda Qanatsiaq, translated by Leah Otak, 16 January 1990, transcript, 6.

32 Margaret Blackman, *During My Time: Florence Edenshaw Davidson, A Haida Woman* (Vancouver: Douglas and McIntyre 1982), 31. But at least Native women during these years gave birth within their own communities, a situation that did not last. With the advent of Western medical care, the percentage of births occurring in hospitals or nursing stations increased. In the Northwest Territories it was 38.9 per cent in 1953; by 1968, 90.6 per cent. Lesley Paulette, 'The Family Centred Maternity Care Project,' in Mary Crnkovich, ed., *'Gossip': A Spoken History of Women in the North* (Ottawa: Canadian Arctic Resources Committee 1990), 77. For a description of the wide belief in the power of menstrual blood (and birth blood), see Janice Delaney, Mary Jane Lupton, and Emily Toth, *The Curse: A Cultural History of Menstruation* (New York: Dutton 1976); Thomas Buckley and Alma Gottleib, eds., *Blood Magic: The Anthropology of Menstruation* (Berkeley: University of California Press 1988; and Penelope Shuttle and Peter Redgrove, *The Wise Wound: Myths, Realities, and Meanings of Menstruation* (New York: Grove Press 1988).

33 H. Gordon Green, *Don't Have Your Baby in the Dory: A Biography of Myra Bennett* (Montreal: Harvest House 1973), 22. Myra Bennett read about this story.

34 Igloolik Oral History Project, computer no. HPU1, tape IE082, interview with Hanna Uyarak, by Rhoda Qanatsiaq, translated by Louis Tapardjuk, 15 January 1990, transcript, 3.

35 See Paulette, 'The Family Centred Maternity Care Project,' 73–4; Hirst, *A Text-Book of Obstetrics*, 170; *Woman's Century*, February 1917, 6.

36 The feminist literature on midwifery usually sees the decline in midwifery as a loss for women. See Dianne Dodd and Deborah Gorham, eds., *Caring and Curing: Historical Perspectives on Women and Healing* (Ottawa: University of Ottawa Press 1994), 6. What I am suggesting is that we need to ask for which women – that is, the degree of loss has be considered and nuanced. Edward Shorter argues that women have never been in total control of birthing, and I agree. Edward Shorter, *A History of Women's Bodies* (New York: Basic Books 1982), 68. Where we differ is that he feels that midwives and medical births exhibit the same degree of control, whereas I would argue that the nature of the control is different and the result of those differences is that, with midwives, women probably feel more sense of control.

37 Mary Rubio and Elizabeth Waterston, eds., *The Selected Journals of Lucy Maud Montgomery*, vol. 2: *1910–1921* (Toronto: Oxford University Press 1987), 99.

38 Laurel Halladay, '"We'll See You Next Year": Maternity Homes in Southern Saskatchewan in the First Half of the Twentieth Century' (MA thesis, Carleton University, 1996), 31.

39 Public Archives of Nova Scotia, Victorian Order of Nurses, RT98, V645, *VON Report*, 1923, 67.

40 Adam H. Wright, *A Textbook of Obstetrics* (New York: D. Appleton 1908), 95.

41 Constance Backhouse, *Petticoats and Prejudice: Women and the Law in Nineteenth-Century Canada* (Toronto: Women's Press 1991), 133.

42 Halladay, 'We'll See You Next Year,' 27–9.

43 For example, James Langstaff attended almost 70 per cent of the births in the Thornhill, Ontario, area; and in the Wakefield area of Quebec most women sought out a doctor for their deliveries. Jacalyn Duffin, *Langstaff: A Nineteenth-Century Medical Life* (Toronto: University of Toronto Press 1993), 180; and Jayne Elliott, '"Endormez-moi!" An Early Twentieth-Century Obstetrical Practice in the Gatineau Valley, Quebec' (MA thesis, Carleton University, 1997), 121.

44 British Columbia Archives, GR706, 'B.C. Commission on Health Insurance, 1919–21,' file 1, 'Recommendations,' 9; GR707, box 2, file 16, 'Evidence on Maternity Sickness,' in *B.C. Royal Commission State Health Insurance and Maternity Benefits* (Victoria: King's Printer 1932), x, 26; National Council of Women, *Yearbook 1923*, 78–9.

45 For women's concerns, see Jutta Mason, 'Midwifery in Canada,' in Sheila Kitzinger, ed., *The Midwife Challenge* (London: Pandora Press 1988), 110, 112; Denyse Baillargeon, 'Care of Mothers and Infants in Montreal between the Wars: The Visiting Nurses of Metropolitan Life, les Gouttes de Lait, and Assistance Maternelle,' in Dodd and Gorham eds., *Caring and Curing*, 175; interview with Grace McKenzie, 8 June 1993.

46 *Annual Report of the Montreal Maternity Hospital*, 1901, 7; ibid., 1916, 27–31; ibid., 1920, 28–30.

47 Ibid., 1905, 23.

48 Elliott, 'Endormez-moi!' 151.

49 See *Nova Scotia Medical Bulletin* 14 (March 1935): 172; *University of Toronto Medical Journal* 15 (March 1938): 225; *CMAJ* 38 (February 1938): 139; *CMAJ* 43 (July 1940): 41.

50 Webster, *A Textbook of Obstetrics*, 228; Fairbairn, *Gynaecology with Obstetrics*, 245.

51 Wright, *A Textbook of Obstetrics*, 104.

52 See David Berry Hart, *Guide to Midwifery* (London: Rebman 1912), 210; DeLee, *The Principles and Practice of Obstetrics*, 290.

53 P. Brooke Bland, *Practical Obstetrics for Students and Practitioners* (Philadel-

phia: F.A. Saunders 1932), 355; *McGill Medical Undergraduate Journal* 3 (April 1934): 197; Samuel S. Peikoff, *Yesterday's Doctor: An Autobiography* (Winnipeg: Prairie Publishing, 1980), 31.

54 Loudon, *Death in Childbirth,* 155.

55 For statistics on place of birth, see *Historical Statistics* B 1–14; *CMAJ* 43 (July 1940): 41; Statistics Canada, *Annual Report of Hospitals 1932–39,* 42; C. Lesley Biggs, 'The Response to Maternal Mortality in Ontario, 1920–1940' (MA thesis, University of Toronto, 1983), 59, 64; Beth Light and Ruth Roach Pierson, eds., *No Easy Road: Women in Canada 1920s to 1960s* (Toronto: New Hogtown Press 1990), 168; J. Oppenheimer, 'Childbirth in Ontario: The Transition from Home to Hospital in the Early Twentieth Century,' *Ontario History* 75 (March 1983): 36; Public Archives of Nova Scotia, RG25, series C, vol. 11(A), Public Health,'Report on the Survey of Hospitals in Nova Scotia, 1949,' 28. By 1940 the hospitalization rate was 84.4 per cent in B.C., 62.2 per cent in Ontario; 72.9 per cent in Alberta, but only 26.2 per cent in P.E.I. and 15.6 per cent in Quebec. Veronica Strong Boag and Kathryn McPherson, 'The Confinement of Women: Childbirth and Hospitalization in Vancouver, 1919–1939,' in Arnup, Lévesque, and Pierson, eds., *Delivering Motherhood,* 78. Some of this variation was based on the economics of building hospitals (or not building them) in isolated areas. Occupational profile also may be linked to some of the regional variations. For example, in 1929, 93.1 per cent of births of fishermen's children were non-institutional but only 43.6 per cent of professionals' children were. *American Journal of Public Health* (1932), 618. This did not necessarily mean a rejection of hospital births by fishermen's families but rather a lack of affordable access to hospital care and even lack of access, since they often lived in small villages.

56 See *CMAJ* 36 (June 1937): 600; *Manitoba Medical Review* 26 (May 1946): 276; William Victor Johnston, *Before the Age of Miracles: Memoirs of a Country Doctor* (Toronto: Fitzhenry & Whiteside, 1972), 35. As women increasingly used hospital services, organizations such as the VON, which had provided childbirth care in conjunction with physicians in the home, found their role shifting from actual childbirth assistance to prenatal and postnatal care. Public Archives of Nova Scotia, Victorian Order of Nurses, RT98, V645, *VON Report,* 1929, 30. The Halifax VON reported that in 1911 just over 28 per cent of its cases were attendance at childbirth, but only 2.5 per cent were in 1946. Public Archives of Nova Scotia, annual reports, VON Halifax, 1911–50. In 1950 the report of the chief superintendent of the VON pointed out that in the last ten years VON nurses had attended 76.5 per cent fewer births. Public Archives of Nova Scotia, Victorian Order of Nurses, RT98, V645, *VON Report,* 1950, 28.

57 For a discussion of such homes, see Elliott, 'Endormez-moi!' 156, and Halladay, 'We'll See You Next Year.'

58 Halladay, 'We'll See You Next Year' 37, 55–7, 74, 95, 128–34, 142.

59 Christine Payeur, 'Maternal Mortality in Quebec from the Medical Perspective and the Women's Point of View, 1890–1950' (MA thesis, Université de Montréal, 1998), 36.

60 *Annual Report of the Vancouver General Hospital*, 1916, 34; Strong-Boag and McPherson, 'The Confinement of Women, 84.

61 *Annual Report of the Royal Victoria Hospital*, 1930, 104.

62 Public Archives of Nova Scotia, RG25, series C, vol. 11(A), Public Health, *Report on the Survey of Hospitals in Nova Scotia under the Federal Health Survey Grant 1949*, 33.

63 David Gagan, *A Necessity among Us: The Owen Sound General and Marine Hospital, 1891–1985* (Toronto: University of Toronto Press 1990), 83; British Columbia Archives, Royal Jubilee Hospital Discharge Books, Add. MS. 313, vol. 73 – calculated from all patients admitted January to April 1927, 1935, and 1945. The Owen Sound Hospital showed similar trends. In 1895–96, 38% of the patients were female, increasing to 42.7% in 1905–6, 53.4% in 1915–16, 55.3% in 1925, 60.7% in 1935–6, and down to 57.9% in 1940–1. The percentage of adult women admitted for pregnancy-related reasons were 12.5%, 12.9%, 13.5% 26.8%, 29.3%, and 45.1%, respectively. Calculations for the Owen Sound Hospital are based on sampling of the patient records of the hospital. Research was generously given to the author by David Gagan.

64 Payeur, 'Maternal Mortality in Quebec,' 20.

65 *Annual Report of the Montreal Maternity Hospital*, 1902, 9; ibid., 1919, 28; calculations based on 4674 cases, 1896–1915, given to author by Suzann Buckley for the Ottawa Maternity Hospital. A similar pattern occurred at the Vancouver General Hospital. See Strong-Boag and McPherson, 'The Confinement of Women,' 84–5.

66 *Annual Report of the Montreal Maternity Hospital* 1902, 9; ibid., 1919, 28.

67 DeLee, *The Principles and Practice of Obstetrics*, 272. See also *Canada Lancet and Practitioner* 78 (April 1932): 115; Davis, ed., *Gynecology and Obstetrics*, vol. 1, chap. 22, 1.

68 Comacchio, *'Nations Are Built of Babies,'* 68. On control, see also Margarete Sandelowski, *Women, Health, and Choice* (Englewood Cliffs, N.J.: Prentice-Hall 1981), 104.

69 Payeur, 'Maternal Mortality in Quebec,' 82.

70 Oxorn, *Harold Benge Atlee M.D.*, 200.

71 *CMAJ* 37, supplement (1937): 60.

72 *CMAJ* 41 (October 1939): 384.

73 Marion O. Robinson, *Give My Heart: The Dr. Marion Hilliard Story* (Garden City, N.Y.: Doubleday 1964), 235.

74 Interview with Isme Southern, 24 August 1993; with Eunice Jordan, 14 July 1993; with Jane Rutherford, 28 July 1993; with Joan Carr, 22 July 1993.

75 C. Levitt et al., *Survey of Routine Maternity Care and Practices in Canadian Hospitals* (Ottawa: Health Canada and Canadian Institute of Child Health 1995), 5, 38.

76 McGill University Archives, *Annual Report of the Royal Victoria Hospital, Montreal*, 1940, 46. For a discussion of women's ambivalent feelings toward giving birth in a hospital, see Payeur, 'Maternal Mortality in Quebec,' 128–9.

77 *CMAJ* 48 (January 1943): 50; Strong-Boag and McPherson, 'The Confinement of Women,' 88.

78 *Canadian Practitioner and Review* 21 (October 1906): 543.

79 Andrée Lévesque, 'Deviants Anonymous: Single Mothers at the Hôpital de la Miséricorde in Montreal, 1929–1939,' in Arnup, Lévesque, and Pierson, eds., *Delivering Motherhood*, 115.

80 Interview with Irma Avery, 24 August 1993, and with Jennie Graham, 29 June 1993.

81 Oxorn, *Harold Benge Atlee M.D.*, 154.

82 Halladay, 'We'll See You Next Year,' 104.

83 *Maclean's*, 1 July 1943, 60; Marie-Josee Blais argues in her 'Le transfert hospitalier de l'accounchement au Québec, 1930–1960' (MA thesis, Université de Montréal, 1996) that women went to hospital because lack of domestic help and lack of space at home, and also for the rest they received in hospital, the medical security it provided, and the comfort of modernity.

84 Light and Pierson, eds., *No Easy Road*, 181. For concerns about crowded homes, see *Annual Report of the Royal Victoria Hospital, Montreal*, 1946, 48; *CMAJ* 34 (April 1936): 441.

85 *Maclean's*, October 1 1945, 58. See also Munro Kerr, with McIntyre and Anderson, *Operative Obstetrics*, 23.

86 *Canadian Hospital* 23 (May 1946): 32. In some hospitals husbands were encouraged to be present. See *Canadian Nurse* 46 (December 1950): 954.

87 *Chatelaine*, October 1931, 53; *McGill Medical Undergraduate Journal* 3 (April 1934): 197; Ryberg, *Health, Sex and Birth Control*, 41–2, 179; Florence H.M. Emory, *Public Health Nursing in Canada* (Toronto: Macmillan 1953), 289. For other support for home births, see *Canada Lancet and Practitioner* 77 (December 1931): 161; DeLee, *The Principles and Practice of Obstetrics*,

272; *Canadian Public Health Journal* 22 (July 1931): 348; *Nova Scotia Medical Bulletin* 10 (July 1931): 424; *Canada Lancet and Practitioner* 77 (December 1931): 161; *Canadian Public Health Journal* 23 (December 1932): 564; *CMAJ* 34 (May 1936): 522; Kerr, with McIntyre and Anderson, *Operative Obstetrics*, 34; Adair, ed., *Obstetrics and Gynecology*, 1: 848.

88 *CMAJ* 14 (June 1924); 495; *Chatelaine*, July 1928, 7; *CMAJ* 33 (December 1935): 673; *Child and Family Welfare* 11 (January 1936): 23; *CMAJ* 41 (October 1939): 382–3; *University of Toronto Medical Journal* 8 (March 1931): 195; *Canadian Public Health Journal* 22 (July 1931): 348; *Nova Scotia Medical Bulletin* 10 (July 1931): 424; *Canada Lancet and Practitioner* 77 (December 1931): 161; Davis, ed., *Gynecology and Obstetrics*, vol. 1, chap. 22, 2.

89 Rhone Rickman Kenneally, in 'The Montreal Maternity, 1842–1926: Evolution of a Hospital' (MA thesis, McGill University, 1983), examines the decline in maternal mortality due to doctors at the hospital adopting antiseptic technique.

90 *Montreal Medical Journal* 36 (June 1906): 396. For a very full description of the preparation of the obstetric patient at Burnside, see *Canadian Practitioner and Review* 21 (October 1906): 543–50; and *Canada Lancet* 40 (November 1906): 218. See also *Montreal Medical Journal* 37 (January 1908): 26; Jellett, *A Manual of Midwifery*, 335; David James Evans, *Obstetrics: A Manual for Students and Practitioners* (Philadelphia: Lea Brothers 1900), 123.

91 *Montreal Medical Journal* 36 (June 1906): 396–7. *Canada Lancet* 40 (November 1906): 218.

92 *Montreal Medical Journal* 36 (June 1906): 396; *Canada Lancet* 33 (March 1900): 389; Jellett, *A Manual of Midwifery*, 335; *Canada Lancet* 40 (November 1906): 218;

93 *Montreal Medical Journal* 36 (June 1906): 397; *Canada Lancet* 40 (November 1906): 218, 223. See also *Montreal Medical Journal* 37 (January 1908): 26.

94 Wright, *A Textbook of Obstetrics*, 95; *Canadian Practitioner and Review* 31 (May 1906): 243; *Saskatchewan Medical Journal* 2 (July 1910): 194.

95 *Canada Lancet* 44 (September 1910): 35–6. See also *Montreal Medical Journal* 37 (January 1908): 26.

96 See McGill University Archives, Montreal General Hospital, RG96, vol. 0421, file 00635, 'Notes on Nursing Obstetrics.'

97 By the end of the century, however, shaving and the use of enemas were no longer routine procedures. In 1993, of the hospitals that responded to a survey on childbirth practices, only 16 per cent reported stipulating shaving and only 11 per cent insisted on an enema/suppository. Levitt et al., *Survey of Routine Maternity Care*, 5, 39.

98 *Canadian Nurse* 23 (September 1927): 463. See also Kathryn Mae

McPherson, 'Skilled Service and Women's Work: Canadian Nursing, 1920–1939' (PhD thesis, Simon Fraser University, 1989), 275–6; Strong-Boag and McPherson, 'The Confinement of Women,' 88.

99 Alvine Cyr Gahagan, *Yes Father: Pioneer Nursing in Alberta* (Manchester, N.H.: Hammer Publications 1979), 89; *Dalhousie Medical Journal* 11 (1937): 33. For descriptions of hospital birth, see Ten Teachers, *Midwifery*, 284; *Hospital, Medical and Nursing World* 30 (September 1926): 65; Strong-Boag and McPherson, 'The Confinement of Women,' 88. One woman recalled that when her brother was born at home during the 1930s that her mother was shaved. Marlene O'Brien, 'A History of Childbirth in Ontario' (student paper, University of Waterloo, November 1994), 9; *CMAJ* 22 (April 1930): 470; Penelope Stewart, 'Infant Feeding in Canada: 1910–1940' (MA thesis, Concordia University, 1982), 118; *CMAJ* 40 (February 1939): 188.

100 *CMAJ* 36 (June 1937): 601. See also *CMAJ* 38 (February 1938): 138; *CMAJ* 37, supplement (1937): 65; *CMAJ* 48 (April 1943): 315; Henricus J. Stander, *Williams Obstetrics: A Textbook for the Use of Students and Practitioners*, 8th ed. (New York: Appleton-Century 1941), 407, 411; Strong-Boag and McPherson, 'The Confinement of Women,' 88. A survey of Canadian hospitals in 1993 revealed that just over half of the responding hospitals insisted that staff wear gowns during vaginal birth, 89 per cent insisted on gloves, and 33 per cent insisted on face masks. Smaller hospitals were more likely to insist on gowns and masks than larger ones. Levitt et al., *Survey of Routine Maternity Care*, 7.

101 Davis, 'Southern Kwakiutl Medicine,' 26–7; Paulette, 'The Family Centred Maternity Care Project,' 73–4.

102 Evans, *Obstetrics*, 128. See also Hart, *Guide to Midwifery*, 210; DeLee, *The Principles and Practice of Obstetrics*, 290; Memorial University of Newfoundland Folklore and Language Archive (MUNFLA), no. 75–21, Mary Harriet Doyle, 'Midwifery in the Community of Calvert on the Southern Shore of Newfoundland,' 17.

103 Wright, *A Textbook of Obstetrics*, 95, 427–9. See also Jellett, *A Manual of Midwifery*, 343; and Hirst, *A Text-Book of Obstetrics*, 181.

104 Fairbairn, *Gynaecology with Obstetrics*, 245; *Canadian Public Health Journal* 23 (March 1942): 121.

105 Dalhousie University, Oxorn Papers, Correspondence, A-M, letter from Martha Crosbie, 2 June 1980.

106 One way that modern critics have made their point is with the following analogy: 'If your husband was told that he had to get an erection and ejaculate within a certain time or he'd be castrated, do you think it would

be easy? To make it easier, perhaps he could have an I.V. put into his arm, be kept in one position, have straps placed around his penis, and be told not to move: He could be checked every few minutes; the sheet could be lifted to see if any "progress" had been made.' As Emily Martin notes, 'This strikes us as ridiculous but ... it may seem appropriate to us when women are placed in a structurally analogous position while giving birth.' Emily Martin, *The Woman in the Body: A Cultural Analysis of Reproduction* (Boston: Beacon Press 1987), 58. See also J. Roberts and C. Mendez-Bauer, 'A Perspective of Maternal Position during Labor,' *Journal of Perinatal Medicine* 8 (1980): 258; and Joyce Roberts, 'Maternal Position during the First Stage of Labour,' in Iain Chalmers, Murray Enkin, and Marc J.N.C. Kevise, eds., *Effective Care in Pregnancy and Childbirth*, vol. 2 (Oxford: Oxford University Press 1989), 883–92. Roberts concludes: 'The available evidence suggests that [the supine position] compromises effective uterine activity, prolongs labour and leads to an increased use of drugs to augment contractions. Women should be encouraged to adopt whatever position they find comfortable during the first stage of labour. Many will choose upright positions to begin with and then adopt lateral recumbent positions as labour becomes more advanced' (890).

107 Levitt, et al., *Survey of Routine Maternity Care*, 7, 56. Small hospitals were less likely to do so.

108 *Dominion Medical Monthly* 17 (October 1901): 182. See also Evans, *Obstetrics*, 138. The recumbent position in Britain was for specialists attending births requiring some form of operative intervention. William Ray Arney, *Power and the Profession of Obstetrics* (Chicago: University of Chicago Press 1982), 62–9.

109 Webster, *A Textbook of Obstetrics*, 235–6.

110 Wright, *A Textbook of Obstetrics*, 101, 110, 118.

111 *Canada Lancet* 40 (November 1906): 218.

112 Edgar, *The Practice of Obstetrics*, 868. For birth position and its association with primitive women, see Arney, *Power and the Profession of Obstetrics*, 62–9.

113 Dianne Dodd, 'Helen MacMurchy: Popular Midwifery and Maternity Services for Canadian Pioneer Women,' in Dodd and Gorham, eds., *Caring and Curing*, 144; Johnstone, *A Text-Book of Midwifery*, 156.

114 Harper, *Clinical Obstetrics*, 43–4 (emphasis in original). When women are interviewed, some surprising results emerge. Gertrude Roswell, for example, entered hospital to have her twins in the 1950s and the nurses actually placed her in a squatting position and had her pant to slow down the birth. Interview with Gertrude Roswell, 16 August 1993.

115 While Mitchell rejected the squat position, he did argue the need for students of medicine to be versatile and to at least see a birth in the left side position before they graduated. *Manitoba Medical Review* 28 (May 1948): 244.

116 Alfred C. Beck, *Obstetrical Practice*, 4th ed. (Baltimore: Williams & Wilkins 1947) 303; Johnstone, *A Text-Book of Midwifery*, 156. See also Roberts and Mendez-Bauer, 'A Perspective of Maternal Position during Labor,' 257.

117 The first stage is the opening of the cervix, accompanied by contractions; the second the passage of the foetus through the birth canal; and the third is the separation and expulsion of the placenta.

118 Calculations based on the patient records of the Ottawa Maternity Hospital given to the author by Suzann Buckley.

119 Wright, *A Textbook of Obstetrics*, 374–5.

120 Dianne Dodd, 'Helen MacMurchy, M.D. (1862–1953): Mothers and Doctors in the "Complete" Canadian Mother's Book' (paper presented to the Canadian Historical Association, Kingston, 1991), 4; James Robert Goodall, *Puerperal Infection* (Montreal 1932), 138–9. A 1993 survey of Canadian hospitals reported that 20 per cent had a policy on how much time should be 'allowed' for the second stage of labour. The mean time was 2.6 hours for primiparous women and 2 hours for multiparous. Levitt et al., *Survey of Routine Maternity Care*, 7.

121 *CMAJ* 42 (June 1940): 562.

122 *Nova Scotia Medical Bulletin* 21 (March 1942): 124. See also *Modern Medicine of Canada* 4 (July 1949): 23.

123 Interviews with Irma Avery and Dorothy Atkinson, 15 June 1993.

124 For a discussion about the development of what was normal in labour, see Jo Murphy-Lawless, *Reading Birth and Death: A History of Obstetric Thinking* (Bloomington: Indiana University Press 1998), chap. 5.

6: Obstetrical Intervention

1 David Berry Hart, *Guide to Midwifery* (London: Rebman 1912), 422.

2 See Margarete Sandelowski, *Women, Health, and Choice* (Englewood Cliffs, N.J.: Prentice-Hall 1981), 104; Robbie E. Davis-Floyd has argued that in modern birth, intervention is designed to counteract and control the natural or the unpredictable and reflects a belief in technology. See her *Birth as an American Rite of Passage* (Berkeley: University of California Press 1992), 2. For an in-depth discussion of control, see William Ray Arney, *Power and the Profession of Obstetrics* (Chicago: University of Chicago Press 1982).

3 Marie Adele Rabesca, Diane Romie, Martha Johnson, and Joan Ryan, *Traditional Dene Medicine*, part 2: *Database* (Lac La Marie, NWT: Traditional Dene Medicine Project 1993), 301; also *Traditional Dene Medicine*, part 1: *Report* (Lac La Marie, NWT: Traditional Dene Medicine Project 1994), 49–50, 55, 106; Marni Elizabeth Davis, 'Southern Kwakiutl Medicine' (MA thesis, Unversity of Victoria, 1977), 27; Laurie Lacey, *Micmac Indian Medicine: Traditional Way of Health* (Antigonish, N.S.: Formac 1977), 41.

4 Memorial University of Newfoundland Folklore and Language Archive (MUNFLA), no. 78–211, Carol Anne Ruby, 'Childbearing and Childbirth in Early Twentieth Century Newfoundland,' 86, 91–2, 95; no. 76-165 Gary Gale, 'Mrs. Susan Eveleigh Midwife,' 12–13; no. 77-247, Linda Pauline Warford, 'Reminiscences of a Midwife of Upper Gullies in Conception Bay South,' 7.

5 *Montreal Medical Journal* 31 (October 1902): 772; *Canada Lancet* 33 (March 1900): 388–9; J. Clifton Edgar, *The Practice of Obstetrics ... for the Use of Students and Practitioners*, 3rd ed. (Philadelphia: Blakiston 1907), 463; *Canadian Medical Association Journal* (*CMAJ*) 38 (February 1938): 140; *CMAJ* 39 (September 1938): 300.

6 David Gollacher has made this analysis with respect to belief in circumcision, but it applies to other aspects of medical practice as well. 'From Ritual to Science: The Medical Transformation of Circumcision in America,' *Journal of Social History* 1 (Fall 1994): 5–36.

7 *Canadian Practitioner and Review* 44 (April 1919): 114. See also *CMAJ* 10 (October 1920): 902.

8 29.5 per cent of Dr Almon's patients had some form of intervention and 33.1 per cent of those who paid did. Calculations based on 312 patients, 1898–1914, Public Archives of Nova Scotia, MG1, no. 12–14, William Bruce Almon Obstetrical Casebook, 1898–1912. Veronica Strong-Boag and Kathryn McPherson, 'The Confinement of Women: Childbirth and Hospitalization in Vancouver, 1919–1939,' in Katherine Arnup, Andrée Lévesque, and Ruth Roach Pierson, eds., *Delivering Motherhood: Maternal Ideologies and Practices in the Nineteenth and Twentieth Centuries* (London: Routledge, 1990), 90–1, 93.

9 McGill University Archives, RG95, vol. 88, Obstetrical Casebook, Royal Victoria Hospital (Montreal Maternity Hospital), patient no. 277, Lorna Moschini, admitted 28 September 1901, discharged 5 January 1902. See also *University of Toronto Medical Journal* 10 (January 1933): 80; *Canadian Public Health Journal* 25 (March 1934); 142; *CMAJ* 34 (May 1936): 520, 526; Marion Hilliard, *A Woman Doctor Looks at Love and Life* (Garden City, N.Y.: Doubleday 1957), 20.

10 *CMAJ* 25 (October 1931): 419.

11 *Alberta Medical Bulletin* 13 (January 1948): 70.

12 *University of Toronto Medical Journal* 15 (March 1938): 225. See also *Manitoba Medical Bulletin* 99 (November 1929): 6; *CMAJ* 34 (May 1936): 520, 526; *Canadian Nurse* 34 (September 1938): 475; *Nova Scotia Medical Bulletin* 21 (March 1942): 125.

13 Queen's University Archives, F.B. Exner, *The Nature of Medical Practice*, 1951, 5. Concerning the problems of intervening and not intervening, seeing birth as pathological or not, see Arney, *Power and the Profession of Obstetrics*, chap. 3, esp. 51–62.

14 *Annual Report of the Montreal Maternity Hospital*, 1914, 23–4.

15 *CMAJ* 14 (August 1924): 704.

16 *CMAJ* 41 (October 1939): 384.

17 Public Archives of Nova Scotia, MG1, no. 12–14, William Bruce Almon Obstetrical Casebook 1898–1912; Strong-Boag and McPherson, 'The Confinement of Women,' 91.

18 Richard W. Wertz and Dorothy C. Wertz, *Lying-In: A History of Childbirth in America* (New York: Schocken Books 1979), 143.

19 Ann Oakley, *The Captured Womb: A History of the Medical Care of Pregnant Women* (Oxford: Basil Blackwell 1984), 84.

20 *Canadian Practitioner and Review* 25 (March 1900): 116.

21 Ibid., 122. See also Adam H. Wright, *A Textbook of Obstetrics* (New York: Appleton 1908), 89; *Canadian Practitioner and Review* 31 (May 1906): 243, and 43 (March 1918): 85; Charles Jewett, ed., *The Practice of Obstetrics*, 2nd ed. (New York: Lea Brothers & Co., 1901), 598; *Canadian Practitioner and Review* 31 (October 1906): 546. Henry Jellett in his 1910 text accused older nurses in Britain of following a labour with their finger in the vagina and even assisting with the dilatation of the os. There is very little evidence that this occurred in the Canadian context. Henry Jellett, *A Manual of Midwifery for Students and Practitioners*, 2nd ed. (London: Bailliere, Tindall and Cox 1910), 343. The concern about infection was not unwarranted. The most common cause of maternal mortality in Quebec was puerperal septicaemia. Christine Payeur, 'Maternal Mortality in Quebec from the Medical Perspective and the Women's Point of View, 1890–1950' (MA thesis, Université de Montréal, 1997), 60.

22 Marie-Aimée Cliche, 'Morale chrétienne et "double standard sexuel": Les filles-mère à l'hôpital de la Miséricorde à Québec 1874–1972,' *Histoire sociale/Social History* 24 (May 1991): 110.

23 *Hospital, Medical and Nursing World* 34 (September 1928): 69. See also *CMAJ* 22 (April 1930): 471; *Canada Lancet and Practitioner* 78 (April 1932): 111;

CMAJ 34 (May 1936): 522; J.S. Fairbairn, *Gynaecology with Obstetrics: A Text-Book for Students and Practitioners* (London: Humphrey Milford, Oxford University Press 1924), 245; *CMAJ* 36 (June 1937): 601.

24 Fred L. Adair, ed., *Obstetrics and Gynecology*, vol. 1 (Philadelphia: Lea & Febiger 1940), 819.

25 My thanks to Dr Murray Enkin for pointing this out.

26 C. Levitt et al., *Survey of Routine Maternity Care and Practices in Canadian Hospitals* (Ottawa: Health Canada and Canadian Institute of Child Health 1995), 5, 55. Thirty-four per cent of the hospitals that responded to a 1993 survey reported having regulations that specified how frequent vaginal examinations could be.

27 *Nova Scotia Medical Bulletin* 16 (February 1938): 156; *University of Toronto Medical Journal* 22 (March 1945): 179; Strong-Boag and McPherson, 'The Confinement of Women,' 91–2.

28 Public Archives of Nova Scotia, MG1, no. 12–14, William Bruce Almon Obstetrical Casebook. Calculations based on 312 cases between 1898 and 1912.

29 *CMAJ* 34 (May 1936): 520.

30 *Annual Report of the Royal Victoria Hospital, Montreal*, 1948, 37.

31 *CMAJ* 48 (January 1943): 49.

32 Jayne Elliott, '"Endormez-moi!": An Early Twentieth-Century Obstetrical Practice in the Gatineau Valley, Quebec' (MA thesis, Carleton University, 1997), 104.

33 Vancouver City Archives, Add. Mss. 16 daybooks, Henri Evariste Langis Obstetrical Records, 1893, 1894, 1903, 1904, based on 72 patients

34 *Canadian Practitioner and Review* 34 (October 1909): 634.

35 *CMAJ* 1 (October 1911): 945–7.

36 Twenty per cent of hospitals responding to a 1993 survey had policies on how long the second stage of labour should last before intervention occurred. Levitt et al., *Survey of Routine Maternity Care*, 7.

37 *Montreal Medical Journal* 31 (October 1902): 772; McGill University Archives, Royal Victoria Hospital (Montreal Maternity Hospital), RG95, vol. 88, Obstetrical Casebook, patient no. 196, Mrs Henderson, admitted 6 February 1902

38 Barton Cooke Hirst, *A Text-Book of Obstetrics*, 7th ed. (Philadelphia: W.B. Saunders 1912), 190; *Canadian Practitioner and Review* 44 (April 1919): 114. Manual dilation was discouraged in the Boston Lying-in Hospital. *CMAJ* 45 (October 1941): 366, and this conservative approach was approved by Ross Mitchell, a Winnipeg physician.

39 Elliott, 'Endormez-moi!' 88, 90.

40 *Dominion Medical Monthly* 17 (October 1901): 183. See also *Canadian Practitioner and Review* 37 (April 1912): 233. This use of ergot seemed to fly in the face of British custom. John S. Haller Jr., 'Smut's Dark Poison: Ergot in History and Medicine,' *Transactions and Studies, College of Physicians of Phildelphia* 3 (March 1981): 75–6.

41 *CMAJ* 3 (September 1913): 739–50. See *Canada Lancet* 48 (January 1915): 285 for a discussion of when to use pituitrin.

42 *CMAJ* 7 (May 1917): 418.

43 *Canadian Practitioner and Review* 43 (March 1918): 85.

44 My thanks to Dr Murray Enkin for this information.

45 Harry Beckman, *Treatment in General Practice* (Philadelphia: W.B. Saunders 1931), 757–8.

46 *CMAJ* 17 (December 1927): 1436. The breakdown of its known use in the 327 cases where it was implicated was as follows: before labour in 5; in the first stage of labour 9; in the second stage of labour 123; in the third stage 32; during the post-partum period 50; and during the operation for caesarian section 11.

47 *CMAJ* 10 (October 1920): 903; *CMAJ* 11 (May 1921): 351; *Manitoba Medical Bulletin* 86 (October 1928): 8–9; *Hospital, Medical and Nursing World* 34 (September 1928): 69; *CMAJ* 13 (September 1923): 679; *Canada Lancet and Practitioner* 71 (October 1928): 123–4; and 70 (May 1928): 166; *Chatelaine*, July 1928, 60. Ian Carr and Robert E. Beamish have argued that before the First World War physicians in Manitoba were interventionist but afterward allowed labour to go on for too long. The medical literature in general does not suggest this. This Manitoba rate may have reflected the predilection of Dr Bjornson, head of the university's Department of Obstetrics. See their *Manitoba Medicine: A Brief History* (Winnipeg: University of Manitoba Press 1999), 114–15.

48 *Nova Scotia Medical Bulletin* 4 (May 1925): 5; *University of Toronto Medical Journal* 3 (May 1926): 304.

49 Beckman, *Treatment in General Practice*, 753–4, 757–8.

50 *University of Toronto Medical Journal* 9 (November 1931): 47, 49. See also *CMAJ* 27 (October 1932): 388; *CMAJ* 34 (January 1936): 49; *University of Toronto Medical Journal* 23 (January 1946): 146; *Manitoba Medical Review* 28 (April 1948): 179; *CMAJ* 48 (April 1943): 316; *Modern Medicine of Canada* 4 (July 1949): 53.

51 Strong-Boag and McPherson, 'The Confinement of Women,' 91. Post-maturity was an indicator, but some hospitals gave women leeway in this regard. When Mrs Gail Saunders entered the Montreal Maternity Hospital on 12 July 1937, estimates were that she was already eleven days overdue

and so had a medical induction of labour with pituitrin. McGill University Archives, Royal Victoria, Montreal Maternity Hospital, Patient records, vol. 120, conf. 22802, Mrs Gail Saunders, admitted 12 July 1937, discharged 24 July 1937; *CMAJ* 46 (February 1942): 156.

52 *CMAJ* 42 (June 1940): 560.

53 Oakley, *The Captured Womb*, 87.

54 *University of Toronto Medical Journal* 10 (January 1933): 80; *Alberta Medical Bulleting* 13 (July 1948): 13.

55 *University of Toronto Medical Journal* 5 (December 1927): 39, 44; *Canadian Nurse* 31 (November 1935): 490.

56 *CMAJ* 21 (July 1929): 64–5. By the late 1940s, the use of the bag seems to have been less popular. But 'large doses of oestrogens' were now being used as an adjunct to induction. *Alberta Medical Bulletin* 13 (January 1948): 69. Rates of induction could vary tremendously. In London, England, the highest rate of one hospital was fourteen times that of the lowest. Oakley, *The Captured Womb*, 88.

57 For an examination of induction in the late twentieth century, see Michel Thiery, Cornelia J. Baines, and Marc J.N.C. Keirse, 'The Development of Methods for Inducing Labour,' 969–80, and Marc J.N.C. Keirse and Iain Chalmers, 'Methods for Inducing Labour,' 1058–79, in Iain Chalmers, Murray Enkin, and Marc J.N.C. Keirse, eds., *Effective Care in Pregnancy and Childbirth*, vol. 2 (Oxford, New York, and Toronto: Oxford University Press 1989). See also Arney, *Power and the Profession of Obstetrics*, 75–85.

58 William Victor Johnston, *Before the Age of Miracles: Memoirs of a Country Doctor* (Toronto: Fitzhenry & Whiteside 1972), 42. See also Victoria General Hospital, Halifax, patient no. 1290, register no. 1218, surgical department, patient Mrs Emily McIsaac, admitted 24 June 1921, discharged 12 July 1921.

59 *Manitoba Medical Review* 28 (April 1948): 179. See also *CMAJ* 22 (April 1930): 471.

60 *CMAJ* 13 (June 1923): 382.

61 Letter from BR, 9 August 1993; Marion O. Robinson, *Give My Heart: The Dr. Marion Hilliard Story* (Garden City, N.Y.: Doubleday 1964), 257; interview with Becki Crawford, 9 July 1993.

62 MUNFLA, no. 75-21, Mary Harriet Doyle, 'Midwifery in the Community of Calvert on the Southern Shore of Newfoundland,' 14; McGill University Archives, Royal Victoria Hospital, RG95, vol. 888, Obstetrical Casebook, patient no. 321, Mrs Roy, admitted 25 March 1902, discharged 26 March 1902; interview with Ruth Howard, 25 July 1993; interview with Jane Rutherford, 28 July 1993.

63 David Berry Hart, *Guide to Midwifery* (London: Rebman 1912), 196.

64 *Canadian Journal of Medicine and Surgery* 22 (August 1908): 79; *Canada Lancet* 50 (January 1916): 218

65 *Canada Lancet* 47 (September 1913): 9.

66 *Canadian Journal of Medicine and Surgery* 20 (September 1906): 176; *Canadian Practitioner and Review* 21 (October 1906): 548.

67 *Weekly Manitoba Liberal* (Portage La Prairie), 29 January 1914, 3.

68 *Canadian Journal of Medicine and Surgery* 24 (August 1908): 69, and 22 (August 1908): 76; *Canadian Practitioner and Review* 25 (March 1900): 116.

69 Joseph B. DeLee, *The Principles and Practice of Obstetrics* (Philadelphia: W.B. Saunders 1913), 293.

70 Calculations for the Ottawa Maternity Hospital based on statistical runs of patient records: 474 cases, provided by Suzann Buckley: Calculations for Kingston General Hospital based on obstetrical patient records from Kingston General Hospital, 6 October 1916 to 5 February 1920. Queen's University Archives, Kingston General Hospital Archives, Doran Case-book, QUA Coll. 500, R200. See also Marie-Aimée Cliche, 'Morale chrétienne et "double standard sexuel,"' 772. The rate in the United States was 50 per cent at the turn of the century, but this figure included both private and hospital practice. Judith Walzer Leavitt, *Brought to Bed: Child-Bearing in America 1750–1950* (New York: Oxford University Press 1986), 121.

71 Jewett, ed., *The Practice of Obstetrics*, 239.

72 *Canadian Practitioner and Review* 31 (January 1906): 9; *Montreal Medical Journal* 31 (October 1902): 772; *Canada Lancet* 47 (September 1913): 7–9, 12. Chloroform never went out of practice. Dr Geggie in his rural practice chose chloroform over other anaesthetics because of its cheapness and its lack of volatility compared to ether. Elliott, 'Endormez-moi!' 94.

73 See *Canadian Practitioner and Review* 32 (September 1907): 553; *Canada Lancet* 47 (September 1913): 9, and 50 (January 1916): 218; *CMAJ* 7 (March 1917): 223; Carl Henry Davis, *Painless Childbirth: Eutocia and Nitrous Oxid-Oxygen Analgesia* (Chicago: Forbes 1917), 5, 130–1. Apparently the focus on heroin began at the beginning of the war. *Canadian Nurse* 16 (August 1920): 470; *Dominion Medical Monthly* 48 (April 1917): 83; *CMAJ* 7 (May 1917): 405–7.

74 *Canada Lancet* 34 (November 1900): 114; Wright, *A Textbook of Obstetrics*, 144; *Canadian Practitioner and Review* 34 (September 1909): 549.

75 *Dominion Medical Monthly* 17 (October 1901): 183.

76 Payeur, 'Maternal Mortality in Quebec,' 104–5.

77 Johnston, *Before the Age of Miracles*, 42; *Canada Lancet* 53 (May 1920): 407.

R.W. Johnstone, *A Text-Book of Midwifery: For Students and Practitioners*
6th ed. (London: A. & C. Black 1934), 151; Ten Teachers, *Midwifery,* 5th ed.
(London: Edward Arnold 1935), 624; Denyse Baillargeon, 'L'encadrement
de la maternité au Québec entre les deux guerres: Les gardes de La
Metropolitaine, les gouttes de lait et l'assistance maternelle,' *Bulletin,
RCHTQ* 47 & 48 (1990): 41; *Canadian Nurse* 16 (August 1920): 470–1; *University of Toronto Medical Journal* 8 (March 1931): 196.

78 Johnstone, *A Text-book of Midwifery,* 151. According to a 1933 text, chloroform was the anaesthetic of choice in Scotland. J.M. Munro Kerr, J. Haig
Ferguson, James Young, and James Hendry, *Combined Textbook of Obstetrics
and Gynaecology for Students and Medical Practitioners,* 2nd ed. (Edinburgh:
E. & S. Livingstone 1933), 350.

79 *Canada Lancet* 53 (May 1920): 406. *Canadian Nurse* 16 (August 1920): 471;
Chatelaine October 1948, 22; interview with Betsy Lawrence, 30 August
1993.

80 *Hospital, Medical and Nursing World* 29 (April 1926): 105.

81 *Canadian Nurse* 23 (September 1927): 462. See also *CMAJ* 28 (January 1933):
44.

82 *University of Toronto Medical Journal* 12 (December 1934): 48–9. See also
Nova Scotia Medical Bulletin 15 (June 1936): 355; Fred L. Adair, ed., *Obstetrics and Gynecology,* vol. 2 (Philadelphia: Lea and Febiger 1940): 781;
Maclean's, 1 October 1945, 11.

83 Irvine Loudon, *Death in Childbirth: An International Study of Maternal Care
and Maternal Mortality 1800–1950* (Oxford: Clarendon Press 1992), 348, and
Margarete Sandelowski, *Pain, Pleasure, and American Childbirth: From the
Twilight Sleep to the Read Method, 1914–1960* (Westport, Conn.: Greenwood
Press 1984), 27.

84 *Saturday Night,* 5 June 1943, 18; *Chatelaine,* November 1943, 13; *University
of Toronto Medical Journal* 21 (January 1944): 146.

85 *Saturday Night,* 5 June 1943, 18. See also *Maclean's,* 15 July 1950, 6. Esther
Jackson wanted a caudal birth and went to a specific physician for that
reason. Still, she found the experience of delivery 'traumatic.' Interview
with Esther Jackson, 14 July 1993.

86 *CMAJ* 59 (December 1948): 558. See also *CMAJ* 58 (February 1948): 147.

87 *Maclean's,* 1 October 1945, 11, 57; *Chatelaine,* November 1943, 13; *Manitoba
Medical Review* 24 (April 1944): 104; *University of Toronto Medical Journal* 21
(January 1944): 158, and 28 (January 1951): 123; *Manitoba Medical Review*
24 (April 1944): 103; *CMAJ* 55 (July 1946): 43; Alfred C. Beck, *Obstetrical
Practice,* 4th ed. (Baltimore: Williams & Wilkins 1947), 895; *Bulletin of the
Academy of Medicine Toronto* 20 (July 1947): 213; *Alberta Medical Bulletin* 13

(January 1948): 69; *CMAJ* 59 (December 1948): 558; *CMAJ* 62 (February 1950): 116.

88 Beck, *Obstetrical Practice*, 894. See also *Alberta Medical Bulletin* 13 (January 1948): 69.

89 *Alberta Medical Bulletin* 15 (October 1950): 9–10.

90 *Nova Scotia Medical Bulletin* 15 (June 1936): 348; Henricus J. Stander, *Williams Obstetrics: A Textbook for the Use of Students and Practitioner*, 8th ed. (New York: Appleton-Century, 1941): 476; *Manitoba Medical Review* 27 (March 1947): 139.

91 *CMAJ* 35 (September 1936): 282.

92 James Winfred Bridges, *Psychology Normal and Abnormal with Special Reference to the Needs of Medical Students and Practitioners* (New York: D. Appleton 1930), 296. See also *CMAJ* 23 (October 1930): 564; *Saturday Night*, 5 June 1943, 18; *Manitoba Medical Review* 27 (March 1947): 139; *CMAJ* 22 (April 1930): 471.

93 *CMAJ* 23 (October 1930): 564; *Saturday Night*, 5 June 1943, 18; *Manitoba Medical Review* 27 (March 1947): 139; *CMAJ* 24 (January 1931): 22.

94 Laurel Halladay, '"We'll See You Next Year": Maternity Homes in Southern Saskatchewan in the First Half of the Twentieth Century' (MA thesis, Carleton University, 1996), 67.

95 Elliott, 'Endormez-moi!' 99, and Payeur, 'Maternal Mortality in Quebec,' 132.

96 Interview with Esther Thomas, 21 July 1993. See also interview with Dorothy Atkinson, 15 June 1993.

97 *Chatelaine*, November 1931, 67.

98 In 1929, 50 per cent of the maternity patients were given chloroform, 25 per cent were given a whiff of it, and 13 per cent were given a general anaesthetic. By 1935, chloroform still dominated, with 67 per cent of patients receiving it, but the use of general anaesthetic had increased to 23 per cent. By 1940, chloroform alone was used in 47 per cent of cases, but mixed with ether was given to another 47 per cent. Queen's University Archives, Kingston General Hospital, Obstetrical Record, Nickle Casebook.

99 Halladay, 'We'll See You Next Year,' 66.

100 Elliott, 'Endormez-moi!' 143–4.

101 *Nova Scotia Medical Bulletin* 13 (May 1934): 279; *CMAJ* 40 (April 1939): 369. See also *Alberta Medical Bulletin* 13 (January 1948): *CMAJ* 59 (September 1948): 225; *CMAJ* 31 (August 1934): 176. Dr Geggie in his practice experimented as well with some of the suggestions made in the medical literature. See Elliott, 'Endormez-moi!' 96–8.

102 Elliott, 'Endormez-moi!' 87, 95.

103 Harry Oxorn, *Harold Benge Atlee M.D.: A Biography* (Hantsport, N.S.: Lancelot Press 1983), 201, 265. For a feminist critique of natural childbirth, see Sandelowski, *Pain, Pleasure, and American Childbirth*, 136. William Ray Arney, in *Power and the Profession of Obstetrics*, has argued that in the 1980s and 1990s, doctors accommodated women in natural childbirth. By taking away the pain of childbirth, doctors had taken away women's involvement. Yet natural childbirth did not give it back to women as much as women thought. Obstetrics reached an accommodation. 'Birth should occur within a flexible system of obstetrical alternatives in which a woman's experience can take prominence against a backdrop of obstetrical expertise and safety' (220).

104 See *Modern Medicine of Canada* 1 (November 1946): 38; *Canadian Nurse* 43 (May 1947): 346–7; *Health* 17 (Sept.–Oct. 1949): 10; *Maclean's*, 15 July 1950, 7. Grantly Dick Read, *Childbirth without Fear: The Principles and Practice of Natural Childbirth* (New York: Harper 1944).

105 Public Archives of Nova Scotia, RG25, vol. 687(1), Department of Health, National Health Grants, H.B. Atlee, 'A Study into the Psychological Effects of Natural Childbirth on Mother and Baby,' 3; *Alberta Medical Bulletin* 14 (July 1949): 12; *Maclean's*, 15 July 1950, 49. See also *McGill Medical Journal* 17 (October 1948): 365.

106 Julie Vandervoort, *Tell the Driver: A Biography of Elinor F.E. Black* (Winnipeg: University of Manitoba 1992), 218–19. The search for a perfect pain reliever has not ended. At the end of the twentieth century increasing numbers of hospitals were reported offering women the opportunity to choose from among many ways of relieving pain, for example, walking and bathing or showering. Of the hospitals that responded to a 1993 survey, 68 per cent used nitrous oxide, 94 per cent offered narcotics, with 40 per cent of the women in these hospitals taking advantage of the offer. Fifty-five per cent of hospitals offered epidural anaesthesia. Levitt et al., *Survey of Routine Maternity Care*, 39–40.

107 *Canadian Practitioner and Review* 40 (January 1915): 24; *Canadian Nurse* 16 (August 1920): 470; Leavitt, *Brought to Bed*, 134. See also Judith Walzer Leavitt, 'Birthing and Anesthesia: The Debate over Twilight Sleep,' in Judith Walzer Leavitt, ed., *Women and Health in America: Historical Readings* (Madison: University of Wisconsin Press 1984), 175–84.

108 Loudon, *Death in Childbirth*, 348.

109 Ibid.

110 *Canadian Practitioner and Review* 34 (February 1909): 101; *Canada Lancet* 47 (September 1913): 9.

111 *Canadian Practitioner and Review* 40 (January 1915): 24; also 40 (February 1915): 79, and 40 (March 1915): 156; *Canada Lancet* 49 (October 1915): 67–73.

112 *Dominion Medical Monthly* 47 (October 1916): 57–8; *CMAJ* 7 (May 1917): 406.

113 *Canada Lancet* 48 (January 1915): 292–3.

114 *Canadian Practitioner and Review* 41 (June 1916): 283–5. See also *Canadian Practitioner and Review* 43 (June 1918): 201–22, and 43 (March 1918): 84.

115 *CMAJ* 6 (February 1916): 97–110.

116 *Canada Lancet* 50 (September 1916): 39–40; *Dominion Medical Monthly* 48 (April 1917): 81–2; *Canadian Practitioner and Review* 43 (March 1918): 84, and 43 (June 1918): 201–2

117 Oxorn, *Harold Benge Atlee M.D.*, 201.

118 *CMAJ* 14 (August 1924): 702. See also Beckman, *Treatment in General Practice*, 774; *Canada Lancet* 53 (May 1920): 409; *CMAJ* 11 (May 1921): 351. Certainly, hyoscine, scopolamine, and other drugs to bring about amnesia continued to be mentioned in descriptions of childbirth, especially in the first stage of labour, but in conjunction with other forms of anaesthesia not associated with the methods of twilight sleep. But occasionally the full process was mentioned as being employed. *University of Toronto Medical Journal* 12 (December 1934): 47; *CMAJ* 33 (November 1935): 485.

119 *CMAJ* 11 (May 1921): 354–5. See also Frederick C. Irving, *A Textbook of Obstetrics: For Students and Practitioners* (New York: Macmillan 1936), 170; F.L. Adair, ed., *Maternal Care and Some Complications* (Chicago: University of Chicago Press 1939), 45–6.

120 Aleck William Bourne, *Synopsis of Midwifery and Gynaecology*, 3rd ed. (Toronto: The Macmillan 1925), 92. See also Johnstone, *A Text-Book of Midwifery*, 152.

121 *Canada Lancet* 53 (May 1920): 406.

122 *CMAJ* 33 (November 1935): 485; *CMAJ* 35 (September 1936): 283; *CMAJ* 37 (November 1937): 472; *CMAJ* 59 (December 1948): 558; *CMAJ* 48 (January 1943): 51; *CMAJ* 19 (September 1928): 293.

123 *CMAJ* 19 (September 1928): 293.

124 *Annual Report of the Montreal Maternity Hospital*, 1901, 7, 9; Jewett, ed., *The Practice of Obstetrics*, 417; *Canadian Practitioner and Review* 31 (January 1906): 9; Hirst, *A Text-Book of Obstetrics*, 822; *Alberta Medical Bulletin* 13 (January 1948): 71.

125 *Montreal Medical Journal* 31 (October 1902): 772; *Canadian Practitioner and Review* 43 (March 1918): 83–4.

126 See *Annual Report of the Montreal Maternity Hospital*, 1901–12; H.L. Burris, *Medical Saga: The Burris Clinic and Early Pioneers* (n.p., n.d.), 88.

127 *Canada Medical Record* 30 (July 1902): 290–1. See also *Canadian Practitioner and Reveiw* 35 (September 1910): 655; *Canada Lancet* 47 (September 1913): 8.

128 *Canada Medical Record* 30 (August 1902): 360–2. Others agreed that forceps were being blamed for too much. See *Canada Lancet* 45 (May 1912): 677–8; *Canadian Practitioner and Review* 29 (March 1904): 109, and 31 (January 1906): 9.

129 *Canadian Practitioner and Review* 28 (January 1903): 38.

130 DeLee, *The Principles and Practice of Obstetrics*, 965. See Judith Walzer Leavitt, '"Science" Enters the Birthing Room: Obstetrics in America since the Eighteenth Century,' *Journal of American History* 70 (September 1983): 298.

131 *Canada Lancet* 37 (August 1904): 1123; *Canadian Practitioner and Review* 35 (September 1910): 655. See also *Canadian Practitioner and Review* 28 (January 1903): 39; *Canada Lancet* 47 (September 1913): 8, 9; *Canada Lancet* 47 (August 1914): 911; *Canadian Nurse* 13 (March 1917): 120–1; *CMAJ* 1 (February 1911): 132.

132 *Canadian Practitioner and Review* 21 (October 1906): 547.

133 *Canada Lancet* 34 (November 1900): 113–14. For varying rates, see *Canada Lancet* 37 (August 1904): 1125. William Almon had a 20 per cent rate. Public Archives of Nova Scotia, William Bruce Almon Obstetrical Casebook, MG1, no. 12–14, calculations based on 312 cases 1898–1912; *CMAJ* 7 (May 1917): 418; *Nova Scotia Medical Bulletin* 19 (May 1931): 322. For a study of a country practice and use of forceps, see *Canadian Practitioner and Review* 31 (January 1906): 6–9; Ottawa Maternity Hospital, calculations for 1912–14 based on 1,001 records, and for 1914–15 on 474 records, provided by Suzann Buckley. In 1919–20 forceps were used on 11 per cent of the patients at Women's College Hospital. Women's College Hospital, *Annual Report*, 1920, 13. James Langstaff's rate in the 1880s was 30 per cent. Jacalyn Duffin, *Langstaff: A Nineteenth-Century Medical Life* (Toronto: University of Toronto Press 1993), 194. In 1900 the estimated rate for forceps use in the United States was 8 per cent. Leavitt, *Brought to Bed*, 121.

134 *Dominion Medical Monthly* 43 (October 1914): 117–18; *CMAJ* 7 (May 1917): 418.

135 *CMAJ* 14 (September 1924): 801.

136 Cynthia Abeele, '"Nations Are Built of Babies": Maternal and Child Welfare in Ontario, 1914–1940' (PhD thesis, University of Guelph, 1987), 180; *Manitoba Medical Bulletin* 86 (October 1928): 8–9. For the link between forceps and maternal death, see *University of Toronto Medical Journal* 8 (March 1931): 196; *Canada Lancet and Practitioner* 78 (April 1932): 111;

University of Toronto Medical Journal 10 (January 1933): 80; *Canadian Nurse* 42 (May 1936): 214.

137 Victoria General Hospital, patient Mrs Mavis Booth, patient no. 801, register no. 700, surgical department, admitted 1 March 1921, discharged 24 March 1921.

138 *Chatelaine*, July 1928, 60; *CMAJ* 19 (August 1928): 231; *Canada Lancet and Practitioner* 70 (May 1928): 166; *CMAJ* 23 (December 1930): 761; Paul T. Harper, *Clinical Obstetrics* (Philadelphia: F.A. Davis 1930), 549; *Canada Lancet and Practitioner* 77 (August 1931); 33–4; *CMAJ* 34 (May 1936): 522; *University of Western Ontario Quarterly* 6 (1936): 28.

139 Atlee, *Grace Maternity Hospital, 1922–1972*, 3. See also *Hospital, Medical and Nursing World* 34 (September 1928): 3, 69; *CMAJ* 22 (April 1930): 471; *Nova Scotia Medical Bulletin* 16 (February 1938): 156. Rayfield Wood in the last journal felt that the prohibition of high forceps was not as clear cut as others suggested. A review of J.M.Munro Kerr's text in the *CMAJ* in 1938 pointed out that the reviewer did not think that Kerr was clear enough in his opinions of high forceps. The reviewer felt that in Kerr's hands it might be safe but this was certainly not the case in others. *CMAJ* 38 (February 1938): 202.

140 *Canada Lancet and Practitioner* 71 (October 1928): 123–4. See also *University of Toronto Medical Journal* 8 (March 1931): 196; *Canada Lancet and Practitioner* 77 (December 1931): 160; Stander, *Williams Obstetrics*, 1169; *Modern Medicine of Canada* 4 (July 1949): 53; *Chatelaine*, July 1928, 60; *Canada Lancet and Practitioner* 70 (May 1928): 166; Kerr et al., *Combined Textbook of Obstetrics and Gynaecology*, 359.

141 Janet McNaughton, 'The Role of the Newfoundland Midwife in Traditional Health Care, 1900 to 1970' (PhD thesis, Memorial University, 1989), 51.

142 Ten Teachers, *Midwifery*, 632. See also J.M. Munro Kerr, with Donald McIntyre and D. Fyfe Anderson, *Operative Obstetrics: A Guide to the Difficulties and Complications of Obstetric Practice*, 4th ed. (London: Bailliere, Tindall and Cox), 471.

143 McGill University Archives, Royal Victoria Hospital, vol. 120, conf. 22818, Mrs Jeanne Mercier, admitted 16 July 1937, and conf. 22802, Mrs Gail Saunders, admitted 12 July 1937; vol. 140, conf. 2615, Mrs Moira Arthurs, admitted 18 May 1939.

144 *CMAJ* 14 (October 1924): 907.

145 Bourne, *Synopsis of Midwifery and Gynaecology*, 91; *CMAJ* 35 (September 1936): 283; *CMAJ* 59 (December 1948): 558.

146 *CMAJ* 19 (September 1928): 293. See also *CMAJ* 33 (November 1935): 485; *CMAJ* 19 (August 1928): 217; *CMAJ* 33 (November 1935): 485.

147 *CMAJ* 31 (August 1934): 177; *CMAJ* 14 (August 1924): 704. For Geggie's and Walmsley's rates, see Elliott, 'Endormez-moi!' 144.

148 *CMAJ* 19 (September 1928): 293; *Manitoba Medical Review* 15 (December 1935): 4. A similar reference to the teaching needs of students increasing forceps rates at the Dalhousie University Public Health Centre Prenatal Clinic was also made. *CMAJ* 41 (October 1939): 384.

149 *CMAJ* 48 (January 1943): 51; *Annual Report of the Royal Victoria Hospital, Montreal,* 1930, 107–9; ibid., 1948, 37; Queen's University Archives, collection 500, vol. R200, Kingston General Hospital, Obstetrical Records, Nickle Casebook 1929–42 (used 1929, 1935, and 1940). Not much changed. Low forceps delivery for Ontario in 1982–3 was 18.9 per cent. C. Lesley Biggs, '"The Case of the Missing Midwives": A History of Midwifery in Ontario from 1795–1900,' in Arnup, Lévesque, and Pierson, eds., *Delivering Motherhood,* 32.

150 Dorothy C. Wertz, 'What Birth Has Done for Doctors: A Historical View,' *Women and Health* 8 (1983): 20.

151 *CMAJ* 19 (August 1928): 231; Loudon, *Death in Childbirth,* 221.

152 *CMAJ* 45 (August 1941): 139.

153 *CMAJ* 59 (December 1948): 558.

154 Strong-Boag and McPherson, 'Confinement of Women,' 91. See also *CMAJ* 48 (January 1943): 49, 51.

155 *CMAJ* 1 (February 1911): 131–2. See also *CMAJ* 1 (February 1911): 132.

156 *Dominion Medical Monthly* 28 (March 1907): 116. See also *Western Canadian Medical Journal* 1 (November 1907): 500.

157 Hirst, *A Text-Book of Obstetrics,* 193; Alfred Lewis Galabin and George Blacker, *The Practice of Midwifery,* 7th ed. (London: J. & A. Churchill, 1910), 648; Jellett, *A Manual of Midwifery,* 1013; *CMAJ* 1 (February 1911): 133.

158 *Montreal Medical Journal* 34 (January 1905): 25–6.

159 David James Evans, *Obstetrics: A Manual for Students and Practitioners* (Philadelphia: Lea Brothers 1900), 361.

160 *CMAJ* 10 (October 1920): 903; MUNFLA, no. 82–326, Barbara Doran, '"There Was No One but Myself": The Life of a Midwife in Outport Newfoundland,' 13; Leavitt, '"Science" Enters the Birthing Room,' 298; *CMAJ* 20 (June 1929): 647; interview with Jennie Graham, 29 June 1993. See also *CMAJ* 14 (October 1924): 906, and 14 (November 1924): 1095; *CMAJ* 45 (October 1941): 366; Harper, *Clinical Obstetrics,* 549; Davis, ed., *Gynecology and Obstetrics,* vol. 1, chap. 22, 8, chap. 6, 31; *CMAJ* 55 (December 1946): 561; *Modern Medicine of Canada* 3 (October 1948): 37.

161 *Maclean's,* 15 July 1950, 49.

162 Ian Graham, *Episiotomy: Challenging Obstetric Interventions* (Oxford: Blackwell Science 1997), 35.

163 *CMAJ* 48 (January 1943): 51.

164 See Strong-Boag and McPherson, 'Confinement of Women,' 95, for details; also *CMAJ* 48 (January 1943): 50.

165 Graham, *Episiotomy*, 46, 51–4.

166 These figures were based on a 1993 survey and analysis of Canadian hospital procedures. The conclusion of the survey was that there was no evidence that episiotomy prevented perineal trauma and the authors advocated it only for specific foetal indications. Levitt et al., *Survey of Routine Maternity Care*, 59. William Ray Arney argues that episiotomies in the United States were done to maintain the woman's vagina in the condition it had been, that is, for better (or tighter) intercourse from the man's perspective. Canadian physicians did not seem to raise this issue. Arney, *Power and the Profession of Obstetrics*, 69–75.

167 Denyse Baillargeon, 'Care of Mothers and Infants in Montreal between the Wars: The Visiting Nurses of Metropolitan Life, les gouttes de lait, and assistance maternelle,' in Dianne Dodd and Deborah Gorham, eds., *Caring and Curing: Historical Perspectives on Women and Healing in Canada* (Ottawa: University of Ottawa Press 1994), 175.

168 *CMAJ* 59 (August 1948): 171.

169 Andrée Lévesque, 'La santé des femmes en période de dépression économique,' *Bulletin, RCHTQ* (été-automne 1990): 16.

170 *Alberta Medical Bulletin* 14 (July 1949): 13.

171 Egbert H. Grandin and George W. Jarman, *A Textbook on Practical Obstetrics* (Philadelphia: F.A. Davis 1901), 204.

172 Haller Jr., 'Smut's Dark Poison,' 75–6.

173 *Dominion Medical Monthly* 14 (March 1900): 143; Jewett, ed., *The Practice of Obstetrics*, 619; *Canadian Practitioner and Review* 28 (January 1903): 22–3; also 34 (February 1909): 98, and 34 (September 1909): 549.

174 Jewett, ed., *The Practice of Obstetrics*, 619. See also *CMAJ* 8 (April 1918): 324.

175 *CMAJ* 4 (July 1914): 589.

176 Leavitt, '"Science" Enters the Birthing Room,' 298; *CMAJ* 11 (May 1921): 354; *CMAJ* 13 (September 1923): 678–9; *CMAJ* 17 (December 1927): 1436; *Canadian Nurse* 23 (September 1927): 463; *CMAJ* 19 (September 1928): 293; *Modern Medicine of Canada* 4 (July 1949): 53.

177 MUNFLA, no. 77-247, Linda Pauline Warford, 'Reminiscences of a Midwife of Upper Gullies in Conception Bay South,' 7.

7: Caesarian Section

1 *Canadian Medical Association Journal (CMAJ)* 56 (February 1947): 170.
2 *Canadian Practitioner and Review* 29 (April 1904): 196–7; *Maritime Medical News* 18 (March 1906): 89; The first c-section in Winnipeg did not occur until 1895. The Montreal Maternity Hospital first referred to c-section in its 1900 *Annual Report*. The patient was removed to another hospital for the surgery since the Montreal Maternity did not have the surgical facilities required. The Victoria General Hospital, Halifax, first mentioned one in 1906–7. *Manitoba Medical Review* 26 (May 1946): 275; *Annual Report of the Montreal Maternity Hospital*, 1900, 11; 'Report of the Commissioners of Public Charities, Victoria General Hospital,' 1906–7, Nova Scotia, *Journals of the House of Assembly*, 1908, appendix 3B, 87. See *Montreal Medical Journal* 36 (January 1907): 31; *Canadian Practitioner and Review* 34 (February 1909): 105; *CMAJ* 5 (November 1915): 968; and *Canada Lancet* 48 (March 1915): 423, for mention of the c-section's popularity. Also *Canadian Practitioner and Review* 43 (June 1918): 202; *Dominion Medical Monthly* 35 (August 1910): 45–6. For a discussion of c-section in the American context, see Joyce Antler and Daniel M. Fox, 'The Movement toward a Safe Maternity: Physician Accountability in New York City, 1915–1940,' *Bulletin of the History of Medicine* 50 (Winter 1976): 576.
3 See *CMAJ* 22 (January 1930): 29; *CMAJ* 39 (December 1938): 527; *CMAJ* 40 (March 1939): 259; *CMAJ* 45 (December 1941): 541; *Manitoba Medical Review* 30 (June–July 1950): 354; J. Clifton Edgar, *The Practice of Obstetrics*, 3rd ed. (Philadelphia: Blakiston 1907), ix; *Maritime Medical News* 22 (December 1910): 370; David Berry Hart, *Guide to Midwifery* (London: Rebman 1912), 408; *Canada Lancet* 44 (February 1911): 456; *Maritime Medical News* 18 (March 1906): 89; *Canadian Practitioner and Review* 34 (February 1909): 105. *CMAJ* 22 (April 1930): 471.
4 *CMAJ* 22 (April 1930): 471, 473; *Canadian Nurse* 26 (July 1930): 362. The number of comments on the ease of the surgery increased greatly, also its spectacular nature. See *CMAJ* 14 (October 1924): 907; Paul T. Harper, *Clinical Obstetrics* (Philadelphia: F.A. Davis 1930), 588–9; Henricus J. Stander, *Williams Obstetrics: A Textbook for the Use of Students and Practitioners*, 7th ed. (New York: D. Appleton-Century 1936), 599; *CMAJ* 45 (December 1941): 541; *Manitoba Medical Review* 30 (June–July 1950): 354; *CMAJ* 30 (May 1934): 498; *CMAJ* 34 (May 1936): 521; *CMAJ* 37 (July 1937): 32; 34; J. Munro Kerr, with Donald McIntyre and D. Fyfe Anderson, *Operative Obstetrics: A Guide to the Difficulties and Complications of Obstetric Practice,*

4th ed. (London: Bailliere, Tindall and Cox 1937), 512; *CMAJ* 40 (March 1939): 259; *Manitoba Medical Review* 21 (April 1941): 67.

5 *CMAJ* 14 (October 1924): 907; P. Brooke Bland, *Practical Obstetrics for Students and Practitioners* (Philadelphia: F.A. Saunders 1932), 615; Harper, *Clinical Obstetrics*, 588–9.

6 *Canadian Public Health Journal* 23 (December 1932): 566. For American figures, see *University of Toronto Medical Journal* 10 (January 1933): 81, and Dorothy C. Wertz, 'What Birth Has Done for Doctors: A Historical View,' *Women and Health* 8 (1983): 20; *Canadian Public Health Journal* 25 (December 1934): 573. For concern about the popularity of c-section, see J.M. Munro Kerr, J. Haig Ferguson, James Young, and James Hendry, *Combined Textbook of Obstetrics and Gynaecology for Students and Medical Practitioners*, 2nd ed. (Edinburgh: E.& S. Livingstone 1933), 631; Stander, *Williams Obstetrics*, 599: *CMAJ* 34 (May 1936): 520; *University of Western Ontario Quarterly* 6 (1936): 26; *CMAJ* 37 (July 1937): 32; *CMAJ* 38 (May 1938): 512; *CMAJ* 40 (March 1939): 259; *CMAJ* 42 (May 1940): 446; William Albert Scott and H. Brookfield Van Wyck, *The Essentials of Obstetrics and Gynecology* (Philadelphia: Lea & Febiger 1946): 228; *CMAJ* 56 (February 1947): 170; *University of Toronto Medical Journal* 10 (January 1933): 81; Bland, *Practical Obstetrics for Students and Practitioners*, 522; *Manitoba Medical Review* 21 (April 1941): 65; Frederick C. Irving, *A Textbook of Obstetrics: For Students and Practitioners* (New York: Macmillan 1936), 452.

7 *CMAJ* 39 (December 1938): 528; *CMAJ* 56 (February 1947): 170.

8 *CMAJ* 14 (October 1924): 903.

9 *Canadian Practitioner and Review* 49 (April 1924): 210. See also *CMAJ* 21 (December 1929): 656; Carl Henry Davis, ed., *Gynecology and Obstetrics*, vol. 1 (Hagerstown, Md: W.F. Prior 1935), chap. 22, 7; *CMAJ* 37 (July 1937): 34.

10 *University of Toronto Medical Journal* 15 (March 1938): 227. See also Harper, *Clinical Obstetrics*, 588–9; Bland, *Practical Obstetrics for Students and Practitioners*, 522. See also *Manitoba Medical Review* 21 (April 1941): 65; Irving, *A Textbook of Obstetrics*, 452.

11 *Canadian Hospital* 16 (September 1939): 38–9.

12 Fredelle Maynard, 'Cesareans: A Better Way to Give Birth?' *Chatelaine*, August 1981, 58; Megan Williams, 'Vaginal Birth after Cesarean,' *Healthsharing* (Winter–Spring 1992): 24. An Ontario study in 1991–2 revealed that c-section rates varied from hospital to hospital, from a low of 6.67 per cent to a high of 32.2 per cent. *Globe and Mail*, 26 May 1994, A2. In the United States, by comparison, the rate reached 25 by 1988. Gregory I. Goyert et al.,

'The Physician Factor in Cesarian Birth Rates,' *New England Journal of Medicine*, 16 March 1989, 706; Janice G. Raymond, *Women as Wombs: Reproductive Technologies and the Battle over Women's Freedom* (San Francisco: Harper 1993), 117.

13 For Royal Victoria Hospital rates, see *CMAJ* 40 (March 1939): 260. Between 1925 and 1939 the rate was 2.97. For Burnside figures, see *CMAJ* 44 (March 1941): 280. For Montreal Maternity figures, see *Annual Report of the Montreal Maternity Hospital*, 1912, 8, and 1915, 23. For Vancouver General figures, see *CMAJ* 48 (January 1943): 49, and Veronica Strong-Boag and Kathryn McPherson, 'The Confinement of Women: Childbirth and Hospitalization in Vancouver, 1919–1939,' in Katherine Arnup, Andrée Lévesque, and Ruth Roach Pierson, eds., *Delivering Motherhood: Maternal Ideologies and Practices in the Nineteenth and Twentieth Centuries* (London: Routledge 1990), 91. For Winnipeg General Hospital figures, see *Manitoba Medical Review* 15 (December 1935): 4; *CMAJ* 39 (December 1938): 528.

14 *CMAJ* 39 (December 1938): 528; *Manitoba Medical Review* 30 (June–July 1950): 354; Harper, *Clinical Obstetrics*, 589.

15 *CMAJ* 45 (August 1941): 139.

16 *Canadian Public Health Journal* 25 (December 1934): 573.

17 *CMAJ* 43 (July 1940): 43; Julie Vandervoort, *Tell the Driver: A Biography of Elinor F.E. Black* (Winnipeg: University of Manitoba Press 1992), 212. American studies in the 1980s revealed a similar class element. Jeffrey B. Gould, Becky Davey, and Randall S. Stafford, 'Socioeconomic Differences in Rates of Cesarean Section,' *New England Journal of Medicine*, 27 July 1989, 233.

18 *CMAJ* 43 (July 1940): 43.

19 *Manitoba Medical Review* 30 (June–July 1950): 357–8.

20 Montreal Maternity Hospital, annual reports, 1901–4. Embryotomy was not the only procedure used in cases of severe disproportion. The physicians could perform a pubiotomy. In attempts to ensure the birth of a live child the physicians would separate the pubic bones of the mother to allow the child to be delivered. David James Evans of the Montreal Maternity Hospital described a case he had in 1906. Patient E.M. aged twenty-four and pregnant for the third time, was admitted to the hospital on 8 September 1906. Previous pregnancies had necessitated craniotomies due to a 'flat rachitic pelvis.' Evans had decided to opt for a c-section, but with the rupturing of the membranes he decided on a pubiotomy instead. Fortunately, mother and child survived the procedure. This was not always the case, since it could result in severe damage to the mother. Because of this and because it necessitated great skill, it was not a common procedure.

Canadian Practitioner and Review 32 (January 1907): 22. See also Canadian Practitioner and Review 34 (February 1909): 104; Maritime Medical News 21 (September 1909): 337; Dominion Medical Monthly 35 (August 1910): 45–6; Maritime Medical News 22 (December 1910): 370; Thomas Watts Eden, A Manual of Midwifery, 4th ed. (Toronto: Macmillan 1915), 721. For a gruesome description of pubiotomy, see Canadian Practitioner and Review 32 (January 1907): 18; Richard C. Norris, ed., An American Text-Book of Obstetrics for Practitioners and Students (Philadelphia: W.B. Saunders, 1895), 917–18; Queen's Medical Quarterly 3 (January 1900): 74.

21 Edgar, The Practice of Obstetrics, ix.
22 Montreal Medical Journal 34 (May 1907): 317. See also Canadian Practitioner and Review 29 (April 1904): 196–7.
23 Hart, Guide to Midwifery, 438.
24 Montreal Medical Journal 34 (May 1907): 318–19.
25 Canada Lancet 43 (April 1910): 577.
26 Maritime Medical News 21 (September 1909): 337; Dominion Medical Monthly 33 (August 1909): 63; Eden, A Manual of Midwifery, 721.
27 CMAJ 16 (February 1924): 119. See also Canada Lancet and Practitioner 64 (March 1925): 116.
28 Manitoba Medical Review 15 (October 1935): 3. See also a case at the Grace Maternity Hospital, Halifax. Nova Scotia Medical Bulletin 19 (June 1940): 365. The records of Dr Geggie's rural Gatineau Valley practice also revealed embryotomies being done well into the 1930s. Jayne Elliott, '"Endormez-moi!" An Early Twentieth-Century Obstetrical Practice in the Gatineau Valley, Quebec' (MA thesis, Carleton University 1997), 105.
29 CMAJ 3 (October 1913): 836.
30 Maritime Medical News 15 (December 1903): 566. See also William Thompson Lusk, The Science and Art of Midwifery, 3rd ed. (New York: D. Appleton 1889), 425; Norris, ed., An American Text-Book of Obstetrics, 917–18; David James Evans, Obstetrics: A Manual for Students and Practitioners (Philadelphia: Lea Brothers 1900), 405. Charles Reed in his 1901 text posited a third scenario – faced with a woman who was unlikely ever to be delivered vaginally, perform a c-section so as to sterilize her at the same time. Reed deemed a present risk acceptable to offset future risks (additional embryotomies). Charles A.L. Reed, ed., A Text-Book of Gynecology (New York: D. Appleton and Company 1901), 464.
31 Reed, ed., A Text-Book of Gynecology, 461; Maritime Medical News 21 (September 1909): 337.
32 J. Clarence Webster, A Textbook of Obstetrics (Philadelphia: W.B. Saunders 1903), 712. See also Hart, Guide to Midwifery, 408.

33 *CMAJ* 3 (October 1913): 836. For an excellent discussion of risk, see Jo Murphy-Lawless, *Reading Birth and Death: A History of Obstetric Thinking* (Bloomington: Indiana University Press 1998), chap. 4; and Patricia A. Kaufert and John O'Neill, 'Analysis of a Dialogue on Risks in Childbirth: Clinicians, Epidemiologists, and Inuit Women,' in Shirley Lindenbaum and Margaret Lock, eds., *Knowledge, Power and Practice: The Anthropology of Medicine and Everyday Life* (Berkeley: University of California Press 1993), 32–54.

34 *Canadian Practitioner and Review* 29 (April 1904): 196–7. See also Webster, *A Textbook of Obstetrics*, 712; *Canada Lancet* 43 (April 1910): 579.

35 *CMAJ* 1 (February 1911): 129.

36 *Maritime Medical News* 18 (March 1906): 89. Reddy felt it was still warranted in cases of eclampsia when the os was not dilated. *CMAJ* 1 (October 1911): 1070. See also Alfred Lewis Galabin and George Blacker, *The Practice of Midwifery*, 7th ed. (London: J. & A. Churchill 1910), 904.

37 *Montreal Medical Journal* 37 (November 1908): 825.

38 *CMAJ* 5 (November 1915): 968. See also *Canadian Practitioner and Review* 47 (April 1922): 142–3.

39 *CMAJ* 14 (October 1924): 907. See also *CMAJ* 42 (May 1940): 446; *CMAJ* 43 (July 1940): 43; *Manitoba Medical Review* 21 (April 1941): 67.

40 *CMAJ* 16 (February 1924): 118.

41 Jo Oppenheimer, 'Childbirth in Ontario: The Transition from Home to Hospital in the Early Twentieth Century,' in Arnup, Lévesque, and Pierson, eds., *Delivering Motherhood*, 66; *Canadian Public Health Journal* 25 (March 1934): 142, and 25 (December 1934): 573. For general figures, see *Canadian Nurse* 27 (June 1932): 289; *CMAJ* 30 (May 1934): 498; *Canadian Public Health Journal* 23 (December 1932): 565–6. See also *Canada Lancet and Practitioner* 64 (March 1925): 116. For Winnipeg General Hospital figures, see *CMAJ* 39 (December 1938): 531.

42 Antler and Fox, 'The Movement Toward a Safe Maternity,' 581–2.

43 Harper, *Clinical Obstetrics*, 593; *Nova Scotia Medical Bulletin* 12 (October 1933): 588. Feminist scholars in recent years have criticized physicians for using the language of economics to justify c-sections, that is, a c-section will guarantee a better product (child). See Helen Bequaert Holmes and Laura M. Purdy, *Feminist Perspectives in Medical Ethics* (Bloomington: University of Indiana Press 1992), 279–80). Physicians in the first half of the twentieth century certainly were not that blatant. Their concern was a live child and a healthy one, and given their experiences before c-sections, their focus was understandable.

44 *Canadian Nurse* 26 (July 1930): 363. See also *CMAJ* 37 (July 1937): 34; *University of Toronto Medical Journal* 15 (March 1938): 227.

45 *CMAJ* 12 (June 1922): 406–7.

46 *CMAJ* 37 (July 1937): 33–4; *University of Toronto Medical Journal* 15 (March 1938): 227.

47 Richard and Dorothy Wertz have argued that c-sections increased in the United States as a result but that statistics failed to reveal any significant saving of infant life. Richard C. Wertz and Dorothy C. Wertz, *Lying-In: A History of Childbirth in American* (New York: Schocken Books 1979), 161.

48 *Bulletin of the Academy of Medicine Toronto* 20 (July 1947): 212.

49 *CMAJ* 43 (July 1940): 43.

50 *Canadian Hospital* 26 (September 1949): 80.

51 *CMAJ* 44 (March 1941): 282; Scott and Van Wyck, *The Essential of Obstetrics and Gynecology*, 228.

52 *CMAJ* 44 (January 1941): 38.

53 Henry Jellett, *A Manual of Midwifery for Students and Practitioners*, 2nd ed. (London: Bailliere, Tindall and Cox 1910), 1096, 1083. See also Hirst, *A Text-Book of Obstetrics*, 868–70.

54 *Canadian Journal of Medicine and Surgery* 33 (June 1913): 403.

55 *CMAJ* 20 (June 1929): 647–8. See also *CMAJ* 14 (October 1924): 903; *CMAJ* 21 (June 1929): 656.

56 *CMAJ* 14 (September 1924): 803. See also *CMAJ* 14 (October 1924): 907; *Canadian Nurse* 34 (December 1938): 700; *CMAJ* 42 (May 1940): 446; Stander, *Williams Obstetrics*, 599; J.S. Fairbairn, *Gynaecology with Obstetrics: A Text-Book for Students and Practitioners* (London: Humphrey Milford, Oxford University Press 1924), 702–3.

57 *Canadian Journal of Medicine and Surgery* 75 (February 1934): 46; *Child and Family Welfare* 11 (November 1935): 14; Fred L. Adair, ed., *Obstetrics and Gynecology*, vol. 1 (Philadelphia: Lea & Febiger 1940), 44; Kerr, with McIntyre and Anderson, *Operative Obstetrics*, 512; *CMAJ* 40 (March 1939): 260; *Manitoba Medical Review* 30 (June–July 1950): 354; Stander, *Williams Obstetrics*, 1145. Dr Nigel Rusted of St John's, Newfoundland, noted that only surgeons performed c-sections. Memorial University of Newfoundland, interview, Dr Nigel Rusted, shelf no. c11362, 21 April 1986, interviewed by Janet McNaughton.

58 Bland, *Practical Obstetrics for Students and Practitioners*, 615.

59 Harper, *Clinical Obstetrics*, 588–9. See also *CMAJ* 40 (March 1939): 259; Scott and Van Wyck, *The Essential of Obstetrics and Gynecology*, 228; *CMAJ* 62 (February 1950): 114; *Manitoba Medical Review* 30 (June–July 1950): 354; *CMAJ* 37 (July 1937): 37; *Canadian Hospital* 16 (September 1939): 38.

60 Lusk, *The Science and Art of Midwifery*, 425; Webster, *A Textbook of Obstetrics*, 712; *Canada Lancet* 43 (December 1909): 275–6, and 44 (June 1911): 771;

Fairbairn, *Gynaecology with Obstetrics*, 702–3; *Canadian Nurse* 27 (March 1931: 130; Stander, *Williams Obstetrics*, 1195.

61 *Montreal Medical Journal* 37 (November 1908): 822. In 1941 a Toronto physician gave almost the same measurements. *CMAJ* 44 (January 1941): 38. See also *Montreal Medical Journal* 34 (May 1907): 317; *CMAJ* 3 (October 1913): 838; *Montreal Medical Journal* 36 (January 1907): 31; *Maritime Medical News* 22 (December 1910): 370.

62 *Canada Medical Record* 30 (October 1902): 434–35; *Montreal Medical Journal* 36 (January 1907): 31. See also *Canada Lancet* 45 (May 1912): 669–700, 702–3, and 44 (June 1911); 722; also *Canada Lancet* 43 (July 1910): 839. For a description of the history of c-section for placenta previa in England and the United States, see Irvine Loudon, *Death in Childbirth: An International Study of Maternal Care and Maternal Mortality 1900–1950* (Oxford: Clarendon Press 1992), 102.

63 *CMAJ* 3 (October 1913): 836; British Medical Association, Nova Scotia Branch, *Minutes*, 18 March 1908, 239.

64 Loudon, *Death in Childbirth*, 102.

65 *Canada Lancet* 43 (April 1910): 572–3; *CMAJ* 1 (October 1911): 1070. See also *Montreal Medical Journal* 36 (January 1907): 31; *CMAJ* 3 (October 1913): 842; *CMAJ* 6 (February 1916): 117; *University of Toronto Medical Bulletin* 1 (April 1913): 60; *Canada Lancet* 44 (February 1911): 456, and 44 (March 1911): 528–9.

66 *Canada Lancet* 44 (March 1911): 528.

67 *Montreal Medical Journal* 34 (May 1907): 317–18. See also *Maritime Medical News* 21 (September 1909): 338.

68 Eden, *A Manual of Midwifery*, 721. See also *Canada Lancet* 48 (March 1915): 423.

69 *CMAJ* 12 (June 1922): 405. See also *CMAJ* 14 (October 1924): 907; *CMAJ* 17 (December 1927): 1435; *Canadian Nurse* 34 (December 1938): 700; *Nova Scotia Medical Bulletin* 12 (October 1933): 588; *Canadian Nurse* 27 (June 1932): 289.

70 *CMAJ* 44 (March 1941): 281–3. Others agreed about heart complications no longer being an indicator. *University of Toronto Medical Journal* 24 (March 1947): 153.

71 *CMAJ* 21 (December 1929): 656.

72 D. Sclater Lewis, *Royal Victoria Hospital, 1887–1947* (Montreal: McGill University Press 1969), 289.

73 William Victor Johnston, *Before the Age of Miracles: Memoirs of a Country Doctor* (Toronto: Fitzhenry & Whiteside 1972), 42.

74 Kitchener-Waterloo Hospital, Mrs Jackson Hover, patient no. 19, entered 2 January 1943.

75 Harold Burrows, *Mistakes and Accidents of Surgery* (Toronto: McClelland and Stewart 1923), 273. For a study of the individualism of practice, see Gregory I. Goyert et al., 'The Physician Factor in Cesarean Birth Rates,' *New England Journal of Medicine*, 16 March 1989, 706.

76 *Nova Scotia Medical Bulletin* 12 (September 1933): 529.

77 *CMAJ* 22 (January 1930): 29; *Nova Scotia Medical Bulletin* 11 (June 1932): 354. For a debate on placenta praevia, see *CMAJ* 37 (July 1937): 34; *CMAJ* 42 (May 1940): 442; *CMAJ* 46 (April 1942): 319; *Bulletin of the Academy of Medicine* 20 (July 1947): 212. For other opinions on rejecting eclampsia as an indicator, see Ten Teachers, *Midwifery*, 5th ed. (London: Edward Arnold 1935), 663; *CMAJ* 30 (May 1934): 498, 500; *CMAJ* 37 (July 1937): 35.

78 *CMAJ* 39 (December 1938): 531.

79 Fairbairn, *Gynaecology with Obstetrics*, 702–3; *CMAJ* 22 (April 1930): 471; *CMAJ* 56 (February 1947): 170.

80 *Dominion Medical Monthly* 35 (August 1910): 45–6; *CMAJ* 34 (May 1936): 520; *CMAJ* 37 (July 1937): 37; *Canadian Nurse* 32 (May 1936): 214; *CMAJ* 14 (October 1924): 907; *Canadian Public Health Journal* 25 (March 1934): 142. See also *Child and Family Welfare* 11 (November 1935): 14; *CMAJ* 43 (July 1940): 43.

81 *CMAJ* 39 (December 1938): 531.

82 One physician interviewed felt that some women requested c-sections because they 'didn't want to go through labour.' Letter to author from Dr BR, 9 August 1993. Maria deKonick, who has studied c-section in Canada in recent years, has noted that the normalization of c-section has been partially a result of women seeing 'in its practice a way of dealing with childbirth which reduces its pain and "their liability" in regard to the perfect child.' Feminist Strategic Health Network, April 1994. On the issue of choice, see Raymond, *Women as Wombs*, x.

83 *CMAJ* 16 (February 1924): 118.

84 *Canadian Practitioner and Review* 47 (April 1922): 142.

85 *CMAJ* 22 (April 1930): 473.

86 Reed, ed., *A Text-Book of Gynecology*, 464.

87 *Montreal Medical Journal* 34 (May 1907): 317, and 37 (November 1908): 823–4; *Canada Lancet* 44 (June 1911): 770.

88 *Montreal Medical Journal* 36 (January 1907): 34.

89 *Canada Lancet* 43 (1910): 591. See also *University of Toronto Medical Bulletin* 1 (April 1913): 60; *CMAJ* 3 (October 1913): 836, 844.

90 *Canadian Practitioner and Review* 36 (May 1911). See also Hirst, *A Text-Book of Obstetrics*, 868–70.

91 Eden, *A Manual of Midwifery*, 734. See also *Nova Scotia Medical Bulletin* 4 (May 1925): 3.

92 *CMAJ* 12 (June 1922): 407. See also *Nova Scotia Medical Bulletin* 8 (1929): 469.

93 *CMAJ* 14 (September 1924): 801; sterilization for women with severe health problems was not an issue. *CMAJ* 17 (December 1927): 1435; Fred L. Adair, ed., *Obstetrics and Gynecology*, vol. 2 (Philadelphia: Lea & Febiger 1940), 834; *CMAJ* 42 (May 1940): 442; *CMAJ* 29 (August 1933): 164; *Canadian Nurse* 34 (December 1938): 700; interview with Drs M and H, Halifax, 29 October 1993; *CMAJ* 30 (May 1934): 498; *CMAJ* 44 (March 1941): 281. In the early 1990s, 40 per cent of c-sections occurred simply because a woman had previously given birth that way. Megan Williams, 'Vaginal Birth after Cesarean,' 24.

94 For discussion of a previous c-section not being an absolute indication for a subsequent c-section, see *CMAJ* 22 (January 1930): 29; Bland *Obstetrics for Students and Practititoners*, 614; *CMAJ* 44 (March 1941): 282. For the importance of seeing each labour on its own merits, see Davis, ed., *Gynecology and Obstetrics*, vol. 2, chap. 4, 7; Stander, *Williams Obstetrics*, 620; *CMAJ* 56 (February 1947): 174; *Manitoba Medical Review* 30 (June–July 1950): 358. For Ross Mitchell's view, see *CMAJ* 39 (December 1938): 529.

95 *Canadian Nurse* 27 (March 1931): 133. See also Harper, *Clinical Obstetrics*, 598; Bland, *Practical Obstetrics for Students and Practitioners*, 614; *CMAJ* 56 (February 1947): 170; Kerr, with McIntyre and Anderson, *Operative Obstetrics*, 533.

96 *CMAJ* 57 (October 1947): 403. It is always dangerous to generalize about a specific group of people. For example, while the Catholic Church frowned on the use of birth control, interviews with some Catholic women have suggested their willingness, in the inter-war period, to use it. See Denyse Baillargeon, *Ménagères au temps de la crise* (Montreal: Éditions Remu-Menage 1991), 102.

97 Ten Teachers, *Midwifery*, 671. See also Kerr, with McIntyre and Anderson, *Operative Obstetrics*, 532; Sir Comyns Berkeley and Victor Bonney, *A Textbook of Gynaecological Surgery*, 4th ed. (London: New York: Cassell 1942), 454.

98 Cynthia Comacchio, in her book *'Nations Are Built of Babies': Saving Ontario's Mothers and Children, 1900–1940* (Montreal: McGill-Queen's University Press 1993), sees the doctor-state relationship as a major theme.

99 *CMAJ* 43 (July 1940): 63.

100 *CMAJ* 44 (March 1941): 281–3.

101 Stander, *Williams Obstetrics*, 617.

102 *CMAJ* 37 (July 1937): 35.

103 Samuel S. Peikoff, *Yesterday's Doctor: An Autobiography* (Winnipeg: Prairie Publishing 1980), 1.
104 *CMAJ* 34 (May 1936): 520.
105 *CMAJ* 37 (July 1937): 34, 37. See also Vandervoort, *Tell the Driver*, 211.
106 *University of Toronto Medical Journal* 10 (January 1933): 80. See also *Canadian Nurse* 32 (May 1936): 214; *CMAJ* 40 (March 1939): 259–60.
107 *CMAJ* 37 (July 1937): 34; *Nova Scotia Medical Bulletin* 19 (June 1940): 363; David Gollacher, 'From Ritual to Science: The Medical Transformation of Circumcision in America,' *Journal of Social History* 1 (Fall 1994): 24.
108 *CMAJ* 117 (August 6 1977): 288.

8: Maternal Mortality and Postnatal Care

1 *Canadian Medical Association Journal (CMAJ)* 29 (August 1933): 159.
2 Helene Laforce, in *Histoire de la sage-femme dans la région de Québec* (Quebec: Institute québécois de recherche sur la culture, Collection: Edmond-de-Nevers no. 4, 1985), argues that maternal mortality rates increased at the turn of the century because of increasing physician control over birth. Edward Shorter argues the opposite – that doctors came to women's rescue. See his *A History of Women's Bodies* (New York: Basic Books 1982).
3 Other causes of underreporting were deficiencies in death certificate forms and also the ability of physicians to classify some maternal deaths in other categories. The 20 to 25 per cent underreporting was based on studies by the Ontario and Dominion governments' departments of health. George Emery, 'Fatal Pregnancies in Ontario, 1920–1935: A Reappraisal of the Published Vital Statistics' (paper presented to the Canadian Historical Association, Victoria, 1990), 1–2, 7, 29–30.
4 *Census*, 1901, 4: 235. The rate peaked between 1910 and 1920. C. Lesley Biggs, 'The Response to Maternal Mortality in Ontario, 1920–1940' (MA thesis, University of Toronto 1983), 25; National Council of Women, *Yearbook 1923*, 60. For 1926 rates, see *CMAJ* 17 (December 1927): 1434; *Manitoba Medical Bulletin* 79 (March 1928): 8; *Canadian Nurse* 24 (April 1928): 180. See Cynthia Abeele, '"Nations Are Built of Babies": Maternal and Child Welfare in Ontario, 1914–1940' (PhD thesis, University of Guelph, 1987), 137–9, appendix 1.2, for the early decades of the century. For American rates, see Joyce Antler and Daniel M. Fox, 'The Movement toward a Safe Maternity: Physician Accountability in New York City, 1915–1940,' *Bulletin of Medical History* 50 (Winter 1976): 574, and Margarete Sandelowski, *Pain, Pleasure, and American Childbirth: From the Twilight Sleep to the Read Method, 1914–1960* (Westport, Conn.: Greenwood Press 1984), 37–8.

5 Ann Oakley, *The Captured Womb: A History of the Medical Care of Pregnant Women* (Oxford: Basil Blackwell 1984), 76.

6 For 1937 rates and those in the 1940s, see Florence H.M. Emory, *Public Health Nursing in Canada* (Toronto: Macmillan 1953), 184; *CMAJ* 46 (January 1942): 1; and Cynthia R. Comacchio, *'Nations Are Built of Babies': Saving Ontario's Mothers and Children 1900–1940* (Montreal: McGill-Queen's University Press 1993), 233. The figures for maternal mortality from 1929 to 1943 are as follows: in 1929, 5.7; 1930, 5.8; 1931, 5.1; 1932, 5.0; 1933, 5.0; 1934, 5.3; 1935, 4.9; 1936, 5.6; 1937, 4.9; 1938, 4.2; 1939, 4.2; 1940, 4.0; 1941, 3.5; 1942, 3.0; and 1943, 2.8. Canadian Youth Commission, *Youth and Health: A Positive Health Programme for Canada* (Toronto: Ryerson Press 1946), 45. The 1926 estimates of women dying between the ages of 15 and 50, were that 11.9 per cent died from pregnancy, 27.2 per cent from TB, 8.6 per cent from cancer, 8.1 per cent from heart conditions, and 4.9 per cent from pneumonia. See *CMAJ* 23 (August 1930): 169, and *Nova Scotia Medical Bulletin* 10 (October 1931): 738–9. At times, heart disease seemed to vie with childbirth for second place. *Chatelaine* 3 (October 1930): 28. When statistics between the 1930s and 1960s are compared, the differences are impressive: in the earlier years maternal mortality accounted for 10–15 per cent of all deaths of women in the childbearing years, but in the later period only 2–3 per cent. The chances of dying in pregnancy fell from one in 150 to one in 3,000. Angus McLaren and Arlene Tigar McLaren, 'Discoveries and Dissimulations: The Impact of Abortion Deaths on Maternal Mortality in British Columbia,' in Katherine Arnup, Andrée Lévesque, and Ruth Roach Pierson, eds., *Delivering Motherhood: Maternal Ideologies and Practices in the Nineteenth and Twentieth Centuries* (London: Routledge 1990), 126.

7 *American Journal of Public Health*, 1932, 625. Manitoba rates revealed variation across ethnic groups. In the late 1930s, the rate for British women was 2.6 per 1000 live births; for Native women it was 7.5, and for Métis 13.2. *Canadian Public Health Journal* 32 (February 1941): 69.

8 *Child and Family Welfare* 11 (November 1935): 11; *Canadian Nurse* 42 (May 1936): 213; *Saturday Night*, 17 April 1937, 39.

9 *Canadian Public Health Journal* 31 (July 1940): 339; Canadian Youth Commission, *Youth and Health*, 46.

10 In 1902 the rate was 1.43 or three deaths out of 209 confinements; in 1905, 0.67; in 1911, 1.137; in 1915, 0.64; in 1920, 0.80. For rates see *Annual Report of the Montreal Maternity Hospital*, 1901, 9; 1902, 10; 1903, 16–17; 1904, 18; 1905, 20–1; 1908, 20; 1909, 21–2; 1911, 24–5; 1912, 13; 1913, 24–5; 1914, 21; 1915, 22–3; 1916, 27; and 1920, 27. In 1926 the rate was 0.33 per cent; it was

0.6 in 1930, 0.79 in 1935, 0.20 in 1940, 0.08 in 1945, and in 1946 had decreased to 0.03 per cent. D. Sclater Lewis, *Royal Victoria Hospital, 1887–1947* (Montreal: McGill University Press 1969), 285; *Annual Report of the Royal Victoria Hospital, Montreal*, 1933, 24; ibid., 1934, 23; ibid., 1948, 35; *Canadian Nurse* 39 (November 1943): 720. For a discussion of maternal mortality at the Montreal Maternity Hospital 1905–9, see *CMAJ* 1 (February 1911): 125–35. For the Vancouver General Hospital, 1933–41, see *CMAJ* 48 (January 1943): 50. The Kingston General Hospital, 1916–20, had a maternal mortality rate of 0.7 per cent (calculations based on patient records). Queen's University Archives, Kingston General Hospital Archives, Doran Case Book, QUA Coll. 500, R200, Operating Room books 1911–50, October 1916 to February 1920, 447 cases.

11 *Annual Report of the Montreal Maternity Hospital*, 1915, 21–4, calculated on the statistics provided; annual report of 1918, 26–7. See also annual report of 1919, 28.

12 H.J.G. Geggie, *The Extra Mile: Medicine in Rural Quebec, 1885–1965* (Ottawa: National Library of Canada 1987), 52; Jayne Elliott, '"Endormez-moi!": An Early Twentieth-Century Obstetrical Practice in the Gatineau Valley, Quebec' (MA thesis, Carleton University 1997), 132.

13 Herbert A. Bruce, *Varied Operations, 1868–1958* (Toronto: Longmans 1958), 112.

14 Penelope Stewart, 'Infant Feeding in Canada: 1910–1940' (MA thesis, Concordia University 1982), 117. For charts on 1927 and 1928 maternal deaths by cause and by whether hospitalized or not, see *American Journal of Public Health* (1932): 618–19. In Manitoba for most of the 1920s, hospital births had three times the mortality rate of non-hospital births. *Manitoba Medical Bulletin* 99 (November 1929): 3. See also *Canadian Public Health Journal* 21 (May 1930): 221; *CMAJ* 21 (October 1929): 450; Jo Oppenheimer, 'Childbirth in Ontario: The Transition from Home to Hospital in the Early Twentieth Century,' in Katherine Arnup, Andrée Lévesque, and Ruth Roach Pierson, eds., *Delivering Motherhood* (London: Routledge 1990), 66; *Canadian Public Health Journal* 25 (December 1934): 572–3; *Canadian Hospital* 11 (December 1934): 20. Studies in the U.S. also confirmed that hospital births in the 1930s were more dangerous than home births. Irvine Loudon, *Death in Childbirth: An International Study of Maternal Care and Maternal Mortality 1800–1950* (Oxford: Clarendon Press 1992), 363–4. Studies in Aberdeen Scotland also confirmed this. *CMAJ* 22 (May 1930): 735.

15 Antler and Fox,' The Movement toward a Safe Maternity,' 582.

16 *Canada Lancet and Practitioner* 77 (December 1931): 161. See also *University of Toronto Medical Journal* 8 (March 1931): 195; *Canadian Public Health*

Journal 22 (July 1931): 348, and 23 (December 1932): 562; *CMAJ* 36 (June 1937): 600, and 43 (July 1940): 41; *Maclean's*, 1 October 1945, 58; *Canada Lancet and Practitioner* 78 (April 1932): 115.

17 Veronica Strong-Boag and Kathryn McPherson, 'The Confinement of Women: Childbirth and Hospitalization in Vancouver, 1919–1939,' in Gillian Creese and Veronica Strong-Boag, eds., *British Columbia Reconsidered: Essays on Women* (Vancouver: Press Gang 1992), 155–6.

18 See *Child and Family Welfare* 11 (November 1935): 11; *Canadian Nurse* 42 (May 1936): 213; *CMAJ* 48 (January 1943): 48; *Canadian Hospital* 23 (May 1946): 31–2; Public Archives of Nova Scotia, *Report on the Survey of Hospitals in Nova Scotia 1949*, 30; *Canadian Hospital* 26 (September 1949): 40; *Bulletin of the Academy of Medicine Toronto* 20 (July 1947): 211.

19 For Seymour and Red Cross hospitals, see Jutta Mason, 'Midwifery in Canada,' in Sheila Kitzinger, ed., *The Midwife Challenge* (London: Pandora Press 1988), 105–6. For rural and urban differences, see Stewart 'Infant Feeding in Canada,' 117; see also *Manitoba Medical Bulletin* 99 (November 1929): 3; *Canadian Public Health Journal* 23 (April 1932): 181; *University of Toronto Medical Journal* 10 (January 1933): 78; Oppenheimer, 'Childbirth in Ontario,' 66; *Canadian Public Health Journal* 25 (December 1934): 571. For a breakdown in maternal mortality rural/urban in Canada, see *Public Health Journal* 16 (September 1925): 412. An embarrassing study in New York City for 1930–3 found that maternal mortality rates were 9.9 per 1000 live births when the woman was cared for by a surgeon, 5.4 when attended by an obstetrician, and the lowest, 1.4, when a midwife attended. Judith Litoff, *American Midwives, 1860 to the Present* (Westport, Conn.: Greenwood Press 1978), 111. When midwives recalled their practices, they took understandable pride pride in mentioning their low maternal mortality rates. For example, a Newfoundland woman who practised from the 1920s onward had helped 323 women with no medical assistance and had not lost one mother or child. Other midwives were not so lucky and had rates comparable to hospital rates. Memorial University of Newfoundland Folklore and Language Archive (MUNFLA), no. 73-160, M. Deanna Emberley, 'Folk Medicine of Newfoundland. Part 1. A Bay de Verde Midwife [Jane Ann Emberley] Part 2. Folk Cures for Common Complaints,' 3; no. 78-119, Larry Harvey, 'Life and Work of Aunt Nora (Lenora) Ellsworth, nee Goodyear, 1877–1951: Her Work as a Healer and Midwife in Carmanville, N.D.B.,' 26–7. Studies outside Canada revealed that midwife-directed birth was safer than physician-directed birth well into the 1930s. Such studies usually involved midwives who had extensive formal training. See also *CMAJ* 21 (October 1929): 448, 449; James Robert Goodall, *Puerperal Infec-*

tion (Montreal 1932), 26; Antler and Fox, 'The Movement toward a Safe Maternity,' 574; *CMAJ* 22 (May 1930): 735; *Chatelaine* 4 (October 1931): 13; *CMAJ* 34 (May 1936): 522.

20 *CMAJ* 19 (September 1928): 293–5. See also *Canadian Journal of Medicine and Surgery* 51 (February 1922): 78; *Manitoba Medical Bulletin* 79 (March 1928): 8. Harold Atlee did the same for the Grace Maternity in Halifax. *Nova Scotia Medical Bulletin* 15 (July 1936); 443. Home births combined with some prenatal care seemed to be among the safest. One organization that was rightly proud of its efforts to improve the lot of women in childbirth was the Victorian Order of Nurses. Its mandate was to provide prenatal supervision in conjunction with a physician's care. Since the nurses had little control over when they were called in, the amount of prenatal care given to any one woman varied. Nor was it possible for a doctor always to be present for the actual birth. Despite these 'problems,' the maternal mortality rate of the VON cases was low. In 1927, for example, the Canadian figure was 5–6 per 1000 live births, but the VON's was 2.5. Dianne Dodd, 'Helen MacMurchy, M.D. (1962–1953): Mothers and Doctors in the "Complete" Canadian Mother's Book' (paper presented to the Canadian Historical Association, Kingston, 1991), 20. See also *Food for Thought* 6 (June 1940): 4–5; *CMAJ* 26 (February 1932): 214; *Child and Family Welfare* 9 (September 1933): 7; *CMAJ* 29 (August 1933): 161; *Child and Family Welfare* 11 (November 1935): 11; *CMAJ* 34 (May 1936): 526; *Canadian Nurse* 42 (May 1936): 213; *American Journal of Public Health* 29 (1939): 249; *Canadian Home Journal*, November 1941, 65; Public Archives of Nova Scotia, *Report of the Chief Superintendent, VON*, 1940, 20.

21 *CMAJ* 22 (April 1930): 470. See also *CMAJ* 27 (July 1932): 114; *Canadian Journal of Medicine and Surgery* 75 (February 1934): 40; *CMAJ* 34 (May 1936): 552; Emory, *Public Health Nursing in Canada*, 284; *Public Health Journal* 10 (September 1919): 411. In 1931, 60,000 women in England and Wales suffered from morbidity of some kind due to childbirth (10 per cent of all mothers). Oakley, *The Captured Womb*, 68.

22 *Annual Report of the Montreal Maternity Hospital*, 1912, 9–10; also the reports for 1914, 21; 1916, 30–1, 27; 1917, 27, 30; 1918, 26–7; 1919, 28–30; and 1920, 27; *Annual Report of the Royal Victoria Hospital*, 1930, 104, and 1935, 113.

23 *CMAJ* 48 (January 1943): 51; *CMAJ* 8 (April 1918): 321; *Canadian Journal of Public Health* 35 (October 1944): 380.

24 *Nova Scotia Medical Bulletin* 9 (1930): 302–3.

25 For general causes, see Emery, 'Fatal Pregnancies in Ontario,' 6; *CMAJ* 21 (October 1929): 448; Antler and Fox, 'The Movement toward a Safe Maternity,' 571. For estimates in the 1920s, see *CMAJ* 17 (December 1927): 1435–

6; for 1932, *Canadian Journal of Medicine and Surgery* 75 (February 1934): 38; and for 1942, *Canadian Journal of Public Health* 35 (May 1944): 176. For a detailed breakdown of maternal mortality and causes 1931–43, see S.A. Cudmore, *A Study in Maternal, Infant and Neo-Natal Mortality in Canada 1926–1940* (Ottawa: King's Printer 1945), 45–6.

26 For Couture, see *Nova Scotia Medical Bulletin* 23 (January 1944): 268; for Blair, see *CMAJ* 52 (February 1945): 166.

27 *Grain Growers' Guide*, 1 October 1937, 37; see also 30 January 1918, 9. Sheilagh L. Steer, 'The Beliefs of Violet McNaughton: Adult Educator 1901–1929' (MEd thesis, University of Saskatchewan, 1979), 92. Similar sentiments were expressed by Nellie McClung in *The Next of Kin: Those Who Wait and Wonder* (Toronto: T. Allen 1917), 108. Some studies have dismissed the degree to which women worried about maternal deaths. Irvine Loudon, in his international study of maternal mortality, pointed out that everyone has heard of someone who has died in a traffic accident, but this does not stop us from driving a car. However, the analogy does not hold. Driving a car is something people can choose to do or not. For the period under study, birth control was illegal, so most women had difficulty avoiding childbirth. Loudon, *Death in Childbirth*, 164. Losing a wife in childbirth was devastating. The gendered separation of tasks meant that most men were not prepared to take on the extra burden of caring for children or the household. Unfortunately, little research on the impact of maternal mortality on the men left behind exists. Most public references focus on men not behaving in the way women wanted Thus, we have instances where women regale one another about men's lack of concern for their wives and their willingness to remarry quickly after their death – replacing them as though they were farm animals. Most often these comments referred to men separated from mainstream society by class or ethnicity. See Marjory Bellamy, 'Beyond the Call of Duty,' *Manitoba Pageant* 20 (Summer 1975): 15; *Chatelaine*, July 1928, 16. For further details on women's reaction to maternal mortality, see Christine Payeur 'Maternal Mortality in Quebec from the Medical Perspective and the Women's Point of View, 1890–1950' (MA thesis, Université de Montréal, 1997), chap. 3; and Judith Walzer Leavitt and Whitney Walton, '"Down to Death's Door": Women's Perception of Childbirth in America,' in Judith Walzer Leavitt, ed., *Women and Health in America: Historical Readings* (Madison: University of Wisconsin Press 1984), 155–65.

28 Arthur W. Beall, *The Living Temple: A Manual on Eugenics for Parents and Teachers* (Whitby, Ont.: A.B. Penhale 1933), 53.

29 *Nova Scotia Medical Bulletin* 10 (May 1931): 268; *CMAJ* 25 (September 1931): 359; *CMAJ* 33, supplement (1935): 26.

30 *CMAJ* 14 (June 1924): 595. See also *CMAJ* 23 (August 1930): 172.

31 Modern studies have suggested that 'streptococcal virulence' increased worldwide in the early decades of the twentieth century, partially accounting for the increased international rate of maternal mortality. Loudon, *Death in Childbirth*, 76–7. This theory is difficult to prove or disprove, but what it fails to address is the variation between countries. It was this variation that physicians in Canada were trying to address. Why was Canada's mortality rate so much higher than that of other countries?

32 *Annual Report of the Montreal Maternity Hospital*, 1901, 9; also the reports for 1902, 10; 1903, 16–17; and 1904, 18. See also *Canada Lancet and National Hygiene* 61 (September 1923): 86; *University of Toronto Medical Journal* 10 (January 1933): 81.

33 *Canadian Nurse* 24 (September 1928): 461. See also W.G. Cosbie, *The Toronto General Hospital, 1819–1965: A Chronicle* (Toronto: Macmillan 1975), 203.

34 McGill University Archives, RG1, Gynaecological Case Charts 1250–99, 1902, Royal Victoria Hospital, patient no. 1255 Mrs Frances Patterson, admitted 4 October 1902.

35 *CMAJ* 17 (December 1927): 1435; *Public Health Journal* 19 (December 1928): 578; *Manitoba Medical Bulletin* 79 (March 1928): 8. As the maternal death rates declined by the late 1930s and early 1940s, particular attention was paid to tuberculosis.

36 *Canada Lancet and Practitioner* 74 (January 1930): 4–5, and 78 (April 1932): 110; *University of Toronto Medical Journal* 10 (January 1933): 81; *Canadian Public Health Journal* 25 (December 1934): 579; *Manitoba Medical Review* 14 (June 1934): 3; *Canadian Public Health Journal* 25 (March 1934): 107; *CMAJ* 33 (December 1935): 672; *Child and Family Welfare* 11 (November 1935): 15; *Canadian Nurse* 42 (May 1936): 215; *Canadian Public Health Journal* 28 (December 1937): 592; *CMAJ* 48 (April 1943): 313. A modern study of historical maternal mortality rates has dismissed first births being a factor. Loudon, *Death in Childbirth*, 251. The age of women giving birth was believed to be increasing due to the delaying of marriage because of the economic problems and the desire of couples to be secure economically before they took on the burden of a family. Christine Payeur has argued that the higher maternal mortality rates in Quebec compared to Ontario after the mid-1930s was due to the larger families in Quebec. She claims that higher parity births (six or more) had maternal mortality rates as high as low ones. Payeur, 'Maternal Mortality in Quebec,' 55.

37 *Canadian Public Health Journal* 23 (April 1932): 181.
38 *Manitoba Medical Bulletin* 99 (November 1929): 4. See also *Canadian Public Health Journal* 23 (December 1932): 562.
39 *CMAJ* 25 (September 1931): 359; *CMAJ* 29 (August 1933): 160.
40 *Manitoba Medical Bulletin* 79 (March 1928): 8.
41 Bellamy 'Beyond the Call of Duty,' 15; *Canadian Journal of Medicine and Surgery* 33 (March 1913): 159; Loudon, *Death in Childbirth*, 379. Contrary to conventional wisdom, analysts of mortality rates in the late twentieth century have suggested that maternal mortality was rather 'insensitive' to improved standards of living and nutrition and a few commentators in the interwar period did as well. George Emery, 'Age-Parity and Marital Status Compositional Influences on the Maternal Mortality Rate in Canada, 1930–1960: A Regional Comparison,' *Histoire sociale/Social History* 25 (November 1992): 230; *Child and Family Welfare* 11 (November 1935): 15; *Canadian Nurse* 42 (May 1936): 215.
42 *CMAJ* 17 (December 1927): 1435; Dianne Dodd, 'Helen MacMurchy: Popular Midwifery and Maternity Services for Canadian Pioneer Women,' in Dianne Dodd and Deborah Gorham, eds., *Caring and Curing: Historical Perspectives on Women and Healing in Canada* (Ottawa: University of Ottawa Press 1994) 152; *CMAJ* 20 (February 1929): 181; Comacchio, 'Nations Are Built of Babies,' 65. *Canadian Public Health Journal* 22 (December 1931): 622. *Canada Lancet and Practitioner* 78 (April 1932): 110; *CMAJ* 29 (August 1933): 160. Occasionally, some argued that the problem was not poverty but too much luxury in the society. *Manitoba Medical Review* 14 (June 1934): 3. Dr Geggie recognized poverty and overwork as factors in maternal mortlaity. He also believed that birth control would help reduce the mortality rates. Elliott, 'Endormez-moi!' 162.
43 *Grain Growers' Guide*, 17 January 1924, 21.
44 British Columbia Archives, GR707, box 2, file 16, 'Evidence on Maternity Sickness,' in *B.C. Royal Commission on State Health Insurance and Maternity Benefits* (Victoria: Kings Printer 1932), x, 26.
45 *Canada Lancet and Practitioner* 74 (April 1932): 110.
46 For example, see *CMAJ* 33 (December 1935): 673.
47 Comacchio, 'Nations Are Built of Babies,' 223. See also *Canadian Public Health Journal* 31 (July 1940): 320.
48 Comacchio, 'Nations Are Built of Babies,' 224; *Canadian Journal of Public Health* 35 (May 1944): 177, 180. See also *Nova Scotia Medical Bulletin* 23 (January 1944): 270; Dominion Bureau of Statistics, Department of National Health and Welfare, *A Study in Maternal, Infant and Neo-Natal Mortality in Canada* (Ottawa: Department of National Health and Welfare

1945), 14; *CMAJ* 62 (February 1950): 109. Poor nutrition was linked to puerperal albuminuria/eclampsia and in the 1930s led to increased maternal mortality rates in Quebec. Payeur, 'Maternal Mortality in Quebec,' 62.

49 Comacchio, *'Nations Are Built of Babies,'* 88. See also *CMAJ* 22 (May 1930): 735; *Canadian Public Health Journal* 22 (December 1931): 622; *CMAJ* 29 (August 1933): 162; *Alberta Medical Bulletin* 1 (January 1936): 27; *CMAJ* 30 (April 1934): 472; *Child and Family Welfare* 11 (November 1935): 12–13; *Canadian Welfare* 16 (January 1941): 16. On the linkage between ignorance and class, see *Alberta Medical Bulletin* 1 (January 1936): 27.

50 *Chatelaine*, July 1928, 61. See also *Canada Lancet and Practitioner* 78 (April 1932): 110.

51 *CMAJ* 35 (November 1936): 572. See also *CMAJ* 17 (December 1927): 1437; *Chatelaine*, July 1928, 6; Comacchio, *'Nations Are Built of Babies,'* 76; *Canadian Home Journal*, November 1931, 80; *CMAJ* 33 (December 1935): 672; *Canadian Nurse* 42 (May 1936): 214; *Canadian Public Health Journal* 31 (July 1940): 320; *Canadian Home Journal*, November 1940, 8.

52 *Canadian Journal of Medicine and Surgery* 33 (March 1913): 159–60.

53 Cosbie, *The Toronto General Hospital*, 204. See also *Canadian Public Health Journal* 22 (July 1931): 347; *CMAJ* 25 (September 1931): 359; *University of Toronto Medical Journal* 10 (January 1933): 81; Stewart, 'Infant Feeding in Canada,' 116; *Canadian Public Health Journal* 25 (March 1934): 107; *Canadian Nurse* 42 (May 1936): 215; *Canadian Public Health Journal* 31 (July 1940): 312, and 32 (February 1941): 59; *Child and Family Welfare* 11 (November 1935): 15.

54 For a discussion of spontaneous and criminal abortions related to maternal mortality, see *CMAJ* 21 (October 1929): 449; Stewart, 'Infant Feeding in Canada,' 116; Comacchio, *'Nations Are Built of Babies,'* 72; *Chatelaine*, October 1931, 13; *Canada Lancet and Practitioner* 78 (April 1932): 110; *Canadian Pubic Health Journal* 25 (March 1934): 142; *CMAJ* 34 (May 1936): 520; *Canadian Public Health Journal* 28 (December 1937): 592; *CMAJ* 43 (July 1940): 39; *CMAJ* 52 (February 1945): 166; Loudon, *Death in Childbirth*, 128–9, 251.

55 Comacchio, *'Nations Are Built of Babies,'* 72; *Child and Family Welfare* 19 (1934): 10. A study in New York in 1933 revealed that 17.5 per cent of the maternal deaths were the result of abortion. Antler and Fox, 'The Movement toward a Safe Matenity,' 581–2. In the mid-1930s, 13 per cent of maternal mortality in England and Wales was the result of abortion deaths, usually following septic infection. Oakley, *The Captured Womb*, 91. For Canadian concern, see *CMAJ* 34 (May 1936): 520; *Canadian Journal of Medicine and Surgery* 75 (February 1934): 38; *Child and Family Welfare* 11 (November 1935): 11; Loudon, *Death in Childbirth*, 107.

56 *Canadian Public Health Journal* 25 (December 1934): 571, and 31 (July 1940): 313; *CMAJ* 34 (May 1936): 526; *Canadian Nurse* 42 (May 1936): 214.

57 *University of Toronto Medical Journal* 15 (March 1938): 221. See also *Food for Thought* 6 (June 1940): 4; *Canadian Public Health Journal* 32 (February 1941): 56.

58 *Manitoba Medical Review* 21 (November 1941): 211; Alfred Henry Tyrer, *Sex, Marriage and Birth Control*, 10th ed. (Toronto: Marriage Welfare Bureau 1943), 67.

59 *Montreal Medical Journal* 34 (January 1905): 24. Irvine Loudon has pointed out that poor obstetric education was an issue for both Britian and the United States as well. Loudon, *Death in Childbirth*, 251, 472.

60 Comacchio, 'Nations Are Built of Babies,' 69.

61 *Canadian Journal of Medicine and Surgery* 31 (April 1912): 218; *Canada Lancet and Practitioner* 78 (April 1932): 115; *Child and Family Welfare* 11 (November 1935): 12–13; *Canada Lancet* 44 (September 1910): 33, 34; *Montreal Medical Journal* 31 (October 1902): 774; *CMAJ* 21 (October 1929): 449. For a study of similar problems in the United States, see Antler and Fox, 'The Movement toward a Safe Maternity,' 569–95.

62 Halifax Medical College calendars, 1900–10; British Columbia Archives, GR1665, box 5, file 5, B.C. Provincial Secretary, 'Inquiry into charges against Dr. Harper Willson, 1909,' 1.

63 *CMAJ* 1 (February 1911): 125–6, 129.

64 *CMAJ* 4 (June 1914): 477. A history of the Toronto General Hospital points out the work done at the Burnside Lying-In Hospital in the 1920s and the fact that its last serious outbreak of puerperal sepsis was early in 1924. Cosbie, *The Toronto General Hospital*, 203.

65 *Canada Lancet and National Hygiene* 60 (March 1923): 86; also 61 (September 1923): 87, 88, and (March 1925); 113; *CMAJ* 19 (September 1928): 293; *Canada Lancet and Practitioner* 70 (May 1928): 166; *CMAJ* 21 (October 1929): 449; *CMAJ* 23 (August 1930): 171; *Canada Lancet and Practitioner* 77 (August 1931): 33–4; *Canadian Public Health Journal* 22 (December 1931): 622; *CMAJ* 34 (May 1936): 522.

66 Peter Ward, ed., *The Mysteries of Montreal: Memoirs of a Midwife by Charlotte Führer* (Vancouver: University of British Columbia Press 1984), 18; and Ian Carr and Robert E. Beamish, *Manitoba Medicine: A Brief History* (Winnipeg: University of Manitoba Press 1999), 116.

67 *Nova Scotia Medical Bulletin* 10 (April 1931): 211. See also *Canadian Public Health Journal* 23 (April 1932) 182.

68 *Canada Lancet and National Hygiene* 61 (September 1923): 87; *CMAJ* 22 (May 1930): 695.

69 Loudon, *Death in Childbirth*, 353.
70 McGill University Archives, Royal Victoria Hospital, RG95, vol. 5, Gynaecology Case Charts, 1903, patient no. 1474, Mrs Stafford Healy, no date of admission. See also J. Clarence Webster, *A Textbook of Obstetrics* (Philadelphia: W.B. Saunders 1903) 641; *Child and Family Welfare* 11 (November 1935): 12–13; J. Clifton Edgar, *The Practice of Obstetrics ... for the Use of Students and Practitioners*, 3rd ed. (Philadelphia: Blakiston 1907), 463; *CMAJ* 1 (February 1911): 129; *Canadian Journal of Medicine and Surgery* 31 (April 1912): 218; *Canadian Practitioner and Review* 38 (February 1913): 89.
71 There was the occasional voice criticizing physicians for not intervening when they should. Edgar, *The Practice of Obstetrics*, 463; *Canada Lancet* (April 1932): 112–14.
72 Dodd, 'Helen MacMurchy,' 151–3; *Canada Lancet and Practitioner* 64 (March 1925): 113. See also *CMAJ* 23 (August 1930): 171; *Canada Lancet and Practitioner* 77 (August 1931): 33–4. Not all were willing to accept the responsibility was the physician's – some blamed the patient. See *CMAJ* 22 (May 1930): 735; *Canada Lancet and National Hygiene* 60 (March 1923): 86; *CMAJ* 13 (April 1923): 253; *Canada Lancet and Practitioner* 64 (March 1925): 113; *CMAJ* 17 (December 1927): 1436; *Manitoba Medical Bulletin* 81 (May 1928): 10, and 86 (October 1928): 8–9; *Canada Lancet and Practitioner* 70 (May 1928): 166; *CMAJ* 21 (October 1929): 449; Julie Vandervoort, *Tell the Driver: A Biography of Elinor F.E. Black, M.D.* (Winnipeg: University of Manitoba Press 1992), 44–5; *Canada Lancet and Practitioner* 77 (December 1931): 160; *Nova Scotia Medical Bulletin* 10 (October 1931): 739; *Canada Lancet and Practitioner* 78 (April 1932): 111–12; *Canadian Public Health Journal* 25 (March 1934): 107; *CMAJ* 30 (April 1934): 472; *Child and Family Welfare* 11 (November 1935): 13–14; *CMAJ* 34 (May 1936): 520, 526; *CMAJ* 40 (March 1939): 260.
73 *CMAJ* 19 (September 1928): 293. For a discussion of hospital births in the United States and the standardization of technique in order to cut back on needless intervention, see Judith Walzer Leavitt, '"Science" Enters the Birthing Room: Obstetrics in America since the Eighteenth Century,' *Journal of American History* 70 (September 1983): 301.
74 Antler and Fox, 'The Movement toward a Safe Maternity,' 581.
75 Oakley, *The Captured Womb*, 72.
76 *Saturday Night*, 3 June 1944, 18; *CMAJ* 54 (May 1946): 493; *Modern Medicine of Canada* 4 (July 1949): 21.
77 *CMAJ* 52 (February 1945): 166.
78 Emery, 'Fatal Pregnancies in Ontario,' 1; Emory, *Public Health Nursing in Canada*, 284; *Canadian Home Journal* 37 (November 1940): 9; *CMAJ* 43 (July

1940): 40–1; Henricus J. Stander, *Williams Obstetrics: A Textbook for the Use of Students and Practitioners*, 8th ed. (New York: Appleton-Century 1941), 1258; *CMAJ* 52 (February 1945): 166; *CMAJ* 57 (September 1947): 208; *Modern Medicine of Canada* 4 (July 1949): 22. In the 1940s, some were giving credit to Vitamin K for the decrease in haemorrhage in birth. *Nova Scotia Medical Bulletin* 23 (January 1944): 268; Dominion Bureau of Statistics, *A Study in Maternal, Infant and Neo-Natal Mortality in Canada*, 14.

79 *CMAJ* 43 (July 1940): 40–1; Mason, 'Midwifery in Canada,' 117; Canadian Youth Commission, *Youth and Health*, 4; *Alberta Medical Bulletin* 13 (January 1948): 71; Some analysts have suggested that the problems themselves had declined, especially the virulence of the streptococcal infection. Loudon, *Death in Childbirth*, 261.

80 Emory, *Public Health Nursing in Canada*, 284; *Canadian Journal of Public Health* 35 (November 1944): 446; *CMAJ* 16 (June 1932): 740; Andrée Lévesque, 'La santé des femmes en periode de dépression économique: L'exemple des patientes de l'hôpital de la Miséricorde à Montréal pendant les années trente (notes de recherche),' *Bulletin, RCHTQ* (Été-automne 1990): 12.

81 *Canada Lancet and National Hygiene* 61 (September 1923): 88. See also *CMAJ* 22 (May 1930): 695; *Canada Lancet* 78 (April 1932): 112–14.

82 Dianne Dodd, 'Advice to Parents: The Blue Books, Helen MacMurchy, M.D. and the Federal Department of Health, 1920–1934, *Canadian Bulletin of Medical History* 8 (1991): 215.

83 Helen MacMurchy, ed., *Handbook of Child Welfare Work in Canada* (Ottawa: King's Printer 1923), 10.

84 Stewart, 'Infant Feeding in Canada,' 117; Dodd, 'Helen MacMurchy,' 151–2; *American Journal of Public Health* 29 (1939): 248; Emory, 'Age-Parity and Marital Status,' 230; Emory, 'Fatal Pregnancies in Ontario.' 1; *CMAJ* 17 (December 1927): 1435–6; *Manitoba Medical Bulletin* 86 (October 1928): 8–9; *Chatelaine* 1 (July 1928): 6; *Public Health Journal* 19 (December 1928): 578; *Manitoba Medical Bulletin* 81 (May 1928): 10–11; National Council of Women, *Yearbook 1923*, 124; *Canada Lancet and Practitioner* 77 (August 1931): 33–4; *Canada Lancet and Practitioner* 78 (April 1932): 109; *Canadian Journal of Medicine and Surgery* 75 (February 1934): 41; *Canadian Public Health Journal* 25 (March 1934): 142; *CMAJ* 33 (December 1935): 672; *CMAJ* 33, supplement (1935), 26; *Canadian Journal of Public Health* 35 (May 1944): 180; Dominion Bureau of Statistics, *A Study in Maternal, Infant and Neo-Natal Mortality in Canada*, 16; Canadian Youth Commission, *Youth and Health*, 4; *CMAJ* 54 (May 1946): 493; *CMAJ* 14 (October 1924): 908; *Child and Family Welfare* 11 (November 1935): 13–12; Cosbie, *The Toronto General*

Hospital, 203; *CMAJ* 13 (April 1923): 253; *Public Health Journal* 14 (June 1923): 243; *CMAJ* 21 (October 1929): 448; *Canada Lancet and Practitioner* 74 (January 1930): 4–5.

85 *Canada Lancet and Practitioner* 70 (May 1928): 167, *Canadian Public Health Journal* 31 (July 1940): 320; *CMAJ* 52 (February 1945): 167. In the United States, physicians felt that hospital birth overcame the problem they saw presented by midwife-directed births, the lack of skill on the part of many general practitioners, and what they saw as the unhygienic conditions of home births. Loudon, *Death in Childbirth*, 339. For support of hospital births in Canada, see Emory, *Public Health Nursing in Canada*, 284; *Canada Lancet and Practitioner* 78 (April 1932): 115; Dominion Bureau of Statistics, *A Study in Maternal, Infant and Neo-Natal Mortality in Canada*, 4; *CMAJ* 52 (February 1945): 166; Canadian Youth Commission, *Youth and Health*, 4; *CMAJ* 54 (May 1946): 493; *CMAJ* 62 (February 1950): 109; Comacchio, 'Nations Are Built of Babies,' 215; *Nova Scotia Medical Bulletin* 23 (January 1944): *Canadian Journal of Public Health* 36 (March 1945): 99.

86 Strong-Boag and McPherson, in 'The Confinement of Women,' 155–6, are careful not to credit the hospitals but rather the introduction of sulpha drugs. Similarly, Jo Oppenheimer argues that improvement in obstetric technique rather than hospitalization accounted for the decline in maternal mortality. Jo Oppenheimer, 'Childbirth in Ontario: The Transition from Home to Hospital in the Early Twentieth Century,' *Ontario History* 75 (March 1983): 36–60. Suzann Buckley disagrees with Oppenheimer and argues that it was improved socio-economic conditions that led to a decline in maternal mortality, not better obstetric technique. Suzann Buckley, 'The Search for the Decline of Maternal Mortality: The Place of Hospital Records,' in Janice Dickin McGinnis and Wendy Mitchinson, eds., *Essays in the History of Canadian Medicine* (Toronto: McClelland and Stewart 1988), 148–63. Danielle Gauvreau credits boh sulpha drugs and socio-economic factors. Danielle Gauvreau, 'Donner la vie et en mourir: La mortalité des femmes en couches au Québec avant 1960,' in Denis D. Cordell et al., *Population, reproduction, sociétés: Perspectives en enjeux de démographie de Montréal* (Montreal: Les presses de l'Université de Montréal 1993), 235–56. Christine Payeur acknowledges a combination of factors but notes that maternal mortality in Quebec had begun to decline before the majority of women gave birth in hospital. Payeur, 'Maternal Mortality in Quebec,' 33–41.

87 See Payeur, 'Maternal Mortality in Quebec,' 136, for women's fatalistic attitude.

88 See note 86, above.

89 Payeur, 'Maternal Mortality in Quebec,' 39.
90 Igloolik Oral History Project, Science Institute of the Northwest Territories, Government of the Northwest Territories, computer no. IE250, tape IE250, interview with Hubert Amarualik by Louis Tapardjuk, translated by Louis Tapardjuk, 31 December 1992, transcript, 20; computer no. RI01, tape IE091, interview with Rosie Iqalliyuq by Eugene Amarualik, translated by Louis Tapardjuk, 14 February 1990, transcript, 8; computer no. (none given), tape IE027, interview with Rosie Iqalijuq by Paul Irngaut and Wim. Rasing, translated by Paul Irngaut, 27 January 1987, transcript 2; computer no. IE085, tape IE085, interview with Sarah Amakllak Haulli by Rhoda Qanatsiaq, translated by Leah Otak, 16 January 1990, transcript 6; computer no. HPU1, tape IE082, interview with Hanna Uyarak by Rhoda Qanatsiaq, translated by Louis Tapardjuk, 15 January 1990, transcript 3.
91 Marie Adele Rabesca, Diane Romie, Martha Johnson, and Joan Ryan, *Traditional Dene Medicine,* part 1: *Report* (Lac La Marie, NWT.: Traditional Dene Medicine Project 1994), 34; Irma Honigmann and John Honigmann, 'Child Rearing Patterns among the Great Whale River Eskimo,' *University of Alaska Anthropological Papers* 2 (1953): 33. See also Margaret Blackman, *During My Time: Florence Edenshaw Davidson, A Haida Woman* (Vancouver: Douglas and McIntyre 1982), 31.
92 Laurel Halladay, '"We'll See You Next Year": Maternity Homes in Southern Saskatchewan in the First Half of the Twentieth Century' (MA thesis, Carleton University, 1996), 112.
93 See Franz Boas, 'The Eskimo of Baffin Island and Hudson Bay,' *Bulletin of the American Museum of Natural History* 15 (1901): 125–6, 143; Igloolik Oral History Project, computer no. IE085, tape IE085, interview with Sarah Amakllak Haulli by Rhoda Qanatsiaq, translated by Leah Otak, 16 January 1990, transcript 6; computer no. (none given) tape IE027, interview with Rosie Iqalijuq by Paul Irngaut and Wim. Rasing, translated by Paul Irngaut, 27 January 1987, transcript; Vilhjalmur Stefansson, 'The Stefansson-Anderson Arctic Expedition of the American Museum: Preliminary Ethnological Report' in *The Anthropological Papers of the American Museum of Natural History* 14, part 1 (New York 1914) 183, 320.
94 Igloolik Oral History Project, computer no. RI01, tape IE091, interview with Rosie Iqalliyuq by Eugene Amarualik, translated by Louis Tapardjuk, 14 February 1990, transcript, 8; Rabesca et al., *Traditional Dene Medicine,* part 1, 34.
95 David James Evans, *Obstetrics: A Manual for Students and Practitioners*

(Philadelphia: Lea Brothers 1900), 152. Webster, *A Textbook of Obstetrics*, 272; Adam H. Wright, *A Textbook of Obstetrics* (New York: D. Appleton 1908), 159.

96 Paul T. Harper, *Clinical Obstetrics* (Philadelphia: F.A. Davis 1930), 56.

97 Wright, *A Textbook of Obstetrics*, 133–4; Janet McNaughton, 'Midwifery, Traditional Obstetric Care and Change in Newfoundland' (paper presented to the Ethnology/Ethnomedicine Group, Memorial University, December 1989), 10–11.

98 *Montreal Medical Journal* 37 (January 1908): 23, and 38 (August 1909): 492; *Canadian Practitioner and Review* 37 (April 1912): 234. See also *CMAJ* 1 (February 1911): 133; *Dominion Medical Monthly* 38 (June 1912): 202.

99 *CMAJ* 14 (October 1924): 906.

100 P. Brooke Bland, *Practical Obstetrics for Students and Practitioners* (Philadelphia: F.A. Saunders 1932), 487; Stander, *Williams Obstetrics*, 496.

101 Alvine Cyr Gahagan, *Yes Father: Pioneer Nursing in Alberta* (Manchester, N.H.: Hammer Publications 1979), 90.

102 Percy E. Ryberg, *Health, Sex and Birth Control* (Toronto: Anchor Press 1942), 179; *Canadian Nurse* 41 (May 1945): 352.

103 William Thompson Lusk, *The Science and Art of Midwifery*, 3rd ed. (New York: D. Appleton 1889), 255; Webster, *A Textbook of Obstetrics*, 270: *Canada Lancet* 40 (November 1906): 219; Joseph B. DeLee, *The Principles and Practice of Obstetrics* (Philadelphia: W.B. Saunders 1913), 326; Wright, *A Textbook of Obstetrics*, 160.

104 *Canada Lancet* 40 (November 1906): 219.

105 Evans, *Obstetrics*, 152–3. See also *Montreal Medical Journal* 37 (January 1908): 33.

106 *Canadian Practitioner and Review* 35 (February 1910): 88–9; *Dominion Medical Monthly* 38 (June 1912): 202; David Berry Hart, *Guide to Midwifery* (London: Rebman Ltd. 1912), 544.

107 *Montreal Medical Journal* 31 (October 1902): 774.

108 *Canada Lancet* 43 (October 1909): 122–3.

109 *Montreal Medical Journal* 38 (August 1909): 491.

110 Hart, *Guide to Midwifery*, 543–4.

111 Thoma Watts Eden, *A Manual of Midwifery* (Toronto: Macmillan Canada 1915), 559.

112 Mary Rubio and Elizabeth Waterson, eds., *The Selected Journals of L.M. Montgomery*, vol. 2: *1910–1921* (Toronto: Oxford University Press 1987), 103.

113 *Woman's Century*, February 1917, 6.

114 Joan Hollobon, *The Lion's Tale: A History of the Wellesley Hospital, 1912–1987* (Toronto: Irwin 1987), 96. The Ottawa Maternity Hospital early in the century kept its patients for approximately fourteen days. Based on 4,674 cases between 1896 and 1915, from research lent to author by Suzann Buckley.

115 *Annual Report of the Montreal Maternity Hospital*, 1918, 26–7. In 1912 the average was 12.1 days. *Annual Report* of 1919, 28.

116 Webster, *A Textbook of Obstetrics*, 270; Wright, *A Textbook of Obstetrics*, 160; *Canadian Practitioner and Review* 44 (April 1919): 116. See also Hart, *Guide to Midwifery*, 544; DeLee, *The Principles and Practice of Obstetrics*, 326.

117 See Egbert H. Grandin and George W. Jarman, *A Textbook on Practical Obstetrics* (Philadelphia: F.A. Davis Company 1901), 254. The norm seemed to be six weeks.

118 *CMAJ* 17 (July 1927): 774; *Manitoba Medical Bulletin* 86 (October 1928): 8; *Dalhousie Medical Journal* 11, 1–3 (1937): 35; F.L. Adair, ed., *Maternal Care and Some Complications* (Chicago: University of Chicago Press 1939), 87; Ryberg *Health, Sex and Birth Control*, 179; *Canadian Nurse* 41 (May 1945): 352; *Canadian Nurse* 43 (May 1947): 356; Alfred Beck, *Obstetrical Practice*, 4th ed. (Baltimore: The Williams & Wilkins Co. 1947), 329.

119 Stewart, 'Infant Feeding in Canada,' 119; *Chatelaine* 5 (May 1932): 24.

120 William Victor Johnston, *Before the Age of Miracles: Memoirs of a Country Doctor* (Toronto: Fitzhenry & Whiteside 1972), 44. Other support for a two-week recuperative period also existed. See *CMAJ* 33 (August 1935): 144; Stander, *Williams Obstetrics*, 449; Elliott, 'Endormez-moi!' 158.

121 *Canadian Nurse* 24 (September 1928): 480; Strong-Boag and McPherson, 'The Confinement of Women,' 167.

122 Comacchio, 'Nations Are Built of Babies,' 169; National Council of Women, *Yearbook 1929*, 126, 128.

123 Bland, *Practical Obstetrics for Students and Practitioners*, 489.

124 R.W. Johnstone, *A Text-Book of Midwifery: For Students and Pracitioners*, 6th ed. (London: A. & C. Black 1934), 211.

125 Ten Teachers, *Midwifery*, 5th ed. (London: Edward Arnold 1935), 529, 531.

126 *CMAJ* 22 (April 1930): 471. See also *CMAJ* 14 (August 1924): 700; *CMAJ* 22 (April 1930): 560; Bland, *Practical Obstetrics for Students and Practitioners*, 489; *CMAJ* 33 (August 1935): 144; *CMAJ* 37 (1937): 66.

127 Stander, *Williams Obstetrics*, 499. See also *Canadian Nurse* 41 (May 1945): 352; *Modern Medicine of Canada* 5 (January 1950): 32; *Journal of Obstetrics and Gynaecology of the British Empire* 60 (1955): 793.

128 Harry Oxorn, *Harold Benge Atlee M.D.: A Biography* (Hantsport, N.S.: Lancelot Press 1983), 117 (emphasis mine).

129 Dalhousie University Archives, Oxorn Papers, H.B. Atlee, *Grace Maternity Hospital, 1922–1972*, 5; *CMAJ* 33 (August 1935): 144–50, and 37 (December 1937): 551. Atlee also began to practise early rising for his abortion cases. *Nova Scotia Medical Bulletin* 26 (February 1947): 41.

130 *Annual Report of the Royal Victoria Hospital, Montreal*, 1948, 18.

131 McNaughton, 'Midwifery, Traditional Obstetric Care and Change in Newfoundland,' 18; *CMAJ* 57 (September 1947): 259, and 22 (April 1930): 471; Edwin Robertson, 'Getting the Patient Out of Bed Early after Child-birth and after Operation,' in *The Book of the Post-Graduate Course* (Kingston: Queen's University 1945).

132 *Maclean's*, 1 July 1943, 12; *Annual Report of the Royal Victoria Hospital, Montreal*, 1947, 18; *Alberta Medical Bulletin* 13 (January 1948): 72; *CMAJ* 59 (August 1948): 170.

133 *CMAJ* 59 (August 1948): 171; Public Archives of Nova Scotia, RG25, series C, vol. 11(A), Public Health, *Report on the Survey of Hospitals in Nova Scotia*, 1949, 31. See also *Chatelaine*, November 1950, 61. By the 1950s some suggestion was that hospitals were keeping patients for only five to seven days. Emory, *Public Health Nursing in Canada*, 287. Geraldine Ransome told of staying in for only four days. Interview with Geraldine Ransome, 16 August 1993. Esther Jackson stayed in five days. Interview with Esther Jackson, 14 July 1993. Bea Leavis stayed in six days. Interview with Bea Leavis, 30 August 1993. Verda McDonald stayed five days and would have stayed longer. Interview with Verda McDonald, 17 July 1993.

134 Interview with Dorothy Atkinson, 15 June 1993; interview with Becki Crawford, 9 July 1993; British Columbia Archives, Provincial Royal Jubilee Hospital, Add. Mss, 313, vol. 242, *Annual Report*, 1949 19.

135 Interview with Joan Carr, 22 July 1993; with Jane Rutherford, 28 July 1993; with Ruth Howard, 25 August 1993; with Betty Mackenzie, 19 August 1993; *Alberta Medical Bulletin* 14 (July 1949): 13; Public Archives of Nova Scotia, Victorian Order of Nurses, RT98, V 645, *Report* 1950, 28; *Journal of Obstetrics and Gynaecology of the British Empire* 60 (1955): 793.

136 Vandervoort, *Tell the Driver*, 221–2.

137 C. Levitt et al., *Survey of Routine Maternity Care and Practices in Canadian Hospitals* (Ottawa: Health Canada and Canadian Institute of Child Health 1995), 8.

138 Johnstone, *A Text-Book of Midwifery*, 211. See also Ten Teachers, *Midwifery*, 531; Stander, *Williams Obstetrics*, 499–500.

139 Ryberg, *Health, Sex and Birth Control*, 179. See also *Canadian Child* 5 (October 1924): 17; *Canadian Nurse* 43 (May 1947): 356.

140 Abeele, 'Nations Are Built of Babies,' 294.

141 *Annual Report of the Montreal Maternity Hospital,* 1907, 23–4. Daily visits by nurses was true of the Burnside as well. *Canadian Nurse* 14 (March 1918): 906.

142 Denyse Baillargeon, 'Care of Mothers and Infants in Montreal between the Wars: The Visiting Nurses of Metropolitan Life, Les Gouttes de Lait, and Assistance Maternelle,' in Gorham and Dodd, eds., *Caring and Curing,* 166.

143 Wright, *A Textbook of Obstetrics,* 154–5. See also Hart, *Guide to Midwifery,* 541–2.

144 *Western Canadian Medical Journal* 3 (July 1909): 311.

145 Bland, *Practical Obstetrics for Students and Practitioners,* 487; *CMAJ* 37, supplement (1937): 65; Frederick C. Irving, *A Textbook of Obstetrics: For Students and Practitioners* (New York: Macmillan 1936), 168.

146 Irving, *A Textbook of Obstetrics,* 177. The number and sequence of visits could vary. See Ten Teachers, *Midwifery,* 527.

147 *Dalhousie Medical Journal* 11, 1–3 (1937): 35; *Annual Report of the Royal Victoria Hospital, Montreal,* 1930, 65, and 1931, 62. For a detailed description of postnatal care and areas of intervention by doctors, see *Alberta Medical Bulletin* 12 (July 1947): 17–18.

148 Baillargeon, 'Care of Mothers and Infants in Montreal between the Wars,' 175.

Illustration Credits

American Authors, ed. Charles Jewett, *The Practice of Obstetrics* (New York: Lea Brothers and Co., 1901), 238: Instrumental puncture of the membranes.

Archives of Women's College Hospital, Toronto: Medical students examining patient, 1950; Happy result of childbirth, 1940; New mother being instructed by nurse.

Alfred C. Beck, *Obstetrical Practice* (Baltimore: The Williams & Williams Co., 1947, 4th ed.), 180: Maternity corset.

P. Brooke Bland, *Practical Obstetrics for Students and Practitioners* (Philadelphia: F.A. Davis Co., 1932), 89, 603: Diagnosis of pregnancy; Classical Caesarian section.

BC Archives: Car bogged down, 1914, H-07229; Maternity Wing, Royal Jubilee Hospital, Victoria, 1946, I-02164 (Duncan Macphail).

Chatelaine, Rogers Publishing Ltd.: Hypnotising for childbirth.

J. Clifton Edgar, *The Practice of Obstetrics Designed for the Use of Students and Practitioners of Medicine* (Philadelphia: P. Blakiston's Son and Co., 1907, 3rd ed.), 1013: Caesarian section in the early years.

Glenbow Archives: Mrs Martin's Nursing Home, 1912.

John W. S. McCullough: Discussion of maternity clothing.

National Archives of Canada: Husband and wife visit the doctor, PA-163733 (Eugene Michael Finn); Ottawa Maternity Hospital, c. 1920, PA-147883; Maternity Hospital, Edmonton, PA-45726 (Albertype Co.); Hospital delivery room, Ottawa General Hospital, 1939, PA-803164 (Eugene Michael Finn); Maternity binders, 1940, PA-803153 (Eugene Michael Finn).

University Health Network: Obstetrical Instrument Case, 1940s; Pregnancy test, 1950; Carsten's pelvimeter, c. 1915; Obstetrical instruments; Braided umbilical tape, c. 1930.

Index

STUDIES IN GENDER AND HISTORY

General editors: Franca Iacovetta and Karen Dubinsky